THE HEART SMART--
SUGAR WISE COOKBOOK

is dedicated to

My husband, Pat, and our grandchildren: Matthew, Jason, Allison, Andrew, Alicia, Sandell and Tory. All have brought great joy into my life.

A special thanks is extended to my sister, Patty Hagerman, for the many hours she spent helping me distribute my first book.

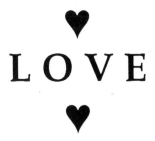

The purpose of this book is to teach people how to prepare food in a more healthful manner and to stimulate an awareness of the importance of good nutrition. Its pages are also extended to the diabetic and include diabetic exchanges along with a breakdown of calories and grams of fat, carbohydrates and protein and milligrams of cholesterol and sodium contained in a recipe serving.

Editor: Patrick Stangl

Copyright 1992
Stangl Publishing Company
Ottumwa, Iowa

First Printing - November 1992
Second Printing - January 1993
Third Printing - October 1994

Library of Congress Catalog Number 92-096978
International Standard Book Number 0-9631854-1-1

All rights reserved. No part of this book may be reproduced in any manner whatsoever without written permission from the publisher, except for the inclusion of brief quotations in a review.

Cover Photo by Jim Hamann

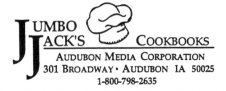

Table of Contents

Introduction	1-24
Substitutes	25-48
Appetizers, Snacks & Beverages	49-72
Breads	73-112
Breakfast, Brunch & Lunch	113-188
Ethnic Foods	189-216
Special Entreés	217-238
Vegetables	239-268
Salads	269-318
Desserts	319-420

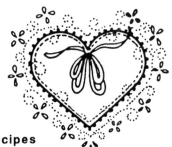

List Your Favorite Recipes

Recipes	Page
_____	_____
_____	_____
_____	_____
_____	_____
_____	_____
_____	_____
_____	_____
_____	_____
_____	_____
_____	_____
_____	_____
_____	_____
_____	_____
_____	_____
_____	_____
_____	_____
_____	_____
_____	_____
_____	_____

Introduction

Introduction

♥ ♥ ♥

The "Heart Smart-Sugar Wise" cookbook continues to put emphasis on fat and cholesterol control just as was done in the "Hold The Fat" cookbook.

This book, however, extends its pages to welcome the diabetic with the inclusion of diabetic exchanges and a breakdown of the grams of carbohydrates and proteins contained in a recipe serving.

More often than not, the diabetic is completely ignored when it comes to cookbooks. Unfortunately, I was not aware of the degree of the unwitting thoughtlessness extended this group of people by the culinary world.

It was not until I developed diabetes myself that I became aware of the lack of good cookbooks available for the diabetic. And even then it didn't dawn on me to share the recipes I developed for myself.

Nutrients and their control are of prime concern to the diabetic when planning meals. A diabetic practicing diet control knows how many calories and how many grams of carbohydrates and protein they are consuming each day.

We all know that the body needs a certain amount of nutrients on a regular basis. However, it would probably be a more healthy world if the population was more aware of how many nutrients the body needs and why it needs them.

CARBOHYDRATES, for instance, is a much needed nutrient. It is the function of the carbohydrate to provide the main supply of fuel to the body.

In the perfect diet the daily consumption of carbohydrates would make up fifty percent of the food consumed each day.

When on a diabetic diet, a range of 40 to 60 percent of carbohydrates is allowed.

The great part about carbohydrates is that they contain only four calories per gram compared to nine calories for a gram of fat.

There are two types of carbohydrates—complex and simple. Simple carbohydrates include the sugar, honey and syrup based foods—foods the sweet-tooth craves.

Simple carbohydrates contain next to no nutrients and are usually discouraged because of their lack of nutrition. It is for this reason that they are often referred to as the "empty food." The diabetic must omit simple carbohydrates from the diet. In place of natural sugar, honey or syrup, artificial sweeteners must be substituted. Natural fruits also help fill the sweet needs.

Too much sugar is not believed to be beneficial in a diet and should be limited by everyone.

FAT is another nutrient we all need on a daily basis. The problem is, one tablespoon of fat per day will supply more than the amount of fat the body needs.

Anything beyond that one tablespoon of fat per day must be stored somewhere in (or on) the body. It's this storage system that accounts for artery blockage and subsequent heart attacks.

The American public has been carrying on a love affair with fat for years, and sadly enough, many are consuming more like a half of cup of fat each day.

Saturated fat is the real culprit. This is the fat found in animal and animal by-products, as well as coconut, coconut oils and palm kernel oil.

The diabetic is restricted to 20 percent fat and under of the daily calories consumed. Not a bad guideline for everyone.

The third nutrient essential to proper body function is PROTEIN. Protein is in charge of the upkeep and maintenance of every tissue in the body.

Protein not only builds muscles, but it is in charge of determining the condition of the hair, enzymes, hemoglobin, hormones, and even insulin.

For the average diet 20 percent protein is suggested. For the diabetic a range of 12 to 20 percent protein is allowed.

Consuming the suggested amount of protein is not difficult when you consider that an ounce of meat or cheese has 7 grams of protein; a cup of cooked beans has between 9 and 14 grams of protein; a slice of bread 2 grams; and an ounce of milk 1 gram of protein.

VITAMINS AND MINERALS are also important nutrients. We all need calcium and iron to keep our bones and blood strong. However, all vitamins and minerals are needed by the body in varying amounts.

One of the best ways to insure you are feeding your body the proper amount of vitamins and minerals is to consume a balanced diet that includes the five major food groups.

It is recommended that Americans consume 2-4 servings of fruit; 3-5 servings of vegetables (include all types); 6-11 servings of bread, cereal and other grains; 5-7 ounces meat; and 2 servings milk, cheese or yogurt. A chart is included in the book showing what constitutes a serving.

Special attention should be paid to the bread, cereal and grain group since it plays a key part to the body's general fitness.

The National Cancer Institute recommends that people consume 10 to 35 grams of fiber per day and that it come from a variety of sources.

It is believed that high fiber diets may prevent or help to lower the rates of colon cancer.

WATER is the most forgotten nutrient. Many people do not even consider water to be a nutrient since it is such an everyday thing to drink water. And since it contains no calories.

Nonetheless, everyone should consume about eight 8-ounce glasses of water per day. Some bodies may even function best on twelve 8-ounce glasses of water per day.

It's not really that difficult to maintain a healthy diet. The most difficult part of it is developing the good habit of eating properly.

The ideal healthy diet is considered to consist of 50 percent carbohydrates; 20 percent protein and 30 percent fat and under.

Due to the diabetic connection in the book, desserts are prepared with an artificial sweetener. In the book, aspertame (Equal) is used with the option of substituting your own favorite sweetener or the amount of sugar it is replacing.

Although aspertame is approved by the Food and Drug Administration as being safe for human consumption, they do recommend that it not be consumed by very small children and by pregnant women.

A sodium breakdown is also included with each recipe. More and more people are becoming aware of the pitfalls of sodium.

It is recommended that the average American limit sodium intake to 1,000 milligrams per 1,000 calories consumed. For those on sodium restricted diets the recommendations are even lower.

Salt has been used in recipes in the book in limited amounts with the option of leaving it out of the recipe. Salt contains 2,134 milligrams of sodium per teaspoon. If you are wise enough to cut salt from the recipe, the sodium breakdown can be adjusted accordingly.

The secret to a healthy diet is balance. Be sure to include foods from all of the food groups in your diet on a daily basis.

And if you balance fat, carbohydrate and protein consumption you are well on your way. It may sound like a big chore, but once you are acquainted with the figures it will become common place.

Being on a 20 percent fat restricted diet does not mean that food with more fat cannot be consumed.

What it means is that at the end of the day your fat consumption should not add up to be more than 20 percent of the calories consumed.

Balance once again. Consume a high fat food at noon and you will have to balance it with a low fat food in the evening.

Being "Heart Smart and Sugar Wise" should add up to a happier, healthier you. At least give it a try.

Bon Appetit!

Taking The Fat Out Of Ground Beef

(statistics used in this article were taken from an article written by Dotty Griffith, Universal Press Syndicate, that appeared in the Des Moines Register.)

The new method of rendering ground beef lean will probably be as difficult for you to accept as it was for me.

I could not believe my eyes when I read of it in the Des Moines Register.

The "Cook And Rinse" method of removing fat from ground beef has been around and accepted for a number of years.

In this method ground beef is crumbled and browned. It is then rinsed under hot water before consumption.

However, in the new "Fat Extraction" method the ground beef is crumbled and browned in oil, then rinsed under boiling water before consumption.

This method was developed by a Boston physician, Dr. Donald Small.

News of the fat extraction method first appeared in the New England Journal of Medicine in 1991 in an article authored by Dr. Small.

Small claimed this method to render ground beef lean, no matter how fat the beginning product. In the end, all ground beef ends up containing only about eight percent fat.

This method also removes more fat and cholesterol than the rinsing method and turns out a ground meat product lower in fat than even ground chicken or turkey.

According to Dr. Small, the oil acts as a solvent to dissolve fat and cholesterol.

A 3.5 ounce serving of the rendered meat has only 144 calories containing only seven grams of fat, 1.4 of which is saturated fat.

That's about half the calories and one-third the fat of regular ground beef. Regular (70 percent lean) ground beef contains 77 percent of its calories from fat. A 3.5 ounce serving has 311 calories and 27 grams of fat. Twelve grams are saturated.

Unable to believe what I had read, I set out to put it to the test. Finding it difficult for me to buy 70 percent ground beef, I purchased 80 percent instead.

I came home and boiled the meat in oil, then rinsed as directed, pressing on the meat to remove the water. Wanting to give it every advantage, I even allowed it to drain in the strainer for 30 minutes before I put it to the test.

I then put the ground meat on a stack of paper towels and stood back to wait on the grease spot to appear. Instead I saw only a water spot. The meat was lean.

That evening my husband and I ate some of the beef. It was so lean that it had a dry taste, but the flavor was still there.

Later I took on the 70 percent lean beef and the results were the same. The only difference was that I had a little less product in the end, since more fat was removed from the beginning product.

On the following page are the two methods for removing some of the fat from ground beef. There is also a chart comparing the two methods.

I now use the fat extraction method. I do several pounds at a time and freeze the rendered lean beef. Not only does it give me an extra lean ground beef, but it gives me an already browned product ready for quick use.

I have not used the rendered ground beef in recipes in the book because I knew there would be many book-users who would not take the time to process the beef.

However, when you do process the beef you can adjust the breakdown figures accordingly and the end results will be a definite plus.

If you think you won't like the taste of the 70 or 80 percent lean ground beef, give it a try. Once the fat is removed from the product, the taste becomes very palatable.

Put extracting fat from beef on your list of things to do when time permits, and reap the benefits of having a lean product on hand ready to use at a moment's notice.

Getting The Fat Out Of Ground Beef

THE FAT EXTRACTION METHOD:

1- Put two cups canola oil into a saucepan and crumble two pounds ground beef into the oil.
2- Heat oil and beef over medium heat to boiling. Cook until meat is brown, mashing with potato masher to crumble. This will take about 5 minutes.
3- Drain meat in colander set over a large bowl or measuring cup. Press down on meat to remove excess oil.
4- Very slowly pour two cups boiling water over meat and allow to drain in bowl or measuring cup.
5- Refrigerate liquid until fat solidifies.
6- Separate fat from bro   Oil can be reused once for fat retraction.
7- Reserve broth and use in recipes calling for beef broth, or freeze in ice cube trays and put in freezer bag for use when sautéing.

This process was developed by Dr. Donald Small.

THE COOK AND RINSE METHOD

1- Brown meat in skillet.
2- Put meat in colander; press down to remove excess fat.
3- Run hot water over meat for a couple of minutes, stirring with a fork for better rinsing and drainage. Running the garbage disposal during this process will help to prevent drainage problems.
4- Allow meat to drain for several minutes before using.

LEAN GROUND BEEF

COMPARING CALORIES, FAT AND CHOLESTEROL IN GROUND BEEF:

GROUND BEEF (3.5 ounces)	TOTAL CALORIES	% OF CALORIES FROM FAT	TOTAL FAT GRAMS	SATUR- ATED FAT GRAMS	CHOLES- TEROL (mg/100 mg)
Regular (70% lean)	311	77%	26.6	12.0	85
Lean (80% lean)	270	69%	20.7	9.3	75
Extra Lean (85% lean)	208	59%	13.9	6.3	69
Super Lean (90% lean)	170	50%	9.6	4.3	NA
Stir-fried, rinsed	160	48%	8.5	3.8	62
Fat extracted beef	144	42%	6.7	1.4	36

SOURCES: PRINTED IN THE DES MOINES REGISTER FROM:
D. M. Small, New England Journal of Medicine, 1991, Vol. 324-73-77
U.S. Dept. of Agriculture Handbook, Composition of Foods No. 8-13;
The Healthy Meat Eater's Cookbook

How Much Fat and Cholesterol Should Be Consumed Daily?

A great deal of research has been done in an attempt to determine the amount of fat and cholesterol to be consumed on a daily basis. Most experts accept the guidelines put out by the American Heart Association as being a reliable dietary guideline. The American Heart Association advises that no more than thirty percent of a person's daily caloric consumption come in the form of fat. Saturated fats, which are found in animal meats and animal by-products, coconut oils, cocoa butter and many hydrogenated shortenings should not exceed ten percent of the daily caloric intake.

One of the best ways to cut saturated fat in the diet is to consume less red meat and eat more poultry, fish and dried beans and peas.

The recommended allowance of fat per day should not exceed 40 grams for women and 60 grams for men. As for cholesterol, it is recommended that no more than 300 milligrams of cholesterol be consumed daily based on no more than 100 milligrams per 1,000 calories.

The following chart shows the amount of fat and cholesterol allowed for the number of calories consumed.

Notes & Recipes

Daily Calories Consumed	30% Daily Calories	Grams of Fat	20% Daily Calories	Grams Of Fat	10% Daily Calories	Grams Of Fat	Daily Mg Cholest. Allowed
1,000	300	33.3	200	22.2	100	11.1	100
1,100	330	36.7	220	24.4	110	12.2	110
1,200	360	40.0*	240	26.7	120	13.3	120
1,300	390	42.2	260	28.9	130	14.4	130
1,400	420	46.7	280	31.1	140	15.6	140
1,500	450	50.0	300	33.3	150	16.7	150
1,600	480	53.3	320	35.6	160	17.8	160
1,700	510	56.7	340	37.8	170	18.9	170
1,800	540	60.0*	360	40.0*	180	20.0	180
1,900	570	63.3	380	42.2	190	21.1	190
2,000	600	66.7	400	44.4	200	22.2	200
2,100	630	70.0	420	46.7	210	23.3	210
2,200	660	73.3	440	48.9	220	24.4	220
2,300	690	76.7	460	51.1	230	25.6	230
2,400	720	80.0	480	53.3	240	26.7	240
2,500	750	83.3	500	55.6	250	27.8	250
2,600	780	86.7	520	57.8	260	28.9	260
2,700	810	90.0	540	60.0*	270	30.0	270
2,800	340	93.3	560	62.2	280	31.1	280
2,900	870	96.7	580	64.4	290	32.2	290
3,000	900	100.0	600	66.7	300	33.3	300

According to the American Heart Association guidelines, no more than 30% of total calories consumed should be fat calories. In instances where there is a health condition involved, a physician may recommend an even lower percentage of calories consumed be made up of fat. The chart shows the amount of calories consumed daily and the grams of fat and the milligrams of cholesterol allowed for calories consumed. Cholesterol is given for 10% of caloires consumed. Fat is given for 10%, 20% and 30% of calories consumed.
*NOTE: It is further recommended that women consume no more than 40 grams of fat per day and men consume no more than 60 grams of fat per day.

Fat Content of Foods

Food Group	Very Low Fat 9% of calories or less	Low Fat 10-29% of calories	Moderate Fat 30-49% of calories	High Fat 50% of calories or more
BEVERAGES	Alcoholic beverages Coffee Fruit drinks Lemonade Tea			
DAIRY PRODUCTS	Cheese (1% butterfat) Dry cottage cheese Egg substitute Egg whites Milk (skim, skim evaporated) Yogurt (home recipe)	Buttermilk Cheese (2-3% butterfat) Cottage cheese (low-fat) Milk (1%) Milk shake (with ice milk & 1% milk) Pudding (tapioca or vanilla, made with 1% milk) Sherbet Yogurt, commercial	Cheese (4-8% butterfat) Cottage cheese (cream style) Chocolate pudding Ice cream Milk (2%) Milk (whole)	Cheese (10% and over) Eggnog Evaporated milk Half & Half cream Non-dairy whipped topping Powdered non-dairy creamer Premium ice cream Sour cream
FATS and OILS				Butter and margarine Lard Oil (safflower, corn, olive sunflower, etc.) Salad dressing Vegetable shortening

Fat Content of Foods

Food Group	Very Low Fat 9% of calories or less	Low Fat 10-29% of calories	Moderate Fat 30-49% of calories	High Fat 50% of calories or more
FRUITS	Apple Apricot Banana Berries Candied fruit plus citron and ginger Cherry Date Fig Fruit cocktail Fruit juices Grapefruit Grapes Kiwi Lemon Mandarin orange Melons Nectarine Orange Peach Pear Pineapple Plum Raisins Rhubarb Tangerine			

Fat Content of Foods

Food Group	Very Low Fat 9% of calories or less	Low Fat 10-29% of calories	Moderate Fat 30-49% of calories	High Fat 50% of calories or more
GRAIN PRODUCTS	Air popped popcorn Angel food cake Bagel Cereal (cooked cream of rice, farina, wheat) Cereal (ready-to-eat) Cornflakes Bran Flakes Grapenuts Rice Krispies Puffed Rice Shredded Wheat Total Wheaties Wheat Chex	Animal crackers Bread (Rye, raisin white, whole wheat) Buns (hamburger or hot dog) Cereal, cooked (oatmeal) Cereal (ready-to-eat) Cheerios, Raisin Bran Dinner rolls Fig bars Graham crackers Melba toast Soda crackers Tortilla (flour) Zwieback	Biscuits Brownies Cakes Cookies (oatmeal, sandwich) Croissant Croutons (home recipe) Fried snack pie Granola Muffin Oil popped popcorn Pancake Sweet rolls Vanilla wafers Waffle	Cheesecake Cookies (chocolate chip, peanut butter) Corn chips Doughnuts Pie crust
LEGUMES, NUTS and SEEDS	Cooked dried beans Carob Lentils Split peas Water chestnuts	Pork and beans	Cooked soybeans	Almonds Cashews Coconut Macadamia nuts Peanuts, dry roasted oil roasted Peanut butter Pecans

Fat Content of Foods

Food Group	Very Low Fat 9% of calories or less	Low Fat 10-29% of calories	Moderate Fat 30-49% of calories	High Fat 50% of calories or more
LEGUMES, NUTS and SEEDS (Continued)				Pistachio nuts Pumpkin seeds Sesame seeds Sunflower seeds Tofu Walnuts (black, California)
MEAT, EGGS, FISH and POULTRY	Egg substitute Egg white Lobster Shrimp, boiled Tuna, water packed	Beef, lean only Flank steak Round steak Clams Corned beef Crab, canned or fresh Fish, baked, broiled or poached Egg substitute, my recipe Oysters, canned or fresh Salmon, fresh Scallops, steamed Turkey, baked or broiled	Beef, lean only Chuck roast Filet mignon Ground round New York strip Porterhouse T-Bone Tenderloin Rump roast Round roast Sirloin Fish, fried Fish sandwich Fish sticks Ham, lean only Hamburger Lamb chop, lean only Liver Macaroni & cheese Pork, lean only, 10% fat Ham, picnic ham	Bacon Bologna Beef, lean & fat Brisket Chuck steak Club steak Ground beef Ground chuck Pot roast Ribeye roast Ribeye steak Standing rib roast Spareribs Pot pies (beef, chicken, tuna) Cheeseburger Deviled ham Eggs, however prepared Hot dogs Lamb chops, lean and fat

Fat Content of Foods

Food Group	Very Low Fat 9% of calories or less	Low Fat 10-29% of calories	Moderate Fat 30-49% of calories	High Fat 50% of calories or more
MEAT, EGGS, FISH and POULTRY (Continued)			Fresh pork, lean only, 13-20% fat Boston butt Roast Chop or loin Shoulder Shrimp, fried Salmon, canned, pink or red Spaghetti & meatballs Trout (Brook) Tuna, oil packed Veal	Pork, lean and fat Fresh 23-30% fat Boston butt Ground Ham, loin picnic Shoulder Spareribs Sausages Luncheon meats Taco Trout (Rainbow)
SOUPS, SAUCES and GRAVIES	Apple butter Apple sauce Barbecue sauce Butterscotch topping Caramel topping Catsup Chili sauce Cranberry sauce Horseradish Marshmallow topping Mustard Soy sauce	Bouillon Gravy (mix) Soups made with water -- Tomato Vegetable beef	Gravy (home recipe) Soups made with milk--skim or 1% White sauce (mix)	Cocoa Mayonnaise Soups made with whole milk All creamed soups Soups made with water -- Cream of chicken Cream of mushroom Cheese sauce Hollandaise Tartar sauce White sauce

Fat Content of Foods

Food Group	Very Low Fat 9% of calories or less	Low Fat 10-29% of calories	Moderate Fat 30-49% of calories	High Fat 50% of calories or more
SOUPS, SAUCES and GRAVIES (Continued)	Strawberry topping Tomato paste Tomato sauce Worcestershire sauce			
SWEETS	Gelatin dessert Gumdrops Honey Jam Jelly Jelly beans Marmalade Marshmallows Mints Popsicle Molasses Syrup	Butterscotch Caramels Fudge 3 Musketeers Tootsie Roll	Malted milk balls Mars candy bar M & M's Raisins, chocolate covered Peanut brittle Snickers	Chocolate bars Chocolate chips Chocolate-coated peanuts Chocolate kisses Mr. Goodbar Nestle's Crunch Peanut Butter Cups
VEGETABLES	Artichoke Beans, green, Italian, kidney, snap & wax Bean sprouts Beets Brussels Sprouts Broccoli Cabbage	Asparagus Spinach	French fries Hash browns Potatoes au gratin Potatoes (scalloped)	French fried onion rings Potato salad Potato chips Olives

Fat Content of Foods

Food Group	Very Low Fat 9% of calories or less	Low Fat 10-29% of calories	Moderate Fat 30-49% of calories	High Fat 50% of calories or more
VEGETABLES (Continued)	Carrot Cauliflower Celery Corn Cucumber Eggplant Lettuce Mushroom Onion Parsley Peas Pepper Pickles Potatoes Baked Boiled Mashed Pumpkin Radishes Squash Sweet Potatoes Tomatoes Turnips Tnip greens Watercrest Yams			

Making the Right Choices

**Breads, Cereals and Other Grain Products
6 to 11 Servings Per Day**

Whole Grain
1/2 c. cooked brown rice
1/2 c. buckwheat grotes
1/2 c. cooked bulgur
1 corn tortilla
4 sm. graham crackers
2 lg. graham crackers
1 ounce granola
1/2 c. cooked oatmeal
1 c. popped corn—no salt or
   fat added
1 slice pumpernickel bread
1 oz. ready-to-eat cereal
4 sm. lowfat rye crackers
1 slice whole wheat bread
1 whole-wheat roll
4 sm. lowfat whole-wheat
   crackers

1/2 c. cooked eggless whole-
   wheat pasta
1/2 c. cooked whole-wheat
   cereals

Enriched
1/2 lowfat bagel
1 small biscuit
1/2 large biscuit
1 sm. piece cornbread
1 sm. corn muffin
1/2 sm. English muffin
1 sm. piece of French bread
1/2 c. cooked grits
1/2 c. hamburger roll
1/2 hot dog bun
1 sm. piece Italian bread
1/2 c. cooked eggless macaroni
1 small muffin
1/2 large muffin
1/2 c. cooked eggless noodles
2 (3") pancakes, fried with
   vegetable spray - no extra fat
   added
1/2 c. cooked eggless pasta
1 oz. ready-to-eat cereal
1/2 c. cooked rice, long grain only
1 slice white bread
1 small white roll

Six to eleven servings may seem a great deal, but it really is not if you select the right foods. A hamburger or hot dog bun counts for two servings. If you're running a little short, feed yourself and family a few whole wheat crackers that are low in fat. Two large crackers or four small crackers is a serving. To help round out the week include rice and pasta on a regular basis. It doesn't take long and takes little effort and planning to make the right choices at meals.

Fruits
2 to 4 Servings Per Day

Citrus, Melons, Berries

1/2 c. cooked or canned blueberries
1 slice (4x8-inch arc) watermelon
1 c. diced watermelon pieces
1 slice (5-inch diameter) cantaloupe
1 c. diced pieces cantaloupe
3/4 c. citrus juices
1/2 c. cooked cranberries
1/2 grapefruit
1 (5") slice honeydew
1 kiwi fruit
1 lemon
1 small orange
1/2 c. cooked raspberries
1/2 c. raw raspberries
1/2 c. fresh strawberries
1 small tangerine

1 small apple
2 small apricots
1 small banana
10 cherries
4 dates
2 figs
3/4 c. fruit juices
10 grapes
1 small nectarine
1 small peach
1 small pear
1/2 c. pineapple
1/2 c. cooked or canned plums
1/4 c. cooked prunes
1/4 c. raisins

Toss freshly peeled bananas in lemon juice
and they will not darken.

Vegetables
3 to 5 Servings Per Day

Dark Green
Beet greens
Broccoli
Chard
Chicory
Collard greens
Dandelion greens
Endive
Escarole
Kale
Mustard greens
Romaine lettuce
Spinach
Turnip greens
Watercress

Select from this group several times per week. 1/2 cup chopped raw or cooked — 1 cup leafy, such as lettuce or spinach.

Deep Yellow
Carrots
Pumpkin
Sweet potatoes
Winter squash

Serve several times each week. 1/2 cup cooked or 1/2 cup raw.

Starchy
Corn
Green peas
Hominy
Lima beans
Potatoes
Rutabaga
Taro

Serve a starch food each day. When fats are decreased, starches should be increased to maintain proper energy (calories).

Marshmallows will not dry out if stored in the freezer.

Dry Beans and Peas (Legumes)

Black beans
Black-eyed peas
Chickpeas (garbanzos)
Kidney beans
Lentils
Lima beans (mature)
Mung beans
Navy beans
Pinto beans
Split peas

These should be served several
times a week—1/2 cup cooked
makes a serving.

Other Vegetables

Artichokes
Asparagus
Bean and alfalfa sprouts
Beets
Brussels Sprouts
Cabbage
Cauliflower
Celery
Chinese cabbage
Cucumbers
Eggplant
Green beans
Green peppers
Lettuce
Mushrooms
Okra
Onions (mature and green)
Radishes
Summer squash
Tomatoes
Turnips
Vegetable juices
Zucchini

Make choices from this list on a
daily basis—1/2 cup raw or cooked
makes a serving.

Meat, Poultry, Fish and Alternates
2 to 3 Servings Per Day
Not to Exceed 5 to 7 Ounces of Meat

Meat
Beef
Ham   Limit to three or four times a week.
Pork
Lamb
Homemade sausage prepared
   with ground round

Poultry
Chicken
Turkey   Serve several times a week.
Turkey sausage (homemade)

Fish
Fish - Any firm fleshed fish   Serve on a regular basis.

Shellfish   Serve only on rare occasions.

Water packed tuna   Serve on a regular basis.
Pink salmon   Serve on a regular basis.

Alternates
Egg whites   Substitute for meals with meat,
Dry beans and peas (legumes)   poultry or fish several times a
Tofu   week. 1/2 cup cooked makes a
                                      serving—2 egg whites makes a
                                      serving.

Milk, Cheese and Yogurt
2 Servings Per Day - 4 for Teens

Lowfat Milk Products
Buttermilk   2 servings per day. 3 for teens
1% or skim milk   and women who are pregnant or
2% milk   breastfeeding. 4 for teens who are
Lowfat plain yogurt   pregnant or breastfeeding.
                                      1 serving equals one cup.

Other Milk Products
American cheese
Cheddar cheese
Chocolate milk
Flavored yogurt   Avoid use of higher fat products.
Fruit yogurt
Process cheeses
Swiss cheese
Whole milk

Fats, Sweets and Alcoholic Beverages
Avoid the following as much as possible.

Fats
Bacon, salt pork	Butter
Cream - dairy and non-dairy	Cream cheese
Lard	Margarine
Mayonnaise	Mayonnaise-type salad dressing
Salad dressing	Shortening
Sour cream	Vegetable oil

Sweets
Candy
Corn syrup
Fruit drinks, ades
Gelatin desserts
Honey
Frosting
Jam, Jelly   Avoid as much as possible.
Maple syrup
Marmalade
Molasses
Popsicles and ices
Sherbets
Soft drinks and colas
Sugar - white and brown

Alcohol
Beer
Liquor   Avoid as much as possible.
Wine

Following A Pattern For Daily Food Choices

	What Counts As A Serving?	Suggested Daily Servings
Breads, Cereals and Other Grain Products-- Whole-grain Enriched	1 slice of bread; 1/2 hamburger bun or English muffin; a small roll or muffin; 3 to 4 small crackers; 2 larger crackers; 1/2 cup cooked cereal, rice or pasta; or 1 (1-ounce) ready-to-eat breakfast cereal.	6 to 11 servings per day. This should include several servings of whole-grain product.
Fruits-- Citrus, melon, berries Other fruits	A piece of whole fruit such as an apple, banana, orange, peach, pear; a grapefruit half; melon wedge; 3/4 cup juice; 1/2 cup berries or 1/2 cup cooked or canned fruit; or 1/4 cup dried fruit.	2 to 4 servings per day.
Vegetables-- Dark-green leafy Deep-yellow Dry beans and peas (legumes) Starchy Other vegetables	1/2 cup of cooked or chopped raw vegetables or 1 cup of leafy raw vegetables such as lettuce or spinach.	3 to 5 servings per day. Include all types on a regular basis. Use dark green leafy vegetables and dry beans and peas several times a week.

Following A Pattern For Daily Food Choices

	What Counts As A Serving?	Suggested Daily Servings
Meats, Poultry, Fish and Alternates-- (Eggs, dry beans and peas, nuts and seeds)	Serving sizes will differ. Amounts should total 5 to 7 ounces of lean meat, fish or poultry per day. A serving of meat the size and thickness of the palm of a woman's hand is about 3 to 5 ounces. Count 1 egg, 1/2 cup cooked dry beans as one ounce of lean meat.	2 to 3 servings per day with a total of no more than five to seven ounces of meat, fish or poultry per day.
Milk, Cheese and Yogurt	1 cup of milk, 8 ounces of yogurt, 1 1/2 ounces natural cheese or 2 ounces of process cheese.	2 servings: Three servings for women who are pregnant or breastfeeding. Four servings for teens who are pregnant or breastfeeding.
Fats, Sweets and Alcoholic Beverages	Fats and sweets should be avoided as much as possible and alcoholic beverages should be consumed with moderation.	

This chart was prepared by the Cooperative Extension Service; Iowa State University, Ames, Iowa. It was prepared to set a daily food choice pattern for Americans who regularly eat foods from all the major food groups listed. Some people such as vegetarians and others may not eat one or more of these types of foods. These people should contact a nutritionist in their community for help in planning food choices.

Substitutes

Substitutes

Within the pages of this chapter lies the key to successfully cooking in a more healthful manner. Many cooking staples are far too high in fat content, especially saturated fat content, to be acceptable in offering recipes that contain no more than thirty percent fat. It is for this reason that these cooking staples have been omitted from this book and substitutes have been offered to take their place.

The substitutes are good tasting and work very well in the recipes. It is not a difficult chore to learn to cook with substitutes. However, the only way they will work is if they are kept in as ready of a supply as ordinary cooking staples. If the pantry shelves and the refrigerator are not supplied with substitutes, most people will not use them.

Using a frozen stock cube for sautéing is no more of a chore than using a tablespoon of margarine as long as the stock cubes are as easy to reach for as the margarine. Using egg substitute will succeed only if it is in easy access as is the egg.

Convenience is the name of the game. Most people are looking for the quick and easy route when it comes to cooking. It is unlikely they will take the time to whip up a substitute when they are in a hurry to prepare the food. For this reason, it is very important that you stroll through the substitute chapter before embarking on more healthful cooking.

As you go through the chapter make a list of the ingredients needed to get set up with the proper substitutes. Purchase what is needed and return home and prepare the substitutes. Only then will you be ready to take full advantage of this book.

Put marbles in the bottom of double boiler. They will
rattle when water level drops too low.

Browned Flour

METHOD NUMBER ONE:

Put flour in a shallow baking dish and put in 350 degree preheated oven 15 to 20 minutes. Watch closely and stir often so it does not over-brown. Browning time depends on amount of flour being browned.

METHOD NUMBER TWO:

Put flour in a heavy-bottomed skillet over medium heat and brown, stirring constantly until flour is light brown.

Browned flour is great for use in sauces and gravies. When using browned flour, it is not necessary to use margarine. If desired, a little margarine can be swirled in before serving, to enhance taste.

Cajun Seasoning
(Recipe contains only a trace of fat)

1/4 c. garlic salt*	1/4 c. dry mustard
1/4 c. garlic powder	1/4 c. thyme
1/2 c. paprika	1/8 c. red pepper
1/4 c. dried basil	1/8 c. black pepper

In a large mixing bowl, put all of ingredients and stir with wire whisk until mixture is of an even color and flavors are distributed throughout. Store in tightly sealed glass container and fill shaker as needed.
Yield: 1 3/4 cups

Approximate Per Teaspoon:
Calories: 4	Carbohydrates: Tr. g
Fat: 0.1 g	Protein: 0.0 g
Cholesterol: 0.0 mg	Sodium: 305 mg

Diabetic Exchanges: Free food in limited amounts
*Garlic powder can be substituted.

Keep red spices (chili powder, paprika and red pepper) in the refrigerator for longer lasting flavor and color.

About Cheeses

Many, many cheeses are filled with saturated fat and must be avoided.

Puréed cottage cheese blends along with the use of "yogurt cheese" will replace many cheese needs in recipes.

More and more fat-free cheeses are appearing on the market. As of yet they are mostly in the sliced American cheese variety, but these can be substituted for other cheeses.

The sliced American cheese that I used in the recipes is a "Free" cheese that contains no fat. It tastes good in the recipes and melts very well.

The cream cheeses that I used in the recipes are the new no-fat cream cheeses that are now in grocery stores. These contain only about 30 calories per ounce and no fat. They work very well.

If you prefer, use the cream cheese substitute for hot and cold dishes. They, too, work well and taste good.

Working around the high fat in many cheeses may take a little longer at the grocery store, but with a little effort you can continue to enjoy the taste of cheese.

Cream Cheese Substitutes

Cream cheese is a very popular cooking ingredient and is used in everything from desserts to casseroles. However, for those who are restricted on fat consumption it is a food they are not allowed to consume. One ounce of cream cheese contains 9.9 grams of fat, 6.0 grams of which is saturated. Even the new "light" cream cheese contains seven grams of fat per ounce with four grams being saturated.

However, fat free cream cheeses are now available. The new "free" cream cheeses do not have quite the same taste and texture as regular cream cheese, but they work well in food preparation. If you prefer, continue to use the cream cheese substitutes in the book.

To scald milk, heat it to just below the boiling point.

Cream Cheese Substitute
for Cold Dishes

(With home recipe yogurt, recipe contains only a trace of fat;
With commercial low-fat yogurt, recipe contains approximately 25% fat)
1 (8 oz.) ctn. plain low-fat yogurt

Secure a piece of cheesecloth or a coffee filter over a glass allowing a pouch to extend down into the glass. Pour yogurt into pouch, cover top with plastic wrap and put in refrigerator for several hours. During the setting time the whey will drain from the yogurt; it will be found in liquid form in the bottom of the glass. The yogurt will now be a more solid product that will perform well in recipes calling for cream cheese. Plain "yogurt cheese" works well in cold dishes.

Yield: 1 cup or 16 tablespoons

Approximate
  Per Tablespoon:
(if using home-recipe yogurt):

Calories: 10	**Carbohydrates: 1 g**
Fat: Tr.	**Protein: 1 g**
Cholesterol: 0.3 mg	**Sodium: 11 mg**

Approximate
  Per Tablespoon:
(If using commercial yogurt):

Calories: 11	**Carbohydrates: 1 g**
Fat: 0.3 g	**Protein: 1 g**
Cholesterol: 1.3 mg	**Sodium: 10 mg**

Diabetic Exchange: Free food when used in limited amounts

When sauteeing always heat pan before adding margarine,
oil or stock. Then food will not stick.

Cream Cheese Substitute
for Hot Dishes

(With home-recipe yogurt, recipe contains only a trace of fat;
With commercial low-fat yogurt,
recipe contains approximately 21% fat)

1 (8 oz.) ctn. plain low-fat   1 scant tsp. cornstarch
    yogurt

Secure a piece of cheesecloth or a coffee filter over a glass allowing a pouch to extend down into the glass. Pour yogurt into the pouch and cover top with plastic wrap. Put in refrigerator for several hours. During this time, the whey will drain from the yogurt' it will be found in liquid form in the bottom of the glass. The yogurt will now be in a more solid form that will perform well in recipes calling for cream cheese. Just before using "yogurt cheese", stir in cornstarch and blend well. This works very well in hot dishes.

Yield: 1 cup or 16 tablespoons

Approximate
   Per Tablespoon:
(if using home-recipe yogurt):

Calories: 12	**Carbohydrates: 1 g**
Fat: Tr.	**Protein: 1 g**
Cholesterol: 0.3 mg	**Sodium: 11 mg**

Approximate
   Per Tablespoon:
(if using commercial yogurt):

Calories: 13	**Carbohydrates: 1g**
Fat: 0.3 g	**Protein: 1 g**
Cholesterol: 1.3 mg	**Sodium: 10 mg**

Diabetic Exchange: Free food when used in limited amounts

Substitute for Cream Soup

Cooking with creamed soups is discouraged due to the fat content of a can of soup along with the heavy sodium content. A can of cream of mushroom soup, for example, contains 8.3 grams of fat. The Casserole Cream Soup Mix contains only 0.9 grams of fat for the equivalent of one can creamed soup. A great saving in fat.

Mix it up and keep it on hand. It's easy to prepare and simple to use in casseroles or any recipe calling for a can of soup. Just use it as you would a can of soup. If the recipe calls for mushroom soup, add a few chopped mushrooms to the cream soup mix. Use as is for chicken or celery soup.

Casserole Cream Soup Mix

(Recipe contains approximately 5% fat)

2 c. instant non-fat dry milk	2 T. dried onion flakes
3/4 c. cornstarch	1/2 tsp. pepper
1/2 c. instant chicken bouillon, low sodium	1 tsp. dried thyme
	1 tsp. dried basil
	1 T. celery salt

Combine all ingredients, mixing very well. Store in airtight container. Makes 3 cups of mix that is equivalent to six 10 1/2-ounce cans of condensed cream soup.

TO USE AS A SUBSTITUTE FOR 1 CAN CREAMED SOUP:

1/2 c. dry soup mix (should be scant 1/2 c.)	1 1/4 c. water

Put soup mix and water in a saucepan and cook over medium heat until thickened. Equivalent to one can condensed cream soup.

This cream soup substitute contains only about one-fourth the fat of regular canned cream soups and will season recipes just as well.

Approximate Per Can:

Calories: 160	Carbohydrates: 27 g
Fat: 0.9 g	Protein: 11 g
Cholesterol: 0.0 mg	Sodium: 2524 mg

Diabetic Exchanges: 1 milk; 2 fruit

For an easy first course, serve cold soup in tall wine glasses before your guests are seated.

Substitute for Heavy or Light Cream

(Recipe contains approximately 3% fat)
Evaporated skim milk

Use cup for cup in recipes calling for heavy or light cream.

Approximate Per Cup:
Calories: 200
Fat: 0.6 g
Cholesterol: 10 mg

Carbohydrates: 2 g
Protein: 1 g
Sodium: 124 mg

Diabetic Exchange: 2 milk

Reduced Fat Spread for Bread

(Recipe contains approximately 67% fat)

1 c. reduced-calorie vegetable spread, no more fat content that 7 grams per tablespoon

2 c. "Free" no-fat, no cholesterol mayonnaise
Butter sprinkles, to taste

In a mixing bowl, whip vegetable spread and mayonnaise until even in texture and color. Add artificial butter sprinkles to taste. Keep in refrigerator.
Yield: 3 cups or 48 tablespoons

Approximate Per Tablespoon:
Calories: 31
Fat: 2.3 g
Cholesterol: 0.0 mg

Carbohydrates: 2 g
Protein: 0 g
Sodium: 172 mg

Diabetic Exchange: 1/2 fat

*Put small containers of yogurt in the freezer
for a healthful frozen dessert.*

Egg Substitute

The undisputed "miracle worker" in the kitchen is the ever ready egg. It thickens puddings, sets custards, stabilizes cakes, binds meatballs and provides mountains of meringue. As a breakfast or brunch food item, it can be fried, boiled, poached, scrambled, stuffed or whipped into a fluffy omelet or a towering soufflé.

Eggs are choked full of vitamins and minerals and they contain a high quality of complete protein. But, lurking behind that innocent looking hard shell is an over-abundance of fat. And in that fat is a substance known as cholesterol—enough to cause many physicians to warn their patients of its hazards.

After extensive research the egg has become more and more suspect of being a heavy contributor to a variety of health problems, including heart attacks. Because of the growing dangers posed by high cholesterol levels, the American Heart Association has even revised its dietary guidelines. They are now advising the American public to eat less fat—less than 30 percent of the daily caloric consumption should come in the form of fat.

Saturated fats, which are found in animal flesh, coconut oils, cocoa butter and palm kernel oils should not exceed ten percent of the daily caloric intake. People are further advised to eat less of cholesterol-rich foods. Daily intake should not exceed 100 milligrams of cholesterol per 1,000 calories, not to exceed 300 milligrams per day.

Neither my husband or myself have been advised to eliminate eggs from our diets, however, we have chosen to use an egg substitute instead of eggs. The egg substitutes in this book were developed by me and will work very well in the recipes in this book. When out of egg substitute, use two egg whites instead of an egg. It will also work.

Be forewarned that it will not be easy in the beginning to discard the egg yolk. At first, when I threw away the yolks I could hardly stand to watch them slide out of sight. That all changes, however, and after a while the regard for them will be no more than the regard of an egg shell.

The recipes in this book have been kitchen tested with egg substitute and no eggs are necessary for any recipe in this book. Once again, the secret to success will be to keep egg substitute on the shelf or in the freezer at all times. If you begin to think fondly of the egg, remember this: one egg yolk has 270 milligrams of cholesterol—more cholesterol than most people are allowed in a day.

Parsley freezes very well.

Egg Substitute
in the Freezer

(Recipe contains approximately 29% fat)

1 dozen egg whites
2 T. canola oil
1 to 2 drops yellow food
  coloring (oil based like
  used for candy melts)

1/2 tsp. baking powder
1/2 c. powdered milk

Put egg whites, oil and food coloring in blender and process until smooth. Slowly add baking powder and powdered milk. One-fourth cup equals 1 egg.
Yield: 2 cups (equivalent to 8 eggs)

Approximate Per 1/4 Cup:
Calories: 56
Fat: 1.8 g
Cholesterol: 0.8 mg

Carbohyrates: 3 g
Protein: 6 g
Sodium: 102 mg

Diabetic Exchanges: 1 vegetable; 1/2 meat

*Always taste cold soups before serving. Cold food
tends to need more seasoning than hot food.*

Egg Substitute
on the Shelf

(Recipe contains approximately 18% fat)

2 c. non-fat dry milk
  granules—use good grade
2 tsp. baking powder
2 T. cornstarch
1 tsp. cream of tartar
	1/4 tsp. yellow food
	  coloring (must have an
	  oil base such as the kind
	  used for candy melts)
	3 T. canola oil

Grind dry milk to a fine powder in a mortar with a pestle, or in a mixing bowl with the back of a heavy tablespoon. Pour powdered milk into a medium bowl and blend in baking powder, cornstarch and cream of tartar. In a cup, mix oil and food coloring. Slowly add milk granules to oil mixture until you have a rather dry mixture. Pour this mixture into remaining milk granules. Grind with a tablespoon until mixture is even in color and fluffy. Store in airtight container. Egg substitute need not be refrigerated, but it will remain fresh longer if refrigerated, if you don't use much of it.

To Use: Mix one tablespoon egg substitute with two tablespoons cool water and blend until smooth. Add two egg whites and mix until smooth and even in color. When prepared as directed above, it is equal to one egg and can be used in most recipes calling for eggs. Egg substitute is great scrambled or used in omelets. For salads, simply scramble and chop up.
Yield: enough for equivalent of 36 eggs

Approximate Per
  Egg Equivalent:
(1 T. egg substitute equals
  2 egg whites):

Calories: 60	Carbohydrates: 4 g
Fat: 1.2 g	Protein: 7 g
Cholesterol: 0.7 mg	Sodium: 124 mg

Diabetic Exchanges: 1 vegetable; 1 meat

If you don't have buttermilk on hand use one tablespoon white vinegar added to one cup milk and allowed to stand for five minutes.

Low Fat Bread Sauce

(Recipe contains approximately 5% fat)

1 whole onion, quartered
1 c. skim milk
1/2 bay leaf
Pinch of white pepper

2 slices reduced-calorie
   bread, reduced to soft
   crumbs
1/8 tsp. salt (opt.)

Put onion, milk, bay leaf and pepper in a saucepan; bring to boil and simmer for five minutes. Strain through sieve and discard solids. Return liquid to saucepan. Add bread crumbs and salt, stirring until smooth.
Yield: About 1 1/2 cups sauce

Approximate Per Half-Cup Sauce:
Calories: 38
Fat: 0.2 g
Cholesterol: 1 mg

Carbohydrates: 6 g
Protein: 3 g
Sodium: 98 mg

Diabetic Exchanges: 1/2 bread

Master Baking Mix Substitute

We all like having a premixed baking or biscuit mix on hand. It has so many uses that it is nice to always have on the shelf. The problem is that commercial master baking mixes have far too much fat in them to be acceptable on a fat restricted diet.

However, the home-style baking mixes can be used at will because the fat is held to thirty percent. It means you don't have to give up the convenience of baking with it. Make up a batch and store it in the refrigerator in an airtight can. It will keep up to 3 months.

Master Baking Mix

(Recipe contains approximately 30% fat)

12 1/2 c. flour (whole wheat,
   unbleached or enriched
   all-purpose)
1/2 c. baking powder*

2 c. non-fat dry milk
   granules
2 tsp. salt (opt.)
1 1/2 c. tub margarine

Blend dry ingredients and cut in margarine. Store in airtight container for 2 to 3 months in the refrigerator.

*If using whole wheat flour, blend flour or half whole wheat and half unbleached, increase baking powder to 3/4 cup.

Approximate Per Cup:
Calories: 573
Fat: 19.4 g
Cholesterol: 1.6 mg

Carbohydrates: 79 g
Protein 13 g
Sodium: 613 mg

Diabetic Exchanges: 5 bread; 4 fat

Olive Oil Substitute

Most people enjoy the taste olive oil lends food. Especially in Italian food or a good tossed salad. However, since it contains over one hundred calories per tablespoon and 14 grams of fat it must be used very sparingly, if at all.

One of the best ways to introduce the olive oil taste to foods without calories and fat is to use the canned olive oil spray. A single serving of olive oil spray (the amount it takes to cover 1/3 of a 10-inch skillet) contains only 2 calories and 1 gram of fat.

For pasta, cook and drain, then spray and toss before putting on serving plate. Use the spray very sparingly. It doesn't take a lot to accomplish the taste. For a salad, try spraying each salad bowl, or the main serving salad bowl, with olive oil before tossing the salad. If not happy with the taste, spray the salad greenery before adding the dressing.

When sautéing with a frozen stock cube, spray the skillet first with the olive oil spray and then melt the cube. This works great and keeps the fat down.

Sausage Patties
(Low-fat)
(Recipe contains approximately 26% fat)

3 lb. ground turkey breast (skin removed)	2 tsp. basil
1 lb. pork tenderloin (lean only), ground	2 tsp. thyme
1 tsp. cumin	2 tsp. sage
1 tsp. marjoram	1 tsp. garlic powder
1 tsp. ground black pepper	1/2 tsp. nutmeg
1 tsp. oregano	1/2 c. whole wheat bread reduced to fine crumbs

Combine all ingredients, blending well. Cover and refrigerate to allow flavors to mingle. Form into 24 patties. Wrap individually in plastic wrap and place in freezing bag. Freeze until ready to use. TO COOK: Brown in nonstick skillet that has been sprayed with cooking spray. Cook until nicely browned, turning often.

Yield: 24 patties

Approximate Per Patty:
Calories: 142
Fat: 4.1 g
Cholesterol: 61 mg

Carbohydrates: 1 g
Protein: 24 g
Sodium: 62 mg

Diabetic Exchanges: 3 meat

Sautéing with Stock

Far too much margarine is used when sautéing. Most cooks think the ingredient being sautéed must swim in butter or margarine in order to come out tasty. The truth is, margarine or butter is really not necessary when sautéing in most cases. A nice hearty stock will do just as well and the dish being prepared will not suffer much from the sacrifice of the oil.

There is a secret to using stock for sautéing. It is important that most liquid is allowed to be absorbed. If this is not happening as it should the heat should be turned up just a bit to hasten the operation.

There are a few recipes where I have used <u>one teaspoon</u> of margarine with my sautéing stock, but only rarely. There is also an occasion or two where I used a little olive oil in certain recipes just to get the olive oil taste into the dish. However, for the most part, only stock is needed. On the following pages are recipes for good stocks. If you don't want to go to the bother (but believe me it is worthwhile), buy a can of consommé even though it is saltier than the homemade stock. It's best not to use bouillon, but in a pinch you can use a couple of tablespoons for sautéing. Best to use low-sodium bouillon.

Again, the secret to success is to keep a supply of the frozen stock cubes on hand. If you are too busy to make stock, buy a can of chicken and a can of beef broth and freeze it into cubes in the ice cube trays.

Frozen Stock Cubes

Make stocks in flavors of your choice. Chill, then de-fat and only then pour them into ice cube trays to freeze. When frozen, transfer them to freezer bags within easy reach. Whenever a recipe calls for sautéing, use a stock cube instead of margarine. It's amazing how much of the fat can be cut in a recipe when this is practiced. And believe me, it works just as well in almost all recipes.

In the following recipes, the stock is simmered down and the end result is a very hearty stock. This makes a very good sautéing frozen stock cube that will add flavor to food. If you are going to use canned broth, it would be wise to simmer it down until it is reduced by about one-third to derive a more hearty broth for the frozen stock cubes.

Serve cold soups in bowls placed in
crushed ice in larger bowls.

Stock

(Recipe contains less than 6% fat)

2 to 3 lb. leftover or fresh
bones
2 1/2 qt. water
2 tsp. seasoned salt (opt.)
3 or 4 c. vegetables—
whatever you have left-
over or in your crisper

1 lg. onion, coarsely
chopped
Bouquet garni (tie 2 tsp.
parsley flakes, 1/2 tsp.
dried basil & 1 bay leaf in
a piece of cheesecloth)

Break or saw bones into the smallest pieces possible and place into a heavy bottomed pan with a tight-fitting lid. Add water and salt. Bring to a boil and simmer 8 to 10 hours. If using fresh bones, brown first. Chop vegetables into small pieces along with onion. After bones have boiled 4 hours, add vegetables and bouquet garni. Boil slowly several hours. Remove from heat and leave covered. Allow to stand 1 hour. Strain through cloth. Refrigerate and allow fat to solidify. Defat and use stock immediately, or freeze for later use.

This stock makes a wonderful base for many soups with the addition of noodles, rice, vegetables, etc. With the use of a little imagination, you can create your own low-fat soups.

Yield: 1 quart

Approximate Per Cup:
Calories: 10
Fat: 0.1 g
Cholesterol: Tr. mg

Carbohydrates: 0 g
Protein: 0 g
Sodium: 0 mg

Diabetic Exchange: Free food in limited amounts

*If you don't have self-rising flour, make your own by combining
1 1/2 teaspoons baking powder and 1/2 teaspoon salt per
one cup all purpose flour.*

Brown Bone Stock

(Recipe contains only a trace of fat—less than 5 %)

3 lb. beef bones
3 sm. onions, quartered
2 carrots, chunked
1 stalk celery, chunked
Bouquet garni (4 sprigs
    parsley, pinch dried
    thyme, pinch basil & 2
    bay leaves tied in a
    cheesecloth pouch)

5 peppercorns
3 qt. water
1 1/2 tsp. salt (opt.)

Wipe bones with paper towel. Don't wash unless a must. Put bones in a large, heavy-bottomed pan over medium heat and fry bones for 10 minutes, or until browned. DO NOT ADD FAT. Stir bones around in pan frequently. DO NOT ALLOW TO BURN. Add vegetables and brown with bones, cooking another 10 to 15 minutes, and stirring very frequently. Add water, bouquet garni, peppercorns and salt. If water level isn't about two-thirds above ingredients, change pans or add a little more water.

Bring to a slow boil. Put lid on pan, covering only half of pan (this allows liquid to reduce) and simmer for 4 to 5 hours. Stock should be strong with a good taste at end of cooking time. If not, allow to continue to simmer. At end of cooking time, this should be a hearty stock, great for sauces and casseroles. If you want a stock for soups, dilute stock with water using one cup water to two cups stock. Or, if you prefer, re-boil bones with fresh vegetables for soup stock.

Strain stock through cheesecloth. You should have about 6 cups of strong brown bone stock. Re-use bones for soup stock if you so desire. Place stock in the refrigerator until any fat that might be present has solidified. Remove fat, then use stock or freeze in ice cube trays and drop a cube or two in casseroles or soups at time of preparation.

Drop in casseroles or soup at will, as it will not affect the fat contained in the recipe. Great way to add extra taste to a recipe without adding countable calories, fat or cholesterol.

Yield: approximately 6 cups stock times 16 tablespoons equals 96 tablespoons or forty-eight 2-tablespoon cubes.

Approximate Per
*   2-Tablespoon Cube:*
Calories: 1
Fat: Tr.
Cholesterol: Tr.

Diabetic Exchange: Free food

Fish Fumet

(Recipe contains less than 6% fat per cup when diluted soup stock; recipe contains only a trace of fat per cube for 2-tablespoon cubes)

2 1/2 to 3 lb. fish bones—
  use bones after fish have
  been filleted. Most fish
  lover's include heads, but
  I've never been inclined
  to do so.
12 c. water
6 stalks celery & leaves,
  chopped

2 lg. onions, chopped
1 clove garlic, chopped
1 lg. carrot, cut in chunks
Bouquet garni (tie 1/2 tsp.
  dried thyme, 1 bay leaf,
  4 sprigs parsley, 1/2 tsp.
  basil & 10 peppercorns
  in cheesecloth)
3 T. lemon juice

Tie the fish bones and scrap meat in a cheesecloth so it will be easy to discard. Put all ingredients, except the lemon juice, in a large heavy-bottomed pot and bring to a boil. Lower heat and simmer for 30 minutes. Put pot in sink and tie cheesecloth containing fish around water spigot. Allow juices to drip into pan for 30 minutes. Squeeze cheesecloth gently before discarding, to further strengthen stock.

Strain stock into a smaller saucepan and discard vegetables and bouquet garni; return to stove. Simmer, uncovered, until reduced by half. Great for sauces and casseroles. For stocks, add 2 cups water for 3 cups stock. Stock must be chilled and defatted before use. Use at will.

Yield: about 6 cups full strength; 9 cups diluted for soup stock

Approximate Per 1 Cup
  Diluted Soup Stock:
Calories: 16
Fat: 0.1 g
Cholesterol: Tr. mg

Diabetic Exchange: Free food

Approximate Per
  2-Tablespoon Cube:
Calories: 2
Fat: Tr. g
Cholesterol: Tr. mg

Diabetic Exchange: Free food

Mixed Stock

*(Recipe contains less than 6% fat as soup base;
recipes contains a trace of fat as a two-tablespoon cube)*

2 to 3 lb. left-over bones—
chicken, steak roast, ham
along with any leftover
meat trimmed of visible
fat (don't be afraid to mix
bones)

6 to 8 c. root vegetables—
carrots, celery, onions or
scrubbed potato peels (it
doesn't matter if they look
shriveled, the flavor is
still there)

Bouquet garni (3 parsley
stalks, pinch of thyme,
pinch of basil & 1 bay
leaf tied in a
cheesecloth bag)

1 tsp. salt (opt.)

3 qt. water

Break or saw bones in small pieces—the more bone exposure, the better the stock. Chop all vegetables coarsely for cut vegetable exposure. Put bones and vegetables in heavy-bottomed kettle and add water and bouquet garni; add salt. Water level should cover vegetables and bones and extend about two-thirds above ingredients. If it doesn't, change pans or add additional water. Half cover pan and simmer 2 hours, or until stock has a strong, good taste. Stock should reduce by one-third. Strain, cool, chill and then defat. Use in sauces and casseroles. For soups, dilute with water—one cup water for two cups stock.

Yield: 2 quarts

*Approximate Per One Cup
Soup Base:*
Calories: 16
Fat: 0.1 g
Cholesterol: Tr. mg

Diabetic Exchange: Free food

*Approximate Per Each
2-Tablespoon Cube:*
Calories: 2
Fat: Tr. g
Cholesterol: Tr. mg

Diabetic Exchange: Free food

Seasoned Crouton Substitutes

Don't fall prey to the commercial seasoned croutons that are in abundance on the grocery shelves. Most are loaded with saturated fats and are not good for you. Besides that, why pay a lot for croutons when they are so easy to prepare yourself? Making your own croutons also gives you the advantage of seasoning them just as your family likes.

Make them when you have a little extra time. Make up a big batch and store them in freezer bags or airtight tins. You'll be surprised at the many uses you'll find for them.

Seasoned Croutons
(Recipe contains approximately 22% fat)

40 slices reduced-calorie bread, cut in 1/4" to 1/2" cubes
Low-fat cooking spray
1/4 c. parsley flakes
2 tsp. garlic powder (opt.)
2 tsp. sweet basil

1 T. poultry seasoning or 1 tsp. sage
1/4 c. celery flakes
1/4 c. minced onion
1/4 c. green pepper flakes
1 T. seasoned salt (opt.)
1 T. onion powder

Cut bread into cubes of desired size and spread out on two baking sheets that have been lined with foil and sprayed with cooking spray. Spray bread cubes as you toss with a fork to allow coating of all sides. Blend remaining ingredients and sprinkle over bread cubes, tossing to coat all sides. Spray lightly one more time, then bake at 250° for at least one hour, stirring frequently. Allow to stand a couple of hours before storing in bags. Store in airtight containers or in freezer bags in the freezer. Use as you would any other croutons. Keep on hand at all times.
Yield: 22 cups

Approximate Per Cup:
Calories: 85
Fat: 2.1 g
Cholesterol: 0.0 mg

Carbohydrates: 22 g
Protein: 4 g
Sodium: 525 mg

Diabetic Exchanges: 1 1/2 bread; 1/2 fat

Sour Cream Substitute

Sour cream is another product that must be avoided because of its high fat content. One ounce of sour cream contains 6 grams of fat, 3.8 grams of which are saturated.

There have been several mock sour cream substitutes to appear in the past few years. Some I have found acceptable, some unacceptable. They all have a little different taste and texture and there are a number of good ones. I prefer to use "yogurt cheese." In recipes where sour cream is given as an ingredient use a low-fat "light" commercial sour cream.

Mock Sour Cream

(Recipe contains approximately 22% fat)

1 c. "yogurt cheese" (see index)

If using in hot dish, use 1 scant teaspoon cornstarch. Stir in cornstarch just before using.

Yield: one cup or 16 tablespoons

Approximate Per Tablespoon:
Calories: 11
Fat: 0.3 g
Cholesterol: 0.9 mg

Carbohydrates: 1 g
Protein: 1 g
Sodium: 10 mg

Diabetic Exchange: Free

Approximate Per Cup:
Calories: 180
Fat: 4.4 g
Cholesterol: 14.0 mg

Carbohydrates: 16 g
Protein: 12 g
Sodium: 159 mg

Diabetic Exchange: 1 milk

Thin White Sauce

(Recipe contains approximately 30% fat)

1 tsp. tub margarine
1 T. flour
1/4 tsp. salt (opt.)

Pinch pepper
1 c. skim milk

Put margarine in the top of a double boiler and, over boiling water, allow margarine to melt. Add flour, salt and pepper, cooking for two minutes and stirring constantly. Remove from stove and very gradually add milk. Return to stove and cook until mixture thickens.

Yield: 1 cup

Approximate Per Tablespoon:
Calories: 9
Fat: 0.3 g
Cholesterol: Tr. g

Carbohydrates: 1 g
Protein: Tr. g
Sodium: 44 mg

Diabetic Exchanges Per 3 Tablespoons: 1/4 milk

Whipped Topping Substitute

Because of the high saturated fat content in most commercial whipped toppings, people on fat restricted diets have been prohibited from using it. This is no longer the case. There are several "light" whipped toppings on the market that have only 0.5 grams of fat per tablespoon. This is acceptable. I used the Estee Brand sugar-free whipped topping in recipes in this book.

If you still prefer to use a substitute instead of a low-fat commercial whipped topping, a Sta-Whip Whipped Topping has been included. It is not all air, as most substitute whipped toppings, but it does not taste like the commercial whipped toppings. However, it has a nice taste and will work in any recipe in this book.

Sugar-Free Whipped Topping

(Recipe contains approximately 3% fat)

3/4 c. "lite" evaporated
  skim milk
2 T. apple juice
  concentrate, thawed

1 tsp. vanilla extract
8 pkg. NutraSweet type
  sweetener

In a deep mixing bowl blend all of listed ingredients, stirring until well blended. Cover bowl with foil and put in freezer for 1 1/2 hours or until partially frozen. Beat with electric beater at high speed for five minutes. Should be very stiff. Serve immediately.

Yield: 8 servings
Serving size: 1/4 cup

Approximate Per Serving:

Calories: 31
Fat: 0.1 g
Cholesterol: 1 g

Carbohydrates: 5 g
Protein: 2 g
Sodium: 12 mg

Diabetic Exchange: 1/2 milk

Try whipping an egg white, adding a little sugar and then adding a mashed banana, beating until smooth. Makes a quick whipped topping replacement.

Sta-Whip Whipped Topping

(Recipe contains approximately 11% fat if regular;
recipe contains approximately 16% fat if sugar-free)

1 (12 oz.) ctn. (1 1/2 c.) 2%
   cream-style cottage cheese
1 (8 oz.) ctn. (1 c.) commercial plain low-fat yogurt

1 sm. pkg. instant vanilla
   pudding, reg. or sugar-
   free

Put cottage cheese and yogurt in blender and process on "whip" speed for 5 minutes. Pour mixture into bowl and add instant dry pudding mix. Beat with an electric beater on high speed for 2 minutes.

This does not taste like other whipped toppings and is not filled with air. It has a superior taste. It will work in any recipe calling for a whipped topping.
Yield: 2 1/2 cups or 40 tablespoons

Approximate Per Recipe:

	Reg.	Sugar-Free		Reg.	Sugar-Free
Calories:	810	550	Carbohydrates:	52 g	34g
Fat:	10.1 g	10.1 g	Protein:	59 g	59 g
Cholesterol:	43.4 mg	43.4 mg	Sodium	1669 mg	1752 mg

Approximate Per Tablespoon:

	Reg.	Sugar-Free		Reg.	Sugar-Free
Calories:	20	14	Carbohydrates:	2 g	1 g
Fat:	0.3 g	0.3 g	Protein:	2 g	2 g
Cholesterol:	1.0 mg	1.0 mg	Sodium	42 mg	44 mg

Diabetic Exchange: 1/4 milk

Whipped Topping Substitute II

(Recipe contains approximately 3% fat)

1 (8 oz.) pkg. fat-free
   cream cheese
1 can evaporated skim
   milk, very cold

2 tsp. vanilla
12 pkt. Equal sweetener,
   or sweetener of choice
   to equal 1/2 c. sugar

In a large mixing bowl beat cream cheese until fluffy—this takes about five minutes. In a second mixing bowl beat evaporated skim milk until it forms peaks. Gradually add sweetener to whipped milk. Beat whipped milk into cream cheese. Put in a container and store in refrigerator.
Yield: About 5 cups

Approximate Per Tablespoon:

Calories: 9	Carbohydrates: 1 g
Fat: Tr. g	Protein: 1 g
Cholesterol: 1 mg	Sodium: 46 mg

Diabetic Exchanges: 1-2 tablespoons free food

"Yogurt Cheese"
(Recipe contains approximately 22% fat)

1 c. plain low-fat yogurt　　　　**1 coffee filter**

Put coffee filter over glass and fasten securely with a rubber band. Cheesecloth works even better. Put yogurt into coffee filter and cover with plastic wrap. Put in refrigerator for several hours to allow whey to drip out of yogurt. This makes a more solid product that will not separate as easily when used in a salad or casserole. If you wish, put whey in a soup, stew or casserole for extra nutrition.

Note: When using "yogurt cheese" in a recipe, measure yogurt before removing whey and use amount of "yogurt cheese" remaining after whey has dripped out. When using "yogurt cheese" in hot dishes, always blend one scant teaspoon of cornstarch into yogurt. This gives the yogurt the courage to stand up in most recipes and not break down.

Approximate Per Tablespoon:

Calories: 9　　　　　　　　　Carbohydrates: 1 g
Fat: 0.2 g　　　　　　　　　Protein: 1 g
Cholesterol: 0.9 mg　　　　　Sodium: 10 mg

Diabetic Exchange: Free food

Approximate Per Cup:

Calories: 144　　　　　　　　Carbohydrates: 16 g
Fat: 3.5 g　　　　　　　　　Protein: 12 g
Cholesterol: 14 mg　　　　　Sodium: 159 mg

Diabetic Exchange: 1 milk

Making Your Own Yogurt

There is nothing difficult about making yogurt. The main thing to remember is that the temperature must be right for the milk to yog. Homemade yogurt is lower in fat than any you can buy, and it costs only pennies a cup. It takes very little time to mix up, and yogs while you're taking care of other chores, or even while you're at work.

When yogurt doesn't yog, it usually means that your heat was not at the proper temperature or that the containers were not properly washed and rinsed. Any kind of milk can be used for yogurt. Experiment and see which flavor you like best. You can also experiment and discover how long you like your yogurt to yog.

Time determines the tartness the yogurt takes on. Once you have learned to make your own yogurt and discovered its many uses, you'll have it on hand in your refrigerator at all times.

Low-Fat Yogurt

(With cool water, recipe contains approximately 7% fat;
with skim milk, recipe contains approximately 6% fat)

2 1/2 c. low-fat dry milk
    granules
4 c. cool water

2 T. yogurt (use a good
    grade of yogurt from a
    previous batch)

OR:

2 c. low-fat dry milk
    granules

4 c. skim milk (for a
    richer yogurt)
2 T. plain yogurt

In a large heavy-bottomed saucepan, blend water (or milk) with dry milk granules. Stir until granules have dissolved. Cook over medium heat to scalding point. Do not boil. Remove from heat and allow to cool until temperature reaches 110° to 115°. Use a candy thermometer to determine proper temperature.

Stir in yogurt, blending until smooth. Pour into containers that have been thoroughly washed and rinsed with boiling water. Use incubation method you prefer.

Incubation: To incubate yogurt, it's necessary to keep the temperature between 90° to 120°. Anything above 120° will kill the yogurt culture. Anything below 90° will more than likely turn into no more than soured milk. For the best yogurt, the temperature should be kept as close to 115° as possible.

If you have a commercial yogurt maker, simply follow the manufacturer's directions for incubation. If you don't have a yogurt maker you will have to improvise the method best for you. This can only be done by experimenting with water and a thermometer until you find a place that will keep yogurt formula at an even temperature as near 115° as possible.

One of the following incubation methods might work for you:

1. Set a pan of water over the pilot light of your stove (if you cook with gas). Put a candy or meat thermometer into the water and leave it for three hours. After three hours, check to see what the temperature is. If the water is over 115°, try placing the pan on a trivet to adjust temperature and run another 3 hour test.

2. Place a pan of water on a trivet over the small burner of an electric stove and set the burner at lowest setting. Insert thermometer and check after three hours. If temperature is within incubation range, this method may be used.

3. Float a casserole dish in a pan of water and set on pilot light on small burner of stove at low setting. Follow described testing procedure above.

Continued on following page.

Continued from preceding page.

4. Place a pan of water on a heating pad and follow testing procedure.

5. Set a pan of water on an electric warming tray set at low setting (or higher, if necessary) and follow testing procedure.

6. Fill a chafing dish with water and follow testing procedure.

Almost any kind of milk can be used for yogurt as long as it is low in fat. If you don't care for the recipes I use, try using evaporated skim milk or combine it with fresh skim milk or low-fat dry milk. Experiment until you get the taste you like best.

Yogurt should yog within five hours. The nearer the temperature is to 115° the faster the formula will yog. If you don't have yogurt within five hours, your temperature is probably below 90° and you'll never have anything more than soured milk.

Yield: each recipe makes 1 quart

Approximate Per 1/2 Cup:
(if cool water is used):

Calories: 77	Carbohydrates: 12 g
Fat: 0.6 g	Protein: 8 g
Cholesterol: 4 mg	Sodium: 126 mg

Approximate Per 1/2 Cup:
(if using skim milk):

Calories: 120	Carbohydrates: 12 g
Fat: 0.8 g	Protein: 8 g
Cholesterol: 6 mg	Sodium: 127 mg

Diabetic Exchange: 1 milk

Appetizers,
Snacks
&
Beverages

Appetizers, Snacks & Beverages

Appetizers

Although we often think of appetizers as being filled with fat, this is not necessarily true. There are many tasty, attractive appetizers that contain acceptable fat levels for the people on fat restricted diets.

It's always a good idea to include an arrangement of fruits and vegetables that can be dipped into a low fat, low calorie dip.

This will not only help anyone on a weight restricted diet, but will also assist anyone who is on a diabetic diet.

The diabetic is allowed only so many food exchanges per day and it is not the wisest thing in the world for them to use these precious exchanges on nibbling food.

By including a tray of vegetables with a low-cal dip, you will allow the diabetic to enjoy the appetizers without wasting food exchanges on them.

When a meal is to follow the appetizers, be sure and keep the appetizers light and serve them for only a short time. An appetizer is meant to only whet the appetite, not satisfy it.

*Avocado Dip: To keep fresh and green,
put pit into dip mix until ready to serve.*

Beef and Bean Dip

(Recipe contains approximately 13% fat)

1/2 lb. ground round	1 tsp. chili powder
1/2 lb. ground turkey breast	1/2 tsp. cumin
1 onion, chopped	6 slices no-fat American
1/2 c. ketchup	cheese, diced
1 (16 oz.) can red kidney	Oven tortilla chips (see
beans, mashed in juice	index)

Brown ground round, turkey breast and onion. Drain off any rendered fat. Add ketchup, mashed beans, chili powder and cumin; heat through. Add cheese and serve with tortilla chips.

Yield: about 6 cups

Approximate Per 1/4 Cup:
Calories: 67
Fat: 1.0 g
Cholesterol: 15 mg
Carbohydrates: 5 g
Protein: 3 g
Sodium: 119 mg

Diabetic Exchanges: 1/4 meat; 1 vegetable; 1/4 fat

Remember that appetites are meant to be whetted by appetizers, not satisfied by them.

A canape or hors d'oeuvre is supposed to be no more than a bite eaten easily out of the hand.

Christmas Eggs

(Recipe contains approximately 26% fat)

8 eggs, boiled, peeled &
    yolks discarded
1 c. cool water
1 drop of green food
    coloring*
1 T. vinegar
1 c. ground lean ham
2 green onions, chopped
    fine

1 T. dill pickle relish
1/4 tsp. dry mustard
2 T. reduced-calorie mayon-
    naise
1/4 tsp. seasoned salt
    (opt.)
4 stuffed green olives

Rinse egg white shells and drop into mixture of water, food coloring and vinegar. Allow to stay until light green egg whites develop. Remove from dye and drain on paper towels. Mix remaining ingredients, except olives. Fill green egg whites with mixture and top with a thin slice of olive.

*At Easter, dye egg white shells several different colors before filling with ham salad.

Yield: 16 filled eggs

Approximate Per Egg Half:
Calories: 24
Fat: 0.7 g
Cholesterol: 7
Carbohydrates: 1
Protein: 2 g
Sodium: 260 mg

Diabetic Exchanges: 1/4 meat; 1/4 vegetable

*Serve soup in a nice wine glass as an
appetizer before guests are seated.*

Easy Elegant Shrimp Dip

(Recipe contains approximately 9% fat)

2 (16 oz.) pkg. shrimp, cleaned & cooked	1/2 tsp. onion powder
1 (8 oz.) pkg. non-fat cream cheese	1/2 tsp. salt (opt.)
	1/4 tsp. pepper
3 T. chili sauce	1/4 tsp. Worcestershire sauce
1 T. lemon juice	1/4 c. skim milk

Put all ingredients, except milk in blender and process until smooth. Add milk, a little at a time, until of a dip consistency (may not need all of milk). Cover and refrigerate for 2 hours or more. Serve with raw vegetables.
Yield: 2 cups

Approximate Per Tablespoon:
Calories: 42
Fat: 0.4 g
Cholesterol: 45 mg
Carbohydrates: 3 g
Protein: 8 g
Sodium: 191 mg

Diabetic Exchanges: 1 meat; 1/4 milk

Make a canape just before serving; food on a piece of limp and soggy toast is an obomination,

Avoid repetition as you would sin; a food included in the first course loses all appeal if encountered again later in the meal.

Holiday Corn Dip

(Recipe contains only a trace of fat)

1 (12 oz.) can Mexi-corn, drained
1 med. fresh tomato, seeded then chopped
1/2 med. green pepper, chopped
1/4 c. sweet onion, chopped
2 jalapeño peppers, seeds discarded & chopped
1 T. light mayonnaise (no fat, no cholesterol)
2 T. reduced-calorie ranch dressing

Put prepared vegetables in a mixing bowl and blend. Stir together mayonnaise and ranch dressing until smooth. Pour over vegetables and blend.

Yield: about 40 tablespoons
Serving size: 1/4 cup

Approximate Per Serving:
Calories: 37
Fat: 0.2 g
Cholesterol: 0.0 g
Carbohydrates: 10 g
Protein: 1 g
Sodium: 161 mg

Diabetic Exchanges: 1 fruit

As with all food, serve hot food hot and cold food cold.
Flavors, like love, are disappointing when lukewarm.

Manhandlers Nachos

(Recipe contains approximately 7% fat)

1/2 lb. turkey sausage (see index)
1/4 tsp. dried basil
1/4 tsp. dried cilantro
1/2 (4 oz.) can green chilies
1/4 c. chopped onion
1/4 c. chopped green pepper
1 (8 oz.) can red kidney beans, drained (1 c.)
1/3 c. chunky salsa (see index)
5 corn tortillas, cut in pie-shaped pieces & baked until crisp
8 oz. no-fat American cheese, diced

Blend turkey sausage, basil, cilantro and green chilies. Add onion and green pepper and put into 1 1/2-quart microwave-safe casserole. Cover with wax paper and microwave 100% power (HIGH) for 4 to 5 minutes or until meat is done. Stir once or twice during cooking. Drain off all rendered fat.

Add beans and salsa and stir to blend. Microwave on HIGH for 2 minutes. Spread half of crisp tortilla chips on large microwave-safe platter and top with half of sausage mixture. Top with half of cheese and cook, uncovered, on HIGH until cheese melts (1 1/2 to 2 1/2 minutes). Repeat layer and cook until cheese melts, giving platter half a turn after 1 minute.

Yield: 16 servings
Serving size: 2 chips

Approximate Per Serving:
Calories: 80
Fat: 0.6 g
Cholesterol: 8 mg
Carbohydrates: 10 g
Protein: 7 g
Sodium: 252 mg

Diabetic Exchanges: 1 meat; 1 fruit

The diabetic should not waste a meat exchange on this appetizer.

Hors d'oeuvres, like any other foods, should have a certain balance. Some should be cold, some hot; some bland, some spicy; some crisp and some soft.

Mexican Dip

(Recipe contains approximately 14% fat)

1/2 lb. ground round	1 pkg. dry taco mix
1/2 lb. ground turkey <u>breast</u>	1/2 tsp. chili powder
1 sm. onion, chopped	1/2 tsp. garlic powder
1 sm. green pepper,	1/4 tsp. cumin
chopped	8 slices no-fat American
1 (8 oz.) can tomato sauce	cheese, diced

In a skillet, brown ground round, turkey, onion and green pepper until pink disappears. Drain any rendered fat. Then stir in remaining ingredients, except cheese, blending well. Pour into serving dish and top with grated cheese. Serve with Home-Style Oven Tortilla Chips (see index).

Yield: about 50 tablespoons
Serving size: 2 tablespoons

Approximate Per Serving:
Calories: 57
Fat: 0.9 g
Cholesterol: 15 mg
Carbohydrates: 3 g
Protein: 7 g
Sodium: 212 mg

Diabetic Exchanges: 1/2 vegetable; 1 meat

Meat exchange is too high to waste on this appetizer for the diabetic.

Use a melon-ball maker to form appetizer-sized meatballs. Dip in cold water occasionally to keep meatballs from sticking.

Nacho Dip Olé

(Recipe contains approximately 8% fat)

1 (15 oz.) can whole
   tomatoes, drained
1 green onion, chopped fine
1 tsp. Worcestershire sauce

2 T. vinegar
1 to 2 pickled jalapeño
   peppers, chopped

Put all of ingredients in a blender and process on low speed for a few seconds—dip should be left a little chunky. Serve with Home-Style Over Tortilla Chips (see index).
Yield: 10 servings with 4 chips
Serving size: 2 tablespoons dip + 4 chips

Approximate Per Serving:
Calories: 57
Fat: 0.5 g
Cholesterol: 0.0 g
Carbohydrates: 7 g
Protein: 1 g
Sodium: 16 mg

Diabetic Exchanges: 1/2 vegetable; 1/2 bread

Oven Tortilla Chips

(Recipe contains approximately 9% fat)

1 pkg. 12 (6") corn tortillas
Vegetable spray

Onion or garlic powder or
   dry taco mix

Cut each tortilla into 6 pie-shaped wedges and lay out onto baking sheet that has been lightly sprayed with cooking oil. Spray tops of tortilla wedges very, very lightly and sprinkle with seasoning of choice. Bake in 400° preheated oven for 8 to 10 minutes or until crisp. DO NOT OVERCOOK.
Yield: 72 chips
Serving size: 6 chips

Approximate Per Serving:
Calories: 72
Fat: 0.7 g
Cholesterol: 0.0 mg
Carbohydrates: 14 g
Protein: 2 g
Sodium: 2 g

Diabetic Exchanges: 1 bread

Potted Herbed Cheese

(Recipe contains approximately 16% fat)

1 lg. clove garlic
1/4 c. packed basil leaves
   or 1 1/2 tsp. dry basil
4 chopped green onion tops
6 stuffed green olives,
   chopped fine

1 c. (1%) low-fat cottage
   cheese, cream-style
1 (3 oz.) pkg. 94% fat-free
   cream cheese (or any
   cream cheese with less
   than a gram of fat per
   ounce)

Put garlic clove in food processor and process 3 to 4 seconds. Add basil, green onion tops and green olives. Process a few seconds on chop speed. Add cheese and use pulse button process until blended but still slightly chunky. Spoon into small decorative dish or crock and chill at least 8 hours. Will keep in airtight container for about a week if refrigerated.

Yield: 1 1/3 cups
Serving size: 1 tablespoon

Approximate Per Serving:
Calories: 17
Fat: 0.3 g
Cholesterol: 10 mg
Carbohydrates: 4 g
Protein: 3 g
Sodium: 128 mg

Diabetic Exchanges: 1/4 milk

Use your imagination. Scorn a food idea copied from
a friend as firmly as you would a copied dress.

Refried Beans

(Recipe contains approximately 6% fat)

2 (15 oz.) cans dark red
    kidney beans
1 (15 oz.) can Great North-
    ern beans
1 frozen chicken stock
    cube, for sautéing (see
    index)

1 med. onion, minced fine
3 cloves garlic, minced
2 tsp. chili powder
1 1/2 tsp. cumin
1/2 tsp. seasoned salt
1 (4 oz.) can green chilies,
    diced very fine

Drain beans and rinse under water. Then allow to drain well so all water disappears. In a small sauté skillet melt frozen stock cube and sauté onions and garlic until liquid disappears. Pour into bowl with beans and add remaining ingredients. Process mixture in food processor for a few seconds. Mixture should be processed only long enough so as to leave it still a little chunky.

This can be served as a bean dip or in any recipe calling for refried beans.

Yield: about 4 cups or 64 tablespoons
Serving size: 1 tablespoon

Approximate Per Serving:
Calories: 16
Fat: 0.1 g
Cholesterol: 0.0 mg
Carbohydrates: 4 g
Protein: 1 g
Sodium: 18 mg

Diabetic Exchanges: 1 vegetable

Always lavish care on garnishing and serve with pride.
After all, love and gaiety are the best sauces for appetite.

Stuffed Mushrooms Florentine

(Recipe contains approximately 25% fat)

20 lg. fresh mushrooms, cleaned & stems removed
1 (10 oz.) pkg. frozen chopped spinach, thawed & well drained
1 c. seasoned croutons, slightly crushed (not too fine) (see index)
Egg substitute to equal 1 egg
1 T. tub margarine, melted
4 slices no-fat American cheese, diced fine
1/4 tsp. pepper
1/2 tsp. garlic salt or powder
1/4 tsp. thyme

Chop mushroom stems very fine and put into mixing bowl. Add remaining ingredients, except mushrooms; blend well. Stuff mushrooms with mixture. Place on ungreased baking sheet and cook in 350° preheated oven for 20 minutes.

Yield: 20 mushrooms
Serving size: 1 mushroom

Approximate Per Serving:
Calories: 33
Fat: 0.9 g
Cholesterol: 1.0 mg
Carbohydrates: 3 g
Protein: 2 g
Sodium: 113 mg

Diabetic Exchanges: 1 vegetable

Plan meals with an eye toward color.
Eye appeal entices good eaters.

Surprise Meatball Skewers

(Recipe contains approximately 27% fat)

1/2 lb. ground round
1/2 lb. ground turkey breast
8 slices non-fat American
  cheese, diced
1/4 c. fine bread crumbs
1 tsp. chili powder
1/2 tsp. minced onion

1/2 tsp. salt (opt.)
1/8 tsp. pepper
Egg substitute to equal
  2 eggs
1/4 c. taco sauce
50 lg. green olives

Blend all ingredients, except olives. Shape into balls. Wrap each ball around olive, reshaping into ball. Place on baking sheet that has been sprayed with cooking oil. Bake in 350° preheated oven for 10 to 12 minutes, or until browned and cooked through. Serve warm on toothpicks as appetizers.

Yield: 50 meatballs
Serving size: 1 meatball

Approximate Per Serving:
Calories: 56
Fat: 1.7 g
Cholesterol: 12 mg
Carbohydrates: 2 g
Protein: 6 g
Sodium: 363 mg

Diabetic Exchanges: 1 meat; 1/2 vegetable

Not a good appetizer for diabetics

*Plan every meal so that you have time to cook
and serve it properly without fuss.*

Sweet and Sour Meatballs

(Recipe contains approximately 11% fat)

2 lb. ground turkey <u>breast</u>
1/4 c. fine saltine cracker
   crumbs (use crackers
   with unsalted tops)
Egg substitute to equal
   2 eggs
1 sm. onion, chopped fine
1/4 sm. green pepper,
   chopped fine

1 tsp. seasoned salt (opt.)
1/4 tsp. pepper
1 (8 oz.) can water chestnuts, chopped fine
1 T. low-sodium soy sauce
1 (12 oz.) jar chili sauce
1 (6 oz.) jar grape jelly

In a large mixing bowl put turkey, crumbs, egg substitute, onion, green pepper, seasoned salt, pepper, water chestnuts and soy sauce; blend well. Chill mixture for at least 2 hours. When chilled, form into 64 bite-size meatballs.

Blend chili sauce and grape jelly, heating until smooth. Put meatballs on baking sheet that has been sprayed with vegetable spray. Brush with sauce and bake 20 to 25 minutes or until meatballs are done. Put meatballs in chafing dish and pour remaining sauce over meatballs.

Yield: 64 meatballs
Serving size: 1 meatball

Approximate Per Serving:
Calories: 40
Fat: 0.5 g
Cholesterol: 11 mg
Carbohydrates: 2 g
Protein: 5 g
Sodium: 85 mg

Diabetic Exchanges: 1/2 meat; 1 vegetable

*Make sure daily meals are adequate by
serving foods from all the food groups.*

Toastada Dip

(Recipe contains approximately 20% fat)

2 c. refried beans (see index)
1/2 tsp. chili powder
2 avocados, peeled & mashed
1/2 c. plain no-fat yogurt
1/4 c. chopped onion
1/2 pkg. dry taco dip

1 c. ripe olives, chopped
2 c. chopped tomatoes
Dash of Tabasco sauce
Dash of lemon juice
1 (4 oz.) can chopped green chilies, drained
2 slices no-fat American cheese, diced

Combine refried beans and chili powder; mix well and set aside. Combine avocados, yogurt, onion and taco dip. Spread bean mixture out on a platter and top with yogurt mixture. Top with a layer of olives. Blend tomatoes, Tabasco and lemon juice. Put on top of olives and top with chilies and then cheese. Serve with Oven Tortilla chips (see index).
Yield: 20 servings

Approximate Per Serving:
Calories: 84
Fat: 1.9 g
Cholesterol: 0.9 mg
Carbohydrates: 16 g
Protein: 6 g
Sodium: 53 mg

Diabetic Exchanges: 1 bread; 1/2 meat

When a recipe calls for sour cream and you are out, use 1/3 cup lemon juice to one cup evaporated skim milk or 1/4 cup lemon juice to 1 cup skim milk or 1 cup "Yougurt cheese," see index, with scant teaspoon of cornstarch added.

Zippy Bean Dip

(Recipe contains approximately 6% fat)

1 (16 oz.) can kidney beans, drained (use dark red)	2 tsp. Worcestershire sauce
	3 T. non-fat mayonnaise
	Juice of 1 lemon
1 clove garlic, minced	1 green onion, minced very fine
1/4 tsp. Tabasco sauce	

Put all ingredients in blender and process until smooth—takes 45 to 60 seconds. Put into serving bowl and serve with raw vegetables. Makes about 2 cups.

Yield: about 2 cups
Serving size: 1 tablespoon

Approximate Per Serving:
Calories: 16
Fat: 0.1 g
Cholesterol: 0.0 mg
Carbohydrates: 3 g
Protein: 1 g
Sodium: 48 mg

Diabetic Exchanges: 1 T. can be considered free food; 1/4 cup equals 1 bread

Save time and money by planning and cooking double quantities. Freeze half for use another day.

Avoid monotony in food as you would the plague.

Snacks

Cereal Party Mix

(Recipe contains approximately 21% fat)

2 T. tub margarine
  (do not use diet)
1/2 tsp. seasoned salt (opt.)
2 tsp. Worcestershire sauce

1 1/2 c. Rice Chex
1 1/2 c. Wheat Chex
1 c. thin pretzel sticks

On a baking sheet, melt margarine and stir in salt and Worcestershire sauce. Add Rice Chex, Wheat Chex and pretzels; stir until evenly coated. Bake in a 250° preheated oven for 45 minutes. Stir every 15 minutes. Spread out on paper towels to cool. Store in airtight container.

Yield: 8 servings
Serving size: 1/2 cup

Approximate Per Serving:
Calories: 177
Fat 4.2 g
Cholesterol 0.0 mg
Carbohydrates: 31 g
Protein: 2 g
Sodium: 532 mg

Diabetic Exchanges: 2 breads; 1 fat

The mold that develops on cheese during storage
is a normal process. Scrape or cut the mold from the surface,
discard it, and use the remainder of the cheese

Jell-O Pops

(Recipe contains approximately 0% fat)

2 c. boiling water
1 (3 oz.) pkg. cherry sugar-
    free flavored gelatin

1 pkg. sugar-free cherry
    Kool-Aid
2 c. cold water

Dissolve gelatin in boiling water. Add Kool-Aid and dissolve. Add cold water. Pour into Dixie Cups (1/4 cup size). Put sticks in to make popsicles. Place in freezer and allow to freeze.

Yield: 18 popsicles
Serving size: 1 popsicle

Approximate Per Serving:
Calories: 4
Fat: 0.0 g
Cholesterol: 0.0 mg
Carbohydrates 0.0 g
Protein: 0.0 g
Sodium: 9 mg

Diabetic Exchanges: Free food

*Serve hot chocolate with a stick of
cinnamon for a stirrer - adds a nice flavor.*

Sweet and Spicy Mexican Mix

(Recipe contains approximately 26% fat)

1 c. light corn syrup
1 c. tub margarine
1/2 c. packed brown sugar
1 pkg. taco seasoning
8 c. Crispix
8 c. corn flakes
8 c. popped popcorn
   (popped with no oil)

6 corn tortillas, torn into
   small pieces, sprayed
   with Pam & baked in
   oven until crisp
2 c. low-salt pretzels

Melt corn syrup, margarine and brown sugar in a saucepan. Add taco seasoning and bring to a full boil, stirring constantly. Pour over cereal mix. Blend well. Spread out on large baking sheet (or two sheets) and bake in 350° preheated oven for 1 hour. Stir every 15 minutes. After 30 minutes switch baking sheet on top shelf to bottom shelf and vice versa.

Yield: about 32 cups
Serving size: 1/2 cup

Approximate Per Serving:
Calories 118
Fat 3.4 g
Cholesterol 0.0 mg
Carbohydrates: 19 g
Protein: 1 g
Sodium: 170 mg

Diabetic Exchanges: 1 1/4 bread

Caution: This has sugar and should not be used by diabetics.

*Freeze leftover tea and coffee in ice cube trays
and use in chilled coffee and tea drinks.*

Beverages

Cranberry Christmas Punch
(Recipe contains approximately 0% fat)

1 (3 oz.) pkg. cherry
    flavored gelatin
1 c. boiling water
2 pkg. lemonade sugar-free
    dry mix sweetened with
    NutraSweet

3 c. cold water
1 (1 qt.) btl. cranberry
    juice cocktail, chilled
    (sugar-free)
1 lg. btl. ginger ale, chilled
    (2 liter), sugar-free

Dissolve gelatin in boiling water; stir in lemonade. Add cold water and cranberry juice. Place in large punch bowl. Just before serving, add ginger ale. Add ice cubes or molded ice ring.

Yield: 15 servings

Approximate Per Serving:
Calories: 23
Fat: 0.0 g
Cholesterol: 0.0 mg
Carbohydrates: 4 g
Protein: Tr.
Sodium: 6 mg

Diabetic Exchanges: 1/2 fruit

Fresh Lemonade
(Recipe contains approximately 8% fat)

1 c. fresh-squeezed
    lemon juice
4 c. water

18 pkt. Equal sweetener, or
    sweetener of choice to
    equal 3/4 c. sugar

Blend all ingredients, chill and serve over ice cubes.

Yield: 4 servings
Serving size: 8 ounces

Approximate Per Serving:
Calories: 31
Fat: 0.3 g
Cholesterol: 0.0 mg
Carbohydrates: 4 g
Protein: Tr. g
Sodium: 13 mg

Diabetic Exchanges: 1/2 fruit

Frozen Banana Daiquiris

(Recipe contains approximately 8% fat)

1 pkg. sugar-free dry
    lemonade mix, sweetener
    included
6 oz. cold water

1 T. rum extract
10 to 15 ice cubes
2 ripe bananas

Combine lemonade, water and rum extract in blender, then slowly add fruit; processing until smooth. Add ice cubes, 2 or 3 at a time, until mixture is slushy.

Yield: 8 servings

Approximate Per Serving:
Calories: 34
Fat: 0.3 g
Cholesterol: 0.0 mg
Carbohydrates: 7 g
Protein: Tr. g
Sodium: 0.0 mg

Diabetic Exchanges: 1 fruit

Holiday Punch

(Recipe contains approximately 0% fat)

1 (3 oz.) pkg. flavored
    gelatin, sugar-free
1 c. boiling water
1 pkg. dry lemonade mix,
    sugar-free (with
    sweetener included)

2 c. cold water
1 (32 oz.) btl. cranberry
    juice, chilled, low
    calorie
1 (28 oz.) btl. ginger ale,
    chilled, sugar-free

Dissolve gelatin in boiling water. Add lemonade granules. Add remaining ingredients. Pour into punch bowl. Add ice ring.

Yield: 12 cups
Serving size: 1 cup

Approximate Per Serving:
Calories: 28
Fat: 0.0 g
Cholesterol: 0.0 mg
Carbohydrates: 4 g
Protein: 1 g
Sodium: 7 mg

Diabetic Exchanges: 1/2 fruit

Hot Spiced Cranberry Punch

(Recipe contains approximately 11% fat)

2 c. cranberry juice,
  low calorie
2 1/2 c. water
12 pkt. Equal sweetener,
  or sweetener of choice
  to equal 1 cup sugar

2 sticks cinnamon
10 whole cloves
1/2 lemon, sliced thin
2 c. freshly-brewed tea
1 c. pineapple juice,
  unsweetened

Combine cranberry juice and water. Add sweetener and stir until dissolved. Add whole spices tied in a bag. Simmer 5 minutes. Add lemon slices, tea and pineapple juice. Serve hot.
Yield: 12 servings

Approximate Per Serving:
Calories: 32
Fat: 0.4 g
Cholesterol: 0.0 mg
Carbohydrates: 6 g
Protein: Tr. g
Sodium: 3 mg

Diabetic Exchanges: 1/2 fruit

Peppermint Refresher

(Recipe contains approximately 3% fat)

1 c. sugar-free, lowfat
  frozen vanilla yogurt
1 c. skim milk

4 sugar-free starlight
  candies

Put all ingredients in a blender and process until smooth. Serve at once.
Yield: 2 servings

Approximate Per Serving:
Calories: 107
Fat 0.7 g
Cholesterol: 5 mg
Carbohydrates: 18 g
Protein: 7 g
Sodium: 10 mg

Diabetic Exchanges: 1 milk; 1/2 fruit

Strawberry-Orange Cooler

(Recipe contains approximately 2% fat)

2 1/2 c. frozen unsweetened
 whole strawberries,
 unthawed
1 c. water
1/3 c. frozen orange juice
 concentrate, unsweet-
 ened, thawed & undiluted

2 pkt. of Equal or sweet-
 ener of choice to equal
 4 tsp. sugar
2 ice cubes

Put all ingredients in an electric blender and process until mixture is smooth. Serve at once.

Yield: 3 servings

Approximate Per Serving:
Calories: 119
Fat: 0.3 g
Cholesterol: 0.0 mg
Carbohydrates: 28 g
Protein: 2 g
Sodium: 2 mg

Diabetic Exchanges: 3 fruits

Sweet and Spicy Tea Mix

(Recipe contains a trace of fat)

3 pkg. sugar-free orange-
 flavored Kool-Aid
6 T. instant tea mix
6 pkt. Equal sweetener, or
 sweetener of choice
 to equal 1/4 c. sugar

1 tsp. ground cinnamon
1/8 tsp. ground cloves
 (opt.)
1/2 tsp. ground allspice

Combine all ingredients, blending well. Store in airtight container.

To Serve: Use 1 tablespoon mix and 6 ounces boiling water. Put mix in cup and add water. Stir until dissolved.

For cool refreshing drink, use chilled water and serve over ice cubes.

Yield: 18 servings

Approximate Per Serving:
Calories: 7
Fat: Tr. g
Cholesterol: 0.0 mg
Carbohydrates: 0.0
Protein: 0.0
Sodium: 0.0

Diabetic Exchanges: Free food in limited amounts

Pumpkin Holiday Shake

*(Serve as a breakfast shake for Thanksgiving
to keep stomachs empty for the big meal)*
(Recipe contains approximately 4% fat)

1 c. cooked pumpkin	1/4 tsp. ginger
1/2 c. skim milk	1 tsp. vanilla
1/8 tsp. salt (opt.)	1/4 c. brown sugar
1/2 tsp. cinnamon	1 1/2 c. nonfat vanilla
1/8 tsp. cardamom	frozen yogurt, sugar-free

Put all ingredients in a blender and process until smooth.
Yield: 3 servings

Approximate Per Serving:
Calories: 183
Fat: 0.8 g
Cholesterol: 9 mg
Carbohydrates: 37 g
Protein: 5 g
Sodium 70 mg

Diabetic Exchanges: 1 milk; 2 1/2 fruit

Purple Passion Shake

(Recipe contains approximately 5% fat)

1 1/2 c. vanilla-flavored yogurt, sugar-free, low-fat	1/2 c. skim milk
	1/2 c. sugar-free frozen grape juice concentrate

Put all ingredients into blender and process until smooth. Serve at once.
Yield: 2 servings

Approximate Per Serving:
Calories: 150
Fat: 0.9 g
Cholesterol: 5 mg
Carbohydrates: 27 g
Protein: 7 g
Sodium: 100 mg

Diabetic Exchanges: 1 milk; 1 1/2 fruit

Spicy Apple Shake

(Recipe contains approximately 4% fat)

1 c. vanilla nonfat, sugar-
free frozen yogurt
1/2 c. skim milk

1/4 c. apple juice concentrate, thawed
1/8 tsp. ground cinnamon
8 ice cubes

Put all ingredients into processor and process until smooth. Serve at once.
Yield: 2 servings

Approximate Per Serving:
Calories: 206
Fat: 0.9 g
Cholesterol: 0.0 mg
Carbohydrates: 44 g
Protein: 5 g
Sodium: 78 mg

Diabetic Exchanges: 1 milk; 3 fruit

Sugar-Free Pineapple Shake

(Recipe contains approximately 4% fat)

1 c. sugar-free, lowfat
vanilla frozen yogurt
1/4 c. unsweetened pine-
apple juice

1 (8 oz.) can pineapple
tidbits, unsweetened,
include juice

Put all ingredients in blender and blend until smooth. Serve at once.
Yield: 2 servings

Approximate Per Serving:
Calories: 162
Fat: 0.7 g
Cholesterol: 3 mg
Carbohydrates: 36 g
Protein: 4 g
Sodium: 47 mg

Diabetic Exchanges: 1/2 milk; 3 fruit

Breads

Breads

Nothing Compares to Homemade Bread

There is nothing more satisfying than removing a golden loaf of bread from the oven.

However, the best reason for baking your own bread is the control you gain over the ingredients that goes into the bread.

For the sodium-restricted it's the best possible way to control the sodium content. Although you can get by without using any salt in bread, there is no disputing that salt does affect the texture of the bread. A dough without salt will not produce the same quality loaf of bread as dough with salt included.

The amount of salt called for in a bread recipe can be reduced without much consequence.

The big consideration when baking bread is the flour used. As we read more and more about putting more fiber in our diets, it only makes sense to use more grains in our bread.

Although using refined white flour is not exactly bad for you, it is not as beneficial as whole grain flours since white flour has been robbed of its bran and germ in the milling process. This cuts the fiber content compared with whole grain flours.

One of the best discoveries I have made is a whole wheat blend flour manufactured by Gold Medal.

It's a special blend of whole wheat and all-purpose enriched flour that can be substituted cup for cup in a recipe. Although I prefer a mix of whole wheat and unbleached flour, there is no disputing that the whole wheat blend flour is great when it comes to converting recipes. It is also an easy way to include more fiber in the diet.

If you have never made bread before don't be afraid to give it a try. It is not as difficult as it is cracked up to be.

The secret is to follow the recipe and do exactly as it instructs. Making bread is an art of patience as it does take a little time to make yeast breads that must be set aside to rise.

However, the presentation of a fresh-baked loaf of bread will not only impress your family, but will give you a feeling of accomplishment that is very satisfying.

Yeast Breads

Cottage Cheese-Dilly Bread

(Recipe contains approximately 27% fat)

1 pkg. dry yeast
1/4 c. warm water
   (110°-115°)
1 c. low-fat cream-style
   cottage cheese
1/4 c. tub margarine
1 T. minced fresh onion
2 tsp. dill seed
1 tsp. salt (opt.)
   (use a little salt)

1/4 tsp. baking soda
Egg substitute to equal
   1 egg
2 1/4 to 2 1/2 c. flour,
   whole wheat blend,
   unbleached or all-
   purpose

Sprinkle yeast over warm water and set aside to sponge. Heat cottage cheese in saucepan over low heat. Stir in tub margarine, onion, dill, salt and baking soda. Add yeast sponge and egg substitute. Add enough flour to make a soft dough; turn out on floured surface and knead in as much flour as needed to make soft elastic dough. Put in bowl that has been sprayed with vegetable oil. Turn once to coat both sides. Set in warm place for 1 hour or until dough doubles. Put into 9x5x3-inch loaf pan that has been sprayed with vegetable oil. Cover and allow to rise 45 minutes. Bake in 350° preheated oven for about 40 minutes. Remove from oven. Brush lightly with margarine and sprinkle with extra dill seeds.
Yield: 1 loaf, 20 slices

Approximate Per Slice:
Calories: 84
Fat: 2.5 g
Cholesterol: 2 mg
Carbohydrates: 12 g
Protein: 2 g
Sodium: 148 mg

Diabetic Exchanges: 1 bread

Have an open mind when baking bread. There are many flours besides white flour that produce delicious bread.

Cracked Wheat Bread

(Recipe contains approximately 10% fat)

1/2 c. cracked wheat (bulgur)	2 T. tub margarine, softened
1 1/2 c. boiling water	2 tsp. salt (opt.)
1 tsp. sugar	2 T. molasses
1/3 c. warm water (115°)	2 T. honey
1 pkg. (1 T.) active dry yeast	1 c. skim milk
	1 c. whole wheat flour
	4 c. all-purpose flour

Put cracked wheat in boiling water and cook for about 10 minutes or until water is absorbed. Stir occasionally. In a large mixing bowl put sugar and water and sprinkle yeast over top. Proof 10 to 15 minutes. Stir margarine, salt, molasses, honey and milk into cracked wheat. Blend well. With a wooden spoon stir in as much of flour as is needed to make a stiff kneadable dough. Turn out onto floured surface and knead a full 10 minutes, working in as much remaining flour as needed. Put smooth and elastic dough into a bowl that has been sprayed with cooking spray. Turn once to coat both sides, then cover with plastic wrap that has been sprayed with cooking spray. Put in warm place to rise until doubled in bulk; about 1 1/2 hours.

Punch dough down; cut dough in half, then put back in bowl, covered, to rest for 10 minutes. Roll each piece of dough out on lightly floured surface, to make a rectangle 6x9-inches. Starting at wide end, roll dough up tightly; pinch seam shut and place in 9x5x3-inch loaf pan that has been sprayed with cooking spray, seam side down. Cover with plastic wrap and allow to rise until doubled in bulk. Bread should be at top of pans when doubled (about 45 to 60 minutes). Bake in 375° preheated oven for 30 to 35 minutes or until done. Bread will have a hollow sound when tapped on the bottom if done.

Yield: 30 slices

Approximate Per Slice:
Calories: 102
Fat: 1.1 g
Cholesterol: 0.0 mg
Carbohydrates: 19 g
Protein: 3 g
Sodium: 90 mg

Diabetic Exchanges: 1 1/2 bread

Fast and Easy Onion Bread

(Recipe contains approximately 12% fat)

1 loaf frozen bread dough   **1 pkg. onion soup mix**

Set bread out to thaw as directed on package. This can be done the night before. Roll dough out on an unfloured surface. Sprinkle half of onion soup mixture over bread and knead until dough is even with soup mix. Repeat with remaining soup mix. Form dough into a loaf and put in 9x5-inch bread pan. Allow to rise, covered with plastic wrap that has been sprayed with cooking spray, for about 2 hours. Bake in 350° preheated oven for 30 to 40 minutes, or until done.

Yield: 14 slices

Approximate Per Slice:
Calories: 90
Fat: 1.2 g
Cholesterol: 0.0 mg
Carbohydrates: 16 g
Protein: 3 g
Sodium: 298 mg

Diabetic Exchanges: 1 bread; 1/4 fat

*Fruit Breads - use orange or pineapple
juice in place of water for added flavor.*

*Always keep in mind that if the liquid in your bread is milk it must be
scalded to halt bacterial action; otherwise your bread may sour.*

Quick Breads

Fresh Blueberry-Banana Bread

(Recipe contains approximately 11% fat)

1 c. fresh blueberries
1 3/4 c. all-purpose flour,
   divided
2 tsp. baking powder
1/4 tsp. baking soda
1/4 tsp. salt (opt.)
1/4 tsp. nutmeg

1/4 c. tub margarine
1/3 c. sugar
Egg substitute to equal
   2 eggs
1 c. very ripe banana,
   mashed
Cooking spray

Sprinkle a little of the flour over blueberries and toss to coat. Set aside. In a small mixing bowl, blend flour, baking powder, baking soda, salt and nutmeg. Set aside. In a second mixing bowl, cream margarine until fluffy and gradually add sugar. Blend well with electric mixer, using medium speed. Add egg substitute 1/4 cup at a time, beating between each addition. Add blueberries. Add flour mixture alternately with mashed banana, mixing with a wooden spoon just until flour is moistened. Do NOT OVERMIX. Spoon batter into loaf pan that has been sprayed with cooking spray. Bake in 350° preheated oven for 45 minutes or until done. Allow to cool in pan 10 minutes before removing. Cool on rack.

Yield: 16 servings

Approximate Per Slice:
Calories: 111
Fat: 1.3 g
Cholesterol: 0.0 mg
Carbohydrates: 18 g
Protein: 4 g
Sodium: 89 mg

Diabetic Exchanges: 1 bread; 1/2 fruit; 1/4 fat

Never be in a hurry when making a yeast bread. The best bread will be the bread that has been given the time to rise slowly.

Multi-Grain Loaf

(Recipe contains approximately 16% fat)

2 c. enriched all-purpose flour	1 T. baking powder
	1/2 tsp. salt
1 c. whole wheat flour	Egg substitute to equal
1/2 c. quick oats	1 egg
2 T. cornmeal	1 1/2 c. skim milk
1/4 c. sugar	2 T. canola oil

Combine flours, oats, cornmeal, sugar, baking powder and salt. Put egg substitute in small mixing bowl and add milk and oil. Add this mixture to dry ingredients. Stir with wooden spoon until just moistened. Pour into an 8-inch round pan that has been sprayed with cooking spray. Bake in 350° preheated oven for 45 minutes or until golden brown. Cool 5 minutes. Remove from pan. Best served warm.

Yield: 16 slices

Approximate Per Slice:
Calories: 133
Fat: 2.4 g
Cholesterol: Tr. mg
Carbohydrates: 24 g
Protein; 4 g
Sodium: 89 mg

Diabetic Exchanges: 1 bread; 1/2 milk; 1/2 fat

There is nothing difficult about making bread. Don't be afraid to give it a try. A yeast dough is one of the most obliging and indestructible material you will ever work with.

Pat's Beer Bread
(Great with pasta)
(Recipe contains approximately 10% fat)

3 c. self-rising flour   1 (12 oz.) can beer
3 T. sugar   1 T. tub margarine

Put flour and sugar in mixing bowl and stir in beer with a fork. Spread in two 7 1/2-inch loaf pans and bake in 350° preheated oven for 30 minutes. Brush tops of bread with margarine and bake another 30 minutes. Remove from pan and cool on rack.

Yield: 2 loaves; 12 slices per loaf

Approximate Per Slice:
Calories: 69
Fat: 0.8 g
Cholesterol: 0.0 mg
Carbohydrates: 13 g
Protein: 2 g
Sodium: 175 mg

Diabetic Exchanges: 1 bread

The yeast that causes bread to rise is a living, breathing thing which must be fed and kept warm.

Proofing water should contain a little sugar or honey to feed the yeast and get maximum performance.

Zucchini Bread

(Recipe contains approximately 28% fat)

2 c. all-purpose flour	1/4 c. canola oil
1 tsp. cinnamon	1/4 c. apple juice
1/2 tsp. nutmeg	concentrate, thawed
1/2 tsp. salt (opt.)	1 1/2 c. tightly-packed,
1 tsp. baking soda	shredded, fresh zucchini
1/2 tsp. baking powder	1/2 c. dates, very finely
Egg substitute to equal	chopped
3 eggs	

In a mixing bowl put flour, cinnamon, nutmeg, salt, baking soda and baking powder. Stir with wire whisk until well blended. Put egg substitute, oil and apple juice concentrate in small bowl and blend. Add to flour mixture along with zucchini. Blend with electric mixer at medium speed until well mixed. Stir in dates. Pour into a 9x5x3-inch loaf pan that has been sprayed with cooking spray. Bake in 375° oven for 45 to 50 minutes or until done. Cake will pull slightly from pan when done. Cool 10 minutes, then remove from pan and cool on rack.

Blend glaze ingredients and drizzle over top of bread after pricking bread with long-tined fork.

GLAZE:

1/2 tsp. cinnamon	3 T. boiling water
16 pkt. Equal	

Yield: 18 servings

Approximate Per Serving:
Calories: 115
Fat: 3.6 g
Cholesterol: 0.0 mg
Carbohydrates: 16 g
Protein: 2 g
Sodium: 74 mg

Diabetic Exchanges: 1 bread; 1 fat

Kneading the dough for a half minute after mixing improves the texture of baking powder biscuits.

Dinner Rolls

Brown and Serve Rolls

(Recipe contains approximately 8% fat)

2 1/4 c. lukewarm water	2 tsp. salt
(110° to 115°)	2 T. tub margarine
3 T. sugar	7 to 7 1/2 c. flour
2 pkg. active dry yeast	

Blend 1/2 cup warm water and sugar. Sprinkle yeast over top. Set aside. In a large bowl put remaining water, salt and margarine. Add yeast sponge. Stir in flour, 1 cup at a time, until you can add no more. Turn out on floured surface and knead in enough flour to make satiny elastic dough. Knead at least 10 minutes. Spray a large bowl with vegetable oil and form dough into a large ball. Put dough in bowl; turn once to coat both sides. Put in warm place and allow to rise until dough is doubled in bulk. Punch down. Turn out on floured surface and divide in 35 to 40 pieces. Knead each piece to work out air, then form into ball and put into muffin tins that have been sprayed with vegetable oil; or make cloverleaf buns by forming each piece in three balls and putting into a muffin tin. Cover and let rise until doubled, about 45 minutes. Bake in a 275° preheated oven 20 to 30 minutes. Do NOT ALLOW ROLLS TO BROWN. Remove from tins and cool on rack. Store in freezer in heavy-duty freezing bag until ready to use.

To serve: Brown rolls in hot 400° preheated oven for 7 to 10 minutes.
Yield: 35 to 40 rolls, depending on size desired

Approximate Per Roll (based on 40 rolls):
Calories: 95
Fat: 0.8 g
Cholesterol: 0.0 mg
Carbohydrates: 19 g
Protein: 4 g
Sodium: 114 mg

Diabetic Exchanges: 1 1/2 breads

A loaf of bread that has been baked to perfection will have shrunk from the sides of the pan; will turn out easily; and when thumped on the bottom will have a hollow sound.

Cottage Rolls

(Recipe contains approximately 6% fat)

1 pkg. (1 T.) active
   dry yeast
	1 tsp. salt (opt.)
	   (needs a little salt)

1/4 c. warm water (110° to 115°)	1/4 tsp. baking soda Egg substitute to equal
1 T. sugar	1 egg

1 c. lowfat cream-style
   cottage cheese, small
   curd
	2 1/2 c. flour, unbleached,
	   whole wheat blend or
	   enriched all-purpose

Put warm water and sugar in saucer and sprinkle yeast over top. Set aside to proof. Warm cottage cheese in a saucepan, then put into mixing bowl. Add salt, soda, egg substitute and 1/2 cup flour. Add yeast sponge and beat with an electric mixer for 2 minutes. With a wooden spoon, gradually stir in remaining flour—enough to make a soft dough. Turn out onto floured surface and knead a full 10 minutes, working in flour as needed. Put dough into bowl that has been sprayed with cooking spray. Cover with plastic wrap that has been sprayed with cooking spray and set in warm place to rise until doubled in bulk—about 1 1/2 hours. Punch down, cover and allow to rest 10 minutes. Turn dough out onto floured surface and shape into balls. Place balls in a 9-inch round baking pan (or pie plate). Cover with plastic wrap and allow to rise until double in bulk—about 30 minutes. Bake in a 350° preheated oven for about 20 minutes or until bread is done. Cool on rack.
Yield: 12 rolls

Approximate Per Roll:
Calories: 123
Fat: 0.6 g
Cholesterol: 16 mg
Carbohydrates: 22 g
Protein: 6 g
Sodium: 260 mg

Diabetic Exchanges: 1/2 milk; 1 bread

Proofing water under 90 degrees will most likely not proof
and over 120 degrees will more than likely kill the yeast.
Keep the water lukewarm - about 110 degrees.

Freeze-Ahead Dinner Rolls

(Recipe contains approximately 18% fat)

5 1/2 to 6 c. flour, whole
   wheat blend, unbleached
   or enriched all-purpose
2 T. sugar
1 tsp. salt (opt.), use at
   least 1/4 tsp. salt

2 pkg. active dry yeast
   (2 T.)
1 1/4 c. water
1/2 c. skim milk
1/3 c. tub margarine
Egg substitute to equal
   2 eggs

In a large mixing bowl, blend 2 cups flour, sugar, salt and dry yeast; set aside. In a saucepan, put water, milk and margarine. Heat, over medium heat, to about 115°. Pour into dry ingredients and beat 2 minutes at medium speed, scraping sides of bowl. Add egg substitute and 1/2 cup flour. Beat at high speed 2 minutes. With a wooden spoon, stir in enough additional flour to make a soft dough. Turn out onto lightly-floured surface and knead 5 minutes or until smooth and elastic, working in as much remaining flour as needed. Cover with plastic wrap and allow to rest for 20 minutes. Punch down, then shape into desired dinner rolls. Place on baking sheets that have been sprayed with vegetable oil. Cover with foil, sealing well, and freeze until firm. Transfer to plastic freezing bags and return to freezer.

To Bake: Remove number desired from freezer bag and place on baking sheet that has been sprayed with vegetable oil. Cover with plastic wrap that has been sprayed with vegetable oil and place in warm place to rise until doubled in bulk, about 1 1/4 hours. Bake in 350° preheated oven for 15 minutes or until golden brown, and until rolls sound hollow when thumped on bottom with finger. Remove from baking sheet and cool on rack.

Yield: 24 rolls

Approximate Per Roll:
Calories: 148
Fat 2.9 g
Cholesterol: Tr. mg
Carbohydrates: 27 g
Protein: 4 g
Sodium: 131 mg

Note: If making cloverleaf rolls, freeze in muffin tins and transfer to freezer bags. When ready to bake, return to muffin tins and bake.

Diabetic Exchanges: 1 3/4 bread; 1/2 fat

Oatmeal Dinner Rolls

(Recipe contains approximately 18% fat)

1 c. quick oatmeal
2 c. boiling water
1 T. honey
1/2 c. lukewarm water
   (110° to 115°)
2 pkg. dry active yeast

3 T. tub margarine
2 T. brown sugar, or
   equivalent artificial
   sweetener
1 tsp. salt (opt.)
Flour as needed (2 to 2 1/2 c.)

Simmer oatmeal in 2 cups boiling water for 1 minute. Cover for 2 minutes, off stove. Put into large mixing bowl until cooled to lukewarm. When oatmeal is lukewarm, put honey and lukewarm water together and sprinkle with yeast. Set aside to proof for 10 minutes. Add yeast sponge, margarine and brown sugar to oatmeal and blend well. Add salt, blend. Add enough flour to make a stiff dough, then turn out onto surface and knead 3 to 10 minutes, adding flour as needed. Put into bowl that has been sprayed with vegetable oil and cover with plastic wrap that has been sprayed with vegetable oil. Put in warm place and allow to rise until double in size. Form into desired shape dinner rolls. Put in muffin tins or on baking sheet and bake in a 350° preheated oven for 20 to 30 minutes.
Yield: 24 rolls

Approximate Per Roll:
Calories 81
Fat: 1.8 g
Cholesterol: 0.0 mg
Carbohydrates: 14 g
Protein: 2 g
Sodium: 107 mg

Diabetic Exchanges: 1 bread

Dip the spoon to be used to measure margarine in hot water first.
The margarine will slip out more easily.

Low Sugar Breakfast Muffins, Sweet Rolls & Coffee Cakes

Blueberry English Muffins

(Recipe contains approximately 13% fat)

1 pkg. active dry yeast
1 c. lukewarm water
  (105° to 115°)
2 T. honey
3 1/2 c. flour, enriched all-
  purpose, whole wheat
  blend, or unbleached

2 T. tub margarine, melted
1/4 tsp. salt (opt.)
1 c. fresh blueberries, can
  use frozen unsweetened,
  thawed & drained
2 T. cornmeal

In a large mixing bowl, put water and honey and sprinkle with dry yeast. Set aside for 10 minutes to proof. To yeast sponge add 2 cups flour, margarine and salt. Blend well. Stir in enough of remaining flour to make a soft dough. Turn dough out onto a lightly-floured surface and gently knead in blueberries. Add more flour to surface, if needed and roll dough to 1/2-inch thickness. Cut dough with 3-inch round cutter. Sprinkle 2 baking sheets lightly with 1 tablespoon cornstarch and place rounds on baking sheets (7 per sheet). Sprinkle tops of English muffins with remaining cornmeal. Cover with plastic wrap that has been sprayed with cooking spray and place in draft-free, warm place until double in size, about 1 hour. Heat an electric skillet to 350°. Transfer muffins to skillet, cooking in 2 to 3 batches, and cook with lid partially on for 5 minutes. Turn, partially cover and cook an additional 8 to 10 minutes. Cool on rack.
Yield: 14 muffins

Approximate Per Muffin:
Calories: 140
Fat: 2.0 g
Cholesterol: 0.0 mg
Carbohydrates: 27 g
Protein: 3 g
Sodium: 60 mg

Diabetic Exchanges: 1 bread; 1 fruit; 1/2 fat

Blueberry Muffins

(Recipe contains approximately 25% fat)

1 1/2 c. enriched all-
   purpose flour
2 tsp. baking powder
1/2 tsp. salt
1/2 tsp. cinnamon
1/2 c. skim milk
Egg substitute to equal
   2 eggs

2 T. canola oil
1/4 c. apple juice concentrate, thawed
1 c. drained, canned-in-
   own-juice blueberries or
1 c. fresh blueberries

GLAZE:

12 pkg. Equal or artificial
   sweetener of choice to
   equal 1/2 c. sugar

1/4 tsp. cinnamon
3 T. boiling water

In a mixing bowl, put flour, baking powder, salt and cinnamon. In a second mixing bowl, combine milk, egg substitute, canola oil and thawed apple juice concentrate. Pour second mixture into dry mixture and blend just until flour is thoroughly moistened. Stir in blueberries. Line 12 muffin cups with paper or foil muffin liners and fill 2/3 full with batter. Bake in 400° preheated oven for 20 to 25 minutes or until done. Remove muffins from tin and prick tops of muffins several times with fork. Mix glaze ingredients and drizzle over muffins.

Yield: 12 muffins

Approximate Per Muffin:
Calories: 101
Fat: 2.8 g
Cholesterol: Tr. mg
Carbohydrates: 14 g
Protein: 3 g
Sodium: 114 mg

Diabetic Exchanges: 1 bread; 1/2 fat

To cut biscuit dough in a hurry, shape dough to conform with the size of a metal ice cube tray with dividers and cut. After baking, biscuits will separate at dividing lines.

Refrigerator Bran Muffins

(Recipe contains approximately 28% fat)

3 c. Bran Buds, 100%
Bran or All-Bran
1 1/2 c. apple juice,
unsweetened
1 1/2 c. unsweetened
applesauce
1/3 c. canola oil
Egg substitute to equal
3 eggs

2 1/2 c. flour, whole wheat
blend, unbleached or
enriched all-purpose
1/3 c. nonfat dry milk
granules
1 T. baking soda
1 tsp. cinnamon
1 tsp. salt (opt.)

In a large mixing bowl, put bran, apple juice, applesauce, oil and egg substitute. Beat with electric mixer at low speed until well blended. Blend flour, dry milk, soda, cinnamon and salt. With a wooden spoon, stir dry mixture into bran mixture, blending until just moistened. This mix can be used immediately or kept in the refrigerator, covered, for up to 3 weeks. If batter becomes a little thick, simply add a small amount of hot water.

To Bake: Line muffin tins with paper liners or spray with cooking spray. Fill half full and bake in 375° preheated oven for 20 to 25 minutes or until done. Serve hot with Strawberry Breakfast Spread. See index.
Yield: 30 muffins

Approximate Per Muffin:
Calories: 98
Fat: 3.1 g
Cholesterol: Tr. mg
Carbohydrates: 18 g
Protein: 3 g
Sodium: 141 mg

Diabetic Exchanges: 1 bread; 1/2 fat

Fresh bread or cake will not crumble if cut with a hot knife.

Breakfast Popovers

(Recipe contains approximately 14% fat)

1 c. flour, whole wheat
   blend, unbleached or
   enriched all-purpose
1/4 tsp. salt (this really
   needs at least a pinch
   of salt)

2 tsp. canola oil
Egg substitute to equal
   2 eggs or 4 egg whites
1/2 c. skim milk
1/2 c. apple juice
   concentrate

Heat oven to 450°, spray muffin tins with cooking spray and put into preheated oven for at least 15 minutes. Put flour and salt in a mixing bowl. Add oil, egg substitute, milk and apple juice concentrate. Beat with an electric mixer, on medium speed, for about 2 minutes. Fill 10 of the muffin cups half full. Bake in preheated oven for 40 minutes. Serve hot.
Yield: 10 popovers

Approximate Per Popover:
Calories: 93
Fat: 1.4 g
Cholesterol: Tr. mg
Carbohydrates: 16 g
Protein: 2 g
Sodium: 50 mg

Diabetic Exchanges: 1 bread; 1/4 fat

If your muffins are sticking to the tin pan, place the hot pan on a wet towel. Muffins will slide right out.

Easy Brown Sugar Rolls

(Recipe contains approximately 18% fat)

1 (1 lb.) loaf frozen bread
   dough, thawed (white
   or wheat)
1/2 c. brown sugar
1/4 c. water

1/2 c. unsweetened
   applesauce
3 T. tub margarine, melted
1 1/2 tsp. cinnamon
2 T. sugar

Put brown sugar and water in a saucepan and bring to a boil over medium heat. Stir in applesauce and simmer for 5 minutes, stirring constantly. Pour mixture into 10-inch, deep pie plate that has been sprayed with cooking oil. Roll bread dough into 9x14-inch rectangle. Spread dough with margarine and sprinkle with cinnamon and sugar. Starting on long side, roll up like a jelly roll and pinch seam so roll will hold. Cut in 12 slices. Arrange slices on top of topping. Allow to rise 40 to 60 minutes until double. Bake in 350° preheated oven for 30 minutes. Let stand 5 minutes, then invert onto serving platter.
Yield: 12 rolls

Approximate Per Roll:
Calories: 199
Fat: 3.9 g
Cholesterol: 0.0 mg
Carbohydrates: 39 g
Protein: 3 g
Sodium: 239 mg

Diabetic Exchanges: 2 breads; 1 fruit; 1 fat

*To substitute for sour milk, add 1 tablespoon vinegar
or lemon juice to enough milk to make one cup.*

Low-Sugar Apple Cinnamon Puffs

(Recipe contains approximately 12% fat)

2 c. all-purpose flour
1 pkg. Quick Rise yeast
2 T. sugar, or equivalent
   sweetener
1/2 tsp. salt
3/4 c. warm water
1 T. canola oil
3 T. unsweetened
   applesauce

Egg substitute to equal
   1 egg
1 c. chopped apples
Cooking spray
1 tsp. cinnamon
6 pkt. Equal sweetener, or
   sweetener of choice to
   equal 1/4 c. sugar

In a large mixing bowl, combine 1 cup flour, yeast, 2 tablespoons sugar and salt. Blend well. Add warm water and oil along with egg substitute and applesauce. Blend at low speed with electric mixer until mixture is moistened. Beat 3 minutes at medium speed. With a wooden spoon, stir in apples and remaining flour to make a soft dough. Spoon into 12 muffin cups that have been sprayed with cooking spray. Cover and allow to rise in warm place until double, about 30 minutes. Bake in 375° preheated oven for 15 to 20 minutes, or until done. Remove from oven and spray tops lightly with cooking spray, then sprinkle a mixture of cinnamon and Equal sweetener over tops.

Yield: 12 puffs

Approximate Per Puff:
Calories: 110
Fat: 1.5 g
Cholesterol: 0.0 mg
Carbohydrates: 20 g
Protein: 3 g
Sodium: 98 mg

Diabetic Exchanges: 1 bread; 1/2 fruit; 1/4 fat

*If out of whole wheat flour use 3/4 cup
cornmeal or 1 1/2 cups ground rolled oats.*

No Knead Cinnamon Rolls

(Recipe contains approximately 10% fat)

1 pkg. active dry yeast	Egg substitute to equal
1/4 c. warm water	1 egg
1 tsp. honey	4 c. flour
1/4 c. sugar	1 c. chopped dates
1 tsp. salt	6 T. apple juice concen-
2 T. tub margarine	trate, thawed
1 c. boiling water	1 tsp. cinnamon
	2 T. water

Dissolve yeast in warm water with 1 teaspoon honey. Set aside to proof. In a large mixing bowl, put sugar, salt and margarine. Add boiling water and allow to cool until lukewarm. Add yeast sponge, egg substitute, and stir in flour. DO NOT KNEAD. Cover and set aside in a warm place for about 2 hours. Divide dough in half. Roll out into 12x9-inch rectangle. Spread 2 tablespoons of thawed apple juice concentrate over each rectangle. Sprinkle with cinnamon and roll up jellyroll fashion. Pinch seam together. Slice each roll into 9 rolls each. In a saucepan, heat 2 tablespoons apple juice concentrate, water and dates until mixture thickens. Put on bottom of 9x13-inch baking dish. Lay rolls on top of mixture. Cover and set aside for 2 hours while rolls rise. Bake in a 400° preheated oven for 12 to 15 minutes or until rolls are done.

Yield: 18 rolls

Approximate Per Roll:
Calories: 159
Fat: 1.7 g
Cholesterol: 0.0 mg
Carbohydrates: 32 g
Protein: 4 g
Sodium: 142 mg

Diabetic Exchanges: 1 1/2 bread; 1 fruit; 1/4 fat

One cup all-purpose flour plus 1 1/2 teaspoons baking powder and 1/2 teaspoon salt can be substituted for 1 cup self-rising flour.

Apple-Oat Coffeecake

(Recipe contains approximately 31% fat)

1 c. oat bran
1/2 c. enriched all-purpose
  flour
2 T. brown sugar, firmly
  packed
1 T. baking powder
1 tsp. ground cinnamon
1/2 tsp. nutmeg
1/3 c. dry nonfat milk
  granules

1/3 c. tub margarine,
  softened
3 egg whites, slightly
  beaten
3/4 c. apple juice
2 tsp. vanilla extract
Cooking spray

In a large mixing bowl, put oat bran, flour, 1 tablespoon brown sugar, baking powder, cinnamon, nutmeg and dry milk granules. Blend with a whisk until even in color. Cut in margarine until mixture resembles coarse meal. In a small bowl, blend egg whites, beat slightly and add apple juice and vanilla. With a wooden spoon, stir into dry mixture just until moistened. Coat an 8-inch round cake pan with cooking spray, lightly, and spoon mixture into pan. Sprinkle with brown sugar. Bake in 375° preheated oven for 30 minutes or until done. Cool in pan on wire rack. Serve just warm.
Yield: 10 servings

Approximate Per Serving:
Calories: 90
Fat: 3.1 g
Cholesterol: Tr. mg
Carbohydrates: 14 g
Protein: 5 g
Sodium: 170 mg

Diabetic Exchanges: 1 bread; 1/2 fat

A 1/4 teaspoon baking soda plus 5/8 teaspoon cream of tartar will substitute for one teaspoon baking powder.

Fig Streusel

(Recipe contains approximately 29% fat)

1/2 c. raw quick-cooking oats	Cooking spray
1/3 c. enriched all-purpose flour	3 c. chopped dried figs
	1/2 tsp. cinnamon
3 T. brown sugar, firmly packed	1/4 c. evaporated skim milk
	Egg substitute to equal 1 egg
3 T. tub margarine, softened	1/2 tsp. vanilla

In a mixing bowl, combine oats, flour and brown sugar. Cut in margarine until you have a meal-like mixture. Spray a 9-inch pie plate with cooking spray and pour half of mixture in bottom of pie plate. Top with chopped figs and sprinkle with cinnamon. Blend milk, egg substitute and vanilla; pour over figs. Top with remaining crumb mixture. Bake in 350° preheated oven for 40 minutes or until nicely browned. Serve warm.

Yield: 8 servings

Approximate Per Serving:
Calories: 164
Fat: 5.3 g
Cholesterol: Tr. mg
Carbohydrates: 29 g
Protein: 4 g
Sodium: 65 mg

Diabetic Exchanges: 1 bread; 1 fruit; 1 fat

To substitute for one cup buttermilk put 1 tablespoon vinegar or lemon juice in measuring cup and fill with skim milk to make one cup.

Biscuits

Angel Biscuits
(Recipe contains approximately 24% fat)

1 pkg. active dry yeast
2 T. warm water (110° to 115°)
1 1/2 tsp. sugar or equivalent sweetener
1 c. nonfat buttermilk

2 1/2 c. enriched all-purpose flour
1 tsp. baking powder
1/2 tsp. salt (opt.)
1/4 tsp. baking soda
3 T. tub margarine
Cooking spray

In a saucer put warm water and sugar. Blend, then sprinkle yeast over top. Set aside 10 minutes to proof. Put buttermilk in bowl and add yeast sponge; set aside. Combine flour, baking powder, salt and baking soda. Cut in margarine until mixture resembles coarse meal. Add buttermilk mixture, stirring with a fork until mixture is moistened. Turn out on lightly-floured surface and knead several times. Roll out to 1/2-inch thickness; cut with a 2 1/2-inch biscuit cutter. Put on baking sheet that has been lightly sprayed with cooking spray. Cover with plastic wrap, sprayed with cooking spray, and set in warm place for 15 minutes. Bake in 400° preheated oven for 10 to 12 minutes or until nicely browned.
Yield: 12 biscuits

Approximate Per Biscuit:
Calories: 133
Fat: 3.5 g
Cholesterol: 1 mg
Carbohydrates: 22 g
Protein: 4 g
Sodium: 152 mg

Diabetic Exchanges: 1 bread; 1/2 milk; 1/2 fat

Four cups sifted all-purpose flour equals one pound of flour.

Baking Powder Biscuits

(Recipe contains approximately 22% fat)

1 c. flour, unbleached,
 whole wheat blend or
 enriched all-purpose
2 tsp. baking powder

1/4 tsp. yeast (1/4 pkg.)
1/4 tsp. salt
1 T. canola oil
6 T. skim milk

Put flour, baking powder, yeast and salt in a small mixing bowl and stir with whisk until well blended. Drizzle oil over top, tossing with fork until oil is evenly distributed. Add milk and stir with wooden spoon until flour is moistened. Turn out onto floured surface and roll to 1/2-inch thickness. Cut with a 2-inch biscuit cutter. Place biscuits on baking sheet that has been sprayed with cooking spray. Cover and allow to rest 15 minutes. Bake in 450° preheated oven for 12 to 15 minutes or until lightly browned.
Yield: 10 biscuits

Approximate Per Biscuit:
Calories 66
Fat 1.6 g
Cholesterol: Tr. mg
Carbohydrates: 10 g
Protein: 2 g
Sodium: 64 mg

Diabetic Exchanges: 3/4 bread; 1/4 fat

*To substitute for one cup light cream, use
one cup undiluted evaporated milk.*

Drop Raisin Biscuits

(Recipe contains approximately 24% fat)

2 c. flour, enriched all-
    purpose or whole wheat
    blend
1 T. baking powder
1 tsp. salt

1/4 c. sugar
1/4 c. tub margarine
1 c. skim milk
1 tsp. cinnamon
1/2 c. raisins

Put flour, baking powder, salt and sugar in mixing bowl and cut in margarine. Toss in milk and fold in cinnamon and raisins. Drop by large tablespoonfuls onto baking sheet that has been lightly sprayed with vegetable oil. Bake in 425° preheated oven for 10 to 12 minutes.
Yield: 12 biscuits

Approximate Per Biscuit:
Calories: 152
Fat: 4.0 g
Cholesterol: Tr. mg
Carbohydrates: 26 g
Protein: 3 g
Sodium: 250 mg

Diabetic Exchanges: 1 3/4 bread; 1 fat

When a recipe calls for one cup of Bisquick, substitute by blending 1 cup flour, 1 1/2 teaspoons baking powder, 1/2 teaspoon salt and 1 tablespoon tub margarine.

Lowfat Baking Powder Biscuits

(Recipe contains approximately 20% fat)

2 c. flour, whole wheat
  blend, unbleached or
  enriched all-purpose
4 tsp. baking powder

1/2 tsp. salt (opt.)
2 T. tub margarine
3/4 c. skim milk

Put flour, baking powder and salt in a mixing bowl and stir with whisk until well blended. Cut in margarine until mixture resembles meal. Add milk slowly, mixing as milk is added. Turn out onto floured surface and roll out to 1/2-inch thickness. Cut with 2-inch biscuit cutter and place on baking sheet. Bake in 400° preheated oven for 15 to 20 minutes or until biscuits are nicely browned.

Yield: 10 biscuits

Approximate Per Biscuit:
Calories: 120
Fat: 2.6 g
Cholesterol: Tr. mg
Carbohydrates: 20 g
Protein: 3 g
Sodium: 169 mg

Diabetic Exchanges: 1 1/4 bread; 1/2 fat

Lowfat Sour Milk Biscuits

(Recipe contains approximately 19% fat)

2 c. flour, unbleached,
  whole wheat blend or
  enriched all-purpose
2 tsp. baking powder

1/2 tsp. salt (opt.) (need a little)
1/2 tsp. baking soda
2 T. tub margarine
1/2 to 3/4 c. sour milk

Sift flour, baking powder and salt into mixing bowl. Cut in margarine. Dissolve baking soda into sour milk and add to flour mixture. Roll on board; cut with biscuit cutter and bake in 400° preheated oven for 10 to 12 minutes.

Yield: 12 biscuits

Approximate Per Biscuit:
Calories: 99
Fat: 2.1 g
Cholesterol: Tr. mg
Carbohydrates: 17 g
Protein: 3 g
Sodium: 108 mg

Diabetic Exchanges: 1 bread; 1/2 fat

Miscellaneous Bread Stuff

Corn Waffle Bread

(Recipe contains approximately 9% fat)

1 can whole kernel corn
    (or 3 ears fresh corn),
    chopped fine
Egg substitute to equal
    3 eggs
3 c. flour, whole wheat blend,
    unbleached or enriched
    all-purpose

2 T. sugar
1 1/2 T. baking powder
1 tsp. salt (opt.)
2 1/4 c. skim milk
1 T. tub margarine, melted

Put corn in mixing bowl and stir in egg substitute. Set aside. In a second mixing bowl, combine flour, sugar, baking powder and salt. Stir flour mixture into corn mixture alternately with milk. Stir in melted margarine. Bake in a preheated waffle iron at moderately-high heat until crisp and golden, using about 1/3 cup batter per batch.
Yield: 15 waffles

Approximate Per Waffle:
Calories: 153
Fat: 1.5 g
Cholesterol: 1 mg
Carbohydrates: 29 g
Protein: 6 g
Sodium: 301 mg

Diabetic Exchanges: 1 1/2 bread; 1 1/2 vegetable; 1/2 fat

Before sifting flour onto wax paper, always crease the paper down the center. This creates a handy pouring spout.

Filled Potato Dumplings

(Recipe contains approximately 9% fat)

2 lb. potatoes, peeled
  & boiled
1 c. ham, lean only, diced
1/4 c. minced onion
Dash of nutmeg
1 1/4 c. flour, whole wheat
  blend, unbleached or
  enriched all-purpose

Egg substitute to equal
  1 egg
1/2 tsp. salt (opt.)
6 c. boiling chicken stock,
  can use low-sodium
  canned stock

While potatoes are cooking, put ham and onions in a skillet and sauté until ham is slightly browned and onions are soft. Spray mixture lightly with cooking spray as it cooks. Add a dash of nutmeg to mixture; blend and set aside to cool. Run potatoes through ricer or food mill (can mash, if preferred) and stir in flour. Add egg substitute and salt; blend until smooth. Turn out on floured surface and knead, adding more flour if needed to make a medium-stiff dough. Form dough into a 2-inch thick roll and cut roll into 10 pieces. Put 1 tablespoon of filling into the center of each piece of dough and roll dough around filling to form an oblong dumpling. Cook the dumplings in boiling stock, about 10 to 12 minutes or until dumplings are cooked through. Transfer dumplings to heated bowl with slotted spoon. Serve immediately.
Yield: 10

Approximate Per Dumpling:
Calories: 136
Fat: 1.4 g
Cholesterol: 11 mg
Carbohydrates: 22 g
Protein: 7 g
Sodium: 379 mg

Diabetic Exchanges: 1 1/2 bread; 1/2 meat

Notch your bread board in inches, so when you roll dough you'll know exactly when you have the size pastry you need.

Lowfat Waffle Garlic Bread
(This bread is delicious)
(Recipe contains approximately 22% fat)

12 slices French bread,
cut very thin (about
1/4" thick)
3 tsp. tub diet margarine,
no more than 7 grams
fat per tablespoon

3 T. no-fat, no cholesterol
mayonnaise
Garlic powder, to taste

Slice bread thin. Blend margarine, mayonnaise and garlic powder; spread very thinly on both sides of bread. Heat waffle iron to waffle setting and put bread in waffle iron. Bake about 4 minutes.
Yield: 6 servings

Approximate Per Serving:
Calories: 89
Fat: 2.2 g
Cholesterol: 0.0 mg
Carbohydrates: 15 g
Protein: 2 g
Sodium: 263 mg

Diabetic Exchanges: 1 bread; 1/2 fat

When chopping dates or other sticky fruits, spray the kitchen shears or chopping blade with cooking spray.

Reservation Flat Bread

(Recipe contains approximately 6% fat)

2 c. enriched all-purpose flour	1/4 c. plain lowfat yogurt
2 tsp. baking powder	Egg substitute to equal 1 egg
1 tsp. sugar	1/4 c. skim milk
1/4 tsp. salt	Cooking spray
1/8 tsp. baking soda	

In a large mixing bowl, put flour, baking powder, sugar, salt and baking soda. Stir with whisk until well blended. Add yogurt, egg substitute and skim milk. Stir just until moistened. Dough should be soft. Turn out onto floured surface and knead until smooth and elastic, 5 to 10 minutes. Spray a mixing bowl with cooking spray. Form dough into ball and place in bowl. Turn once to coat both sides. Cover with plastic wrap that has been sprayed with cooking spray. Place in warm place out of any drafts and allow to rise for 3 hours. Punch dough down and divide into 8 equal portions. On a lightly-floured surface, roll each portion into a 4-inch circle that is about 1/4-inch thick. Place on preheated baking sheets and bake in 450° preheated oven for about 6 minutes or until bread is lightly browned. Cool on rack.
Yield: 8 servings

Approximate Per Serving:
Calories: 132
Fat: 0.9 g
Cholesterol: 2 mg
Carbohydrates: 25 g
Protein: 5 g
Sodium: 97 mg

Diabetic Exchanges: 1 1/2 bread; 1/4 milk

When baking, put all ingredients needed to the left of the mixing bowl. As you add the various ingredients, set each container to the right of the bowl. If interrupted, you will know how far you have gone.

Shish-Ka-Bread

(Recipe contains approximately 8% fat)

8 thick slices French bread
3 slices non-fat
American cheese
1 T. lowfat vegetable
spread (no more than
7 grams fat per tablespoon)

1/2 tsp. garlic powder or
garlic salt
Cooking spray

Spread 6 slices of French bread lightly with vegetable spread and put half slice of cheese on each slice of bread. Stack slices in stacks of 3 slices each. Top each stack with plain slice of bread. Cut each stack into 8 squares. Thread 2 square stacks on 8 bamboo 6-inch skewers. Spray with vegetable spray. Put on baking sheet sprayed with vegetable spray and bake in 400° preheated oven (or cook on barbecue grill) for 10 to 15 minutes or until Skish-Ka-Bread is nicely browned.
Yield: 8 servings

Approximate Per Serving:
Calories: 127
Fat: 1.1 g
Cholesterol: 2 mg
Carbohydrates: 20 g
Protein: 5 g
Sodium: 381 mg

Diabetic Exchanges: 1 1/4 bread; 1/2 meat

To make hot-roll mix or bread dough rise quickly, set the bowl of dough on a heating pad and turn the heat indicator to low. The dough rises in no time.

No End Bread Sticks

(These are great served with soup, stew or salads)
(Recipe contains approximately 14% fat)

1/2 c. lukewarm water	1 1/2 tsp. salt
1/2 c. lukewarm skim milk	3 1/2 c. flour, whole wheat
1/4 tsp. sugar	blend, unbleached or
3 pkg. (3 T.) active dry	enriched all-purpose
yeast	2 egg whites
2 T. tub margarine	2 tsp. sesame seeds
4 tsp. sugar	

Put lukewarm water and lukewarm skim milk in a small mixing bowl. Stir in 1/4 teaspoon sugar. Sprinkle yeast over top and set aside to sponge for about 10 minutes. In a large mixing bowl, put margarine, 4 teaspoons sugar, salt and flour. Make a well in flour mixture and pour yeast sponge into well. Stir the mixture until you have a stiff dough. Turn dough out onto a floured surface and knead for 10 minutes or until dough is smooth and elastic. Form dough into a ball and put into bowl that has been liberally sprayed with cooking spray. Turn once to coat both sides. Cover with plastic wrap that has been sprayed with cooking spray. Set in warm place for 45 minutes or until dough has doubled in bulk. Punch down dough and divide into 12 pieces. Cover with sprayed wrap and allow to rest for 10 minutes, then roll each portion into a 16-inch stick, rolling on a floured surface. Place on baking sheet 2 inches apart. Brush the sticks with egg white; sprinkle with sesame seeds. Allow to rise for 10 minutes. Bake sticks in 400° preheated oven for 15 minutes or until well browned. Cool on racks and store in tightly covered container.

Yield: 12 sticks

Approximate Per Stick:
Calories: 170
Fat: 2.7 g
Cholesterol: Tr. mg
Carbohydrates: 31 g
Protein: 2 g
Sodium: 305 mg

Diabetic Exchanges: 2 breads, 1/2 fat

Whole Wheat Pizza Crust

(Recipe contains approximately 22% fat)

2 c. whole wheat flour
1 pkg. dry yeast
1/4 tsp. salt (opt.)

1 c. hot water
1 T. canola oil
1 T. honey

Blend flour, dry yeast and salt. Add hot water, oil and honey. Blend. Cover and allow to stand 10 minutes. Spread over large pizza pan of 10x15-inch baking pan. Add toppings and bake in 425° preheated oven for 15 to 20 minutes.
Yield: 8 servings

Approximate Per Serving (crust only):
Calories: 126
Fat: 2.4 g
Cholesterol: 0.0 mg
Carbohydrates: 24 g
Protein: 4 g
Sodium: 68 mg

Diabetic Exchanges: 1 1/2 bread; 1/2 fat

To reheat a few muffins, put them into an egg poacher.

After washing raisins for use in baking, dry them in a salad spinner. They will instantly shed their water.

Yeast Dumplings

(Recipe contains approximately 12% fat)

1/2 pkg. active dry yeast
2 T. warm water
1/4 tsp. sugar
2 c. flour, whole wheat
    blend, unbleached or
    enriched all-purpose
1 tsp. sugar

1/2 tsp. salt
1/2 c. scalded milk, cooled
    to lukewarm
1 T. tub margarine, melted
Egg substitute to equal
    1 egg

In a small saucer, put warm water and sugar and sprinkle yeast over top. Set aside to proof for 10 minutes. In a mixing bowl, put flour, 1 teaspoon sugar and salt. Blend. Stir in yeast sponge, cooled milk, margarine and egg substitute. Turn dough out onto lightly-floured surface and knead for 10 minutes or until smooth and elastic. Form dough into ball and put into bowl that has been sprayed with cooking spray. Turn once to coat both sides; cover with plastic wrap that has been sprayed with cooking spray; set in warm place to rise for about 45 minutes or until double in bulk. Punch dough down and let rest 10 minutes. Turn dough out onto lightly-floured surface and form into a cylinder about 2 inches in diameter. Cut cylinder into 8 slices and form into ball. Place on baking sheet that has been sprayed with cooking spray. Let rise for 20 minutes; turn and allow to rise 25 minutes. Should be doubled in bulk. Drop dumplings into large kettle of simmering stock and cook, covered, for 15 to 18 minutes. Remove dumplings with slotted spoon to warm serving dish. Serve immediately.
Yield: 8 servings

Approximately Per Serving:
Calories: 142
Fat: 1.9 g
Cholesterol: Tr. mg
Carbohydrates: 25 g
Protein: 5 g
Sodium: 172 mg

Diabetic Exchanges: 1 bread; 1 vegetable; 1 fat

Store flour sifter in a plastic bag to keep flour contained.

Spreads

Blueberry Preserves
(Recipe contains approximately 8% fat)

1 c. fresh or frozen blueberries, unsweetened
1 tsp. low-calorie pectin
(this pectin is for pre-
serves & jellies made
with artificial sweetener)

6 pkt. Equal sweetener

Put berries in top of double boiler and cook until berries are soft and juicy. Add pectin. Blend well and cook until thickened. Remove from heat and add sweetener. Keep refrigerated.
Yield: 3/4 cup

Approximate Per Tablespoon:
Calories: 12
Fat: 0.1 mg
Cholesterol: 0.0 mg
Carbohydrates: 2 g
Protein: Tr. g
Sodium: 1 mg

Diabetic Exchanges: 1/4 fruit

Freeze fresh fruit intended for preserves and make up the preserves when it's convenient.

Mock Pear Butter

(Recipe contains approximately 7% fat)

1 tsp. unflavored gelatin	1 c. cooked pears, puréed
2 T. apple juice concentrate, unsweetened	6 pkt. Equal sweetener, or sweetener of choice

Put apple juice concentrate in saucepan and heat over low heat until melted. Remove from heat and sprinkle unflavored gelatin over juice. Allow to stand for 2 minutes. Cook over low heat, stirring constantly until gelatin is dissolved. Remove from heat and stir in puréed pears. Add sweetener; blend well. Refrigerate for at least 6 hours. Use within a week.

Yield: 1 cup

Approximate Per Tablespoon:
Calories: 13
Fat: 0.1 g
Cholesterol: 0.0 mg
Carbohydrates: 2 g
Protein: 1 g
Sodium: 19 mg

Diabetic Exchanges: 1/4 fruit

Sprinkle orange, lemon, lime or pineapple juice on cut fruit to prevent fruit from turning brown.

Peach Breakfast Spread

(Recipe contains only a trace of fat)

2 T. orange juice concen-
    trate, thawed
1 tsp. unflavored gelatin
1 c. puréed fresh peaches,
    peeled & pitted (can use
    drained, frozen or canned
    unsweetened peaches)

6 pkg. Equal sweetener,
    or artificial sweetener
    of choice

Put orange juice concentrate in saucepan, over low heat, and cook until melted. Sprinkle with unflavored gelatin. Remove from heat for 2 minutes to allow gelatin to soften. Return to heat and cook, stirring constantly, over low heat until mixture comes to a boil. Remove from heat and stir in puréed peaches. Add sweetener; blend well and refrigerate 6 hours before using.
Yield: 1 cup

Approximate Per Tablespoon:
Calories: 12
Fat: Tr. g
Cholesterol: 0.0 mg
Carbohydrates: 3 g
Protein: Tr. g
Sodium: 1 mg

Diabetic Exchanges: 1/4 fruit

Canning for Diabetics - Instead of using a sugar and water syrup, use a water and liquid sweetener to taste.

Raspberry Preserves

(Recipe contains only a trace of fat)

1 c. fresh or frozen raspberries, unsweetened
1 tsp. low-calorie pectin (the
type made for use with
artificial sweetener)

6 pkt. Equal sweetener,
or sweetener of choice,
to equal 1/2 cup sugar

Put berries in top of double boiler and cook until berries are soft and juicy. Add pectin. Blend well and cook until thickened. Remove from heat and add sweetener. Keep refrigerated.
Yield: 3/4 cup

Approximate Per Tablespoon:
Calories: 10
Fat: Tr. g
Cholesterol: 0.0 mg
Carbohydrates: 1 g
Protein: Tr. g
Sodium: 0.0 mg

Diabetic Exchanges: Free food in limited amounts

*When jam, jelly, syrup or honey crystals on top, place
in a pan of simmering water to dissolve.*

Strawberry Breakfast Spread

(Recipe contains only a trace of fat)

2 T. orange juice concentrate, thawed
1 tsp. unflavored gelatin
1 c. puréed fresh strawberries (can be unsweetened frozen berries)

6 pkt. Equal sweetener, or sweetener of choice to equal to 1/4 c. sugar

Put orange juice concentrate in a saucepan over low heat and cook until melted. Sprinkle with unflavored gelatin. Remove from heat for 2 minutes to allow gelatin to soften. Return to heat and cook, stirring constantly, over low heat, until mixture comes to a boil. Remove from heat and stir strawberries into mixture. Add sweetener, blending well. Refrigerate 6 hours. Use within a week.

Yield: 1 cup

Approximate Per Tablespoon:
Calories: 9
Fat: Tr. g
Cholesterol: 0.0 mg
Carbohydrates: 2 g
Protein: Tr. g
Sodium: Tr. mg

Diabetic Exchanges: Free in very limited amounts

Using standard measuring utensils will result in a better finished product.

Strawberry Preserves

(Recipe contains only a trace of fat)

1 c. fresh or frozen straw- berries, unsweetened 1 tsp. low-calorie pectin (the type specially made for sugar-free preserves)	6 pkt. Equal sweetener, or sweetener of choice to equal 1/4 c. sugar

Put berries in top of double boiler and cook until berries are soft and juicy. Add pectin. Blend well and cook until thickened. Remove from heat and add sweetener. Keep refrigerated.

Yield: 3/4 cup

Approximate Per Tablespoon:
Calories: 10
Fat: Tr. g
Cholesterol: 0.0 mg
Carbohydrates: 1 g
Protein: Tr. g
Sodium: Tr. mg

Diabetic Exchanges: Free food in limited amounts

Notes & Recipes

Breakfast,
Brunch
&
Lunch

Breakfast, Brunch & Lunch

Coping With the First Two Meals of the Day

Coping with the breakfast meal can sometimes be a chore when there is company around.

A family, for the most part, has already established a breakfast eating pattern. It's usually only when company is on hand that breakfast becomes a matter of concern.

Breakfast is usually the light meal of the day for many. A bowl of cereal and a glass of juice is a great way to start the day. However, if this is not exactly what you want to serve company there are other choices.

Pancakes, waffles and French toast are always good choices as long as the fat content is kept in tow. In the recipes in this book the sugar content has also been controlled.

A muffin, particularly a bran muffin, is a good choice. If you prefer to serve sweet rolls, use one of the lower-in-sugar sweet rolls.

Then there is brunch. Brunch is the meal that fits in to serve for a combination breakfast and lunch. A quiche or egg casserole fits the bill here.

For the lunch meal, there is more variety. Choose among soups, sandwiches, potato entrées and lunch entrées. Unless you plan for this to be the big meal of the day don't over-stuff at lunch. Dinner still has to roll around.

The breakfast, brunch and luncheon meals should be kept simple and easy to prepare. They should be light meals with little variety. A sandwich and cup of soup—a cup of soup and a salad—a luncheon entry with a piece of bread and a fruit. Don't overfill the stomach the first 2 meals of the day.

Omelets. Add water instead of milk to egg substitute.
It makes the omelet lighter and fluffier.

Breakfast

Breakfast in a Biscuit

(Recipe contains approximately 27% fat)

1 recipe baking powder
  biscuits, see index
10 thin slices Canadian
  Bacon (about 1 oz. each)

Egg substitute to equal
  6 eggs (see index)

Prepare biscuits. Heat Canadian Bacon in foil in the oven or in plastic wrap in the microwave. Scramble egg substitute. Put a slice of Canadian bacon on ten biscuit halves. Add egg substitute and top with top half of biscuit.
Yield: 10 servings

Approximate Per Serving:
Calories: 141
Fat: 4.3 g
Cholesterol: 14 mg
Carbohydrates: 23 g
Protein: 9 g
Sodium: 450 mg

Diabetic Exchanges: 3/4 bread; 1 milk; 1/2 fat

Rub your pancake griddle with a little bag of salt instead of grease. The pancakes will not stick and the salt will prevent smoke and odor.

Meal on a Muffin

(Recipe contains approximately 23% fat)

3 English muffins, split in half	1/2 c. chopped onion
1 T. no-fat mayonnaise	1/4 c. chopped green pepper
6 (2 oz.) slices ham, lean only	6 lg. mushroom slices
6 slices no-fat American cheese	Vegetable oil spray

Spread mayonnaise on split English muffin halves and top with ham slice and then slice of cheese. Tuck ham and cheese under so it fits muffin. Sprinkle with onion and green pepper and top with mushroom slice. Spray with vegetable oil. Place in a shallow baking dish that has been sprayed with vegetable oil. Bake in 350° oven for 20 to 25 minutes or until cheese melts. **Yield: 6 servings**

Approximate Per Serving:
Calories: 210
Fat: 4.7 g
Cholesterol: 49 mg
Carbohydrates: 19 g
Protein: 22 g
Sodium: 1,317 mg

Diabetic Exchanges: 1 bread; 2 meat; 1/2 milk

If you admit egg substitute to equal one egg in a recipe increase the liquid in the recipe by one fourth cup.

Great Oatmeal Pancakes

(Recipe contains approximately 13% fat)

1 1/2 c. rolled oats
2 c. buttermilk
Egg substitute to equal
   2 eggs

3/4 c. flour, whole wheat blend,
   unbleached or enriched
   all-purpose
1 tsp. sugar
1/2 tsp. salt
2 tsp. baking powder

Put oats in mixing bowl and add buttermilk and egg substitute. Blend well. Sift together flour, sugar, salt and baking powder; add to mixture. Drop by teaspoon onto hot griddle that has been sprayed with cooking oil. Serve warm, topped with 1 tablespoon sugar-free apple pie filling; see index.
Yield: 16 pancakes

Approximate Per Pancake:
Calories: 71
Fat: 1.0 g
Cholesterol: 1 mg
Carbohydrates: 11 g
Protein: 3 g
Sodium: 113 mg

Diabetic Exchanges (for two pancakes): 3/4 bread

You can use 1 1/3 cup brown sugar or 1 1/2 cup powdered sugar for 1 cup granulated sugar.

Oatmeal Pancakes with Fruit

(Recipe contains approximately 12% fat)

Egg substitute to
  equal 2 eggs
2 1/4 c. buttermilk
2 tsp. canola oil
1/4 c. unsweetened
  applesauce

1 c. rolled oats
1 1/2 c. flour
1 tsp. baking soda
1 T. sugar or equivalent
  artificial sweetener

Combine egg substitute, buttermilk, oil and applesauce in a large mixing bowl. Blend well. Add remaining ingredients. Blend well. Cook on griddle sprayed with cooking spray.

TOPPING:

1 c. fresh or unsweet-
  ened strawberries,
  mashed
2 tsp. cornstarch
1 T. water

1 to 2 drops red food
  coloring
6 pkt. Equal or sweetener
  of choice to equal 1/4 c.
  sugar

Put strawberries in small saucepan. Blend cornstarch and water and add to berries. Cook over medium heat until mixture thickens and clears. Remove from stove and cool slightly. Add sweetener. Serve over pancakes.

Yield: 6 servings

Approximate Per Serving:
Calories: 265
Fat: 3.5 g
Cholesterol: 4 mg
Carbohydrates: 45 g
Protein: 11 g
Sodium: 131 mg

Diabetic Exchanges: 2 milk; 1 bread; 1/2 fruit; 1/2 fat

*When out of cornstarch for thickening, use 2 tablespoons
of flour for one tablespoon cornstarch.*

Tender Lowfat Pancakes

(Recipe contains approximately 12% fat)

3/4 c. enriched all-purpose flour	Egg substitute to equal 1 egg
2 tsp. baking powder	1/2 c. plain nonfat yogurt
1 tsp. sugar or equivalent sweetener	1/4 c. sparkling water*
	1/4 tsp. salt (opt.)
	Cooking spray

Combine flour, baking powder and sugar. Add egg substitute, yogurt, sparkling water and salt. Stir with wooden spoon just until flour mixture is moistened. If you have a few lumps don't worry about it. Spray a nonstick skillet or griddle with cooking spray and pour 3 tablespoons of batter for each pancake. Cook until top is covered with bubbles. Turn and cook second side. Serve immediately.

Yield: 8 (4-inch) pancakes

Approximate Per Pancake:
Calories: 65
Fat: 0.9 g
Cholesterol: 1 mg
Carbohydrates: 11 g
Protein: 3 g
Sodium: 97 mg

Diabetic Exchanges: 1 bread

*The addition of sparkling water to both pancakes and waffles makes them more tender.

*If a recipe calls for honey and you have none, substitute
1 1/4 cup sugar with 1/4 cup apple juice or water.*

Whole Wheat Pancakes

(Recipe contains approximately 15% fat)

1/2 c. whole wheat flour
1/4 c. enriched all-purpose
  flour
2 tsp. baking powder
1 tsp. honey
Egg substitute to equal
  1 egg

1/2 c. plain lowfat yogurt
1/4 c. sparkling water (this
  makes pancakes more
  tender)
1 tsp. tub margarine,
  melted

In a large mixing bowl, put flours and baking powder. Mix with wire whisk until even in color. In a small bowl, combine honey, egg substitute, yogurt, sparkling water and margarine. Blend. Make a well in flour mixture and pour mixture into well. Stir with wooden spoon just until flour mixture is moistened. Don't worry if there are a few lumps. They will bake out. Cook pancakes on hot griddle or nonstick skillet sprayed with cooking spray, using 3 tablespoons of batter for each pancake.
Yield: 8 (4-inch) pancakes

Approximate Per Pancake:
Calories: 65
Fat: 1.1 g
Cholesterol: 1 mg
Carbohydrates: 10 g
Protein: 3 g
Sodium: 44 mg

Diabetic Exchanges: 3/4 bread; 1/4 fat

*To make a nice butter substitute, blend 1 cup
tub margarine, 1/3 cup canola oil and 1/2 cup buttermilk.
Beat until liquid is absorbed and refrigerate.*

Oven French Toast

(Recipe contains approximately 10% fat)

1 loaf French bread,
  sliced thick
Egg substitute to equal
  10 eggs
1 c. evaporated skim milk
1/4 tsp. nutmeg
1/4 tsp. cinnamon
1/4 tsp. mace

1/2 c. apple juice concentrate, melted
1 T. flour
2 c. Delicious apples,
  peeled & sliced thin
1/2 tsp. cinnamon
12 pkt. Equal sweetener, or
  sweetener of choice to
  equal 1/2 cup sugar

Spray a 9x13x2-inch casserole with cooking spray and lay bread slices in bottom of dish. Blend egg substitute, milk, nutmeg, cinnamon and mace. Pour mixture slowly over bread. Cover and refrigerate overnight. In a bowl, put apple juice concentrate and stir in flour. Add apple slices and cinnamon. Spoon over bread and put into 375° preheated oven for 50 to 60 minutes or until puffed and brown. Cover with foil once they reach the desired degree of browness. Remove from oven and sprinkle with Equal. Serve at once.
Yield: 6 servings

Approximate Per Serving:
Calories: 207
Fat: 2.3 g
Cholesterol: 1 mg
Carbohydrates: 30 g
Protein: 10 g
Sodium: 306 mg

Diabetic Exchanges: 1 bread; 1 milk; 1 fat

If you drop an egg on the floor, sprinkle it heavily with salt;
after 5 to 10 minutes sweep the dried egg into the dustpan.

Stuffed French Toast

(Recipe contains approximately 9% fat)

1 loaf French bread, cut into 1 1/2" thick slices

FILLING:
1 c. raisins, ground
1/2 c. dried apricots,
chopped very fine
1/2 c. chopped dates,
ground
1 to 3 T. orange juice to
moisten

For filling mix all ingredients together. Using a sharp serrated knife, make a pocket in the center of each piece of bread. Stuff filling in pocket and set aside.

BATTER:
Egg substitute to equal
4 eggs
1/2 c. skim milk
1 tsp. cinnamon
1 tsp. vanilla
1/4 tsp. nutmeg
2 T. sugar

Blend all batter ingredients and dip bread in batter to coat both sides. Spray hot skillet with cooking spray and fry bread.

GLAZE:
1/2 c. orange juice
1 jar apricot preserves,
natural fruit, no sugar
added

Heat orange juice and preserves and pour small amount over French toast.

Yield: 12 slices

Approximate Per Slice:
Calories: 210
Fat: 2.1 g
Cholesterol: Tr. mg
Carbohydrates: 35 g
Protein: 6 g
Sodium: 24 mg

Diabetic Exchanges: 2 bread; 1/2 milk; 1/2 fat

Extra Tender Waffles

(Recipe contains approximately 19% fat)

1 3/4 c. flour, sift 3 times
  before measuring
2 tsp. baking powder
1/2 tsp. salt (opt.)
1 T. sugar

Egg substitute to equal
  2 eggs
2 T. tub margarine
1 c. skim milk
1/2 c. sparkling water
3 egg whites

Blend sifted flour, baking powder, salt and sugar in a large mixing bowl. Make a well in flour mixture and put egg substitute, margarine, skim milk and sparkling water in hole. With swift strokes, combine liquid ingredients with dry ingredients. Blend just until dry ingredients are moist. Batter will not be smooth. Don't worry about lumps. They will bake out. Beat egg whites just until stiff. Fold into batter just until blended. Heat waffle iron, spray with cooking spray. Cover about 2/3 of waffle iron with batter (center part of iron); close lid and allow about 4 minutes for waffles to bake. Some waffle irons are slower than others and it may take 5 to 6 minutes. Experiment until you are familiar with your waffle iron.

Yield: 6 waffles (this is 6 batches on waffle maker)

Approximate Per Waffle:
Calories: 218
Fat: 4.6
Cholesterol: 1 mg
Carbohydrates: 32
Protein: 13 g
Sodium: 325 mg

Diabetic Exchanges: 1 1/2 bread; 1 milk; 1/2 meat; 1/4 fat

*When a recipe calls for one cup egg whites, use
8 to 10 egg whites depending on size of eggs.*

French Toast Waffles

(Recipe contains approximately 24% fat)

Egg substitute to equal	**Dash of salt**
1 egg	**1 tsp. sugar**
1/4 c. skim milk	**1/4 tsp. nutmeg**
2 tsp. tub margarine, melted	**6 slices bread, crusts removed**

Blend egg substitute, milk, margarine, salt, sugar and nutmeg. Stir well to blend. Dip bread, on both sides, into mixture and bake in waffle iron.
Yield: 6 waffles

Approximate Per Waffle:
Calories: 93
Fat: 2.5 g
Cholesterol: Tr. mg
Carbohydrates: 13 g
Protein: 4 g
Sodium: 210 mg

Diabetic Exchanges: 1 bread; 1/2 fat

Granola—Low Sugar

(Recipe contains approximately 14% fat)

6 c. rolled oats	1 c. chopped dried pineapple
1 c. nonfat dry milk	1/2 c. honey
granules	2 T. canola oil
1 1/2 c. chopped dates	1 c. raisins

Put rolled oats on a large baking sheet and bake in 300° preheated oven for 15 minutes, stirring often. Remove from oven and stir in dry milk, chopped dates and dried pineapple. Heat honey and oil until honey becomes thin. Drizzle over oat mixture, tossing to coat evenly. Return to oven and bake 20 to 25 minutes, stirring every 7 to 8 minutes. Remove from oven and stir in raisins. Pour out onto sheets of wax paper to cool. Store in airtight container in refrigerator.
Yield: about 5 cups

Approximate Per 1/4 Cup Serving:
Calories: 102
Fat: 1.6 g
Cholesterol: 1 mg
Carbohydrates: 19 g
Protein: 4 g
Sodium: 19 mg

Diabetic Exchanges: 1 bread; 1/4 milk; 1/4 fruit

Granola—Sugar-Free

(Recipe contains approximately 13% fat)

6 c. rolled oats
1 c. nonfat dry milk granules
1 c. chopped dates
1 c. chopped dried apricots
Cooking spray to equal a
   12-second-count spray
1 c. raisins

12 pkt. Equal sweetener or sweetener of choice to equal 1/2 cup sugar (do not use sugar in this. If sweeter granola is desired use sweetened version of granola, Granola Low Sugar, see index)

Put oats on a baking sheet and bake in 300° preheated oven for 15 minutes, stirring often. Remove from oven and stir in dry milk granules, blending well. Stir in dates and apricots. Using a fork to toss, spray mixture with cooking spray for a 12-second-count, tossing as you spray. Put back into oven and bake 20 to 25 minutes or until oats are nicely browned. Stir every 7 to 8 minutes to prevent burning. Remove from oven and stir in raisins. Sprinkle with sweetener and blend. Turn out onto sheets of wax paper to cool. Store in airtight container in the refrigerator.
Yield: about 10 cups

Approximate Per 1/4 Cup:
Calories: 88
Fat: 1.3 g
Cholesterol: 0.0 mg
Carbohydrates: 17 g
Protein: 4 g
Sodium: 20 mg

Diabetic Exchanges: 1/2 bread; 1 fruit; 1/4 fat

*One orange will yield 6-8 tablespoons juice,
depending on size of orange.*

Apple Syrup—Sugar Free

(Recipe contains approximately 11% fat)

1/3 c. apple juice concentrate	**1/2 c. applesauce, unsweetened** **1/4 tsp. cinnamon**

Melt apple juice concentrate in saucepan over low heat. Add applesauce and stir until blended and heated through. Add cinnamon. Serve hot over pancakes or waffles.

Yield: 3/4 cup

Approximate Per Tablespoon:
Calories: 50
Fat: 0.6 g
Cholesterol: 0.0 mg
Carbohydrates: 15 g
Protein: Tr. g
Sodium: 1 mg

Diabetic Exchanges: 1 fruit

Apricot Syrup For Pancakes, Waffles or Ice Cream

(Recipe contains approximately 4% fat)

1 c. pure apricot jam **(no pectin or sugar** **added)**	**2 T. water** **2 T. dark rum (alcohol will** **cook out of rum)**

Put all of the ingredients in a saucepan and melt jam, cooking until mixture comes to a boil. Remove from heat and strain through cheese-cloth or fine sieve. Serve hot.

Yield: 1 1/4 cups

Approximate Per Tablespoon:
Calories: 24
Fat: 0.1 g
Cholesterol: 0.0 mg
Carbohydrates: 5 g
Protein: Tr. g
Sodium: Tr. g

Diabetic Exchanges: 1/2 fruit

Blackberry Syrup for Pancakes, Waffles or Ice Cream

(Recipe contains approximately 9% fat)

1 c. blackberry pure jam,
  no sugar or pectin added

2 T. water

Put jam and water in a saucepan and melt jam, cooking until mixture comes to a boil. Remove from heat and strain through cheesecloth or fine sieve. Serve over pancakes, waffles or ice cream.

Yield: 1 cup

Approximate Per Tablespoon:
Calories: 19
Fat: 0.2 g
Cholesterol: 0.0 mg
Carbohydrates: 4 g
Protein: 0.0 g
Sodium: 0.0 mg

Diabetic Exchanges: 1/2 fruit

Quick Maple Syrup

(Recipe contains approximately 0% fat)

2 1/2 c. sugar
1 c. hot water

1 1/2 tsp. maple flavoring

Bring water and sugar to rolling boil. When sugar has dissolved and mixture is boiling, remove from stove and add maple flavoring. Serve hot.

Yield: 2 cups

Approximate Per Tablespoon:
Calories: 60
Fat: 0.0 g
Cholesterol: 0.0 mg
Carbohydrates: 16 g
Protein: 0.0 g
Sodium: 0.0 mg

Cannot be used on a diabetic diet

Maple Cinnamon Syrup—Low Sugar

(Recipe contains approximately 26% fat)

2 T. firmly-packed
  brown sugar
1 tsp. cornstarch
1/4 tsp. cinnamon
2/3 c. skim milk

1 T. reduce-calorie margarine
1/4 tsp. maple flavoring
3 pkt. Equal sweetener, or
  sweetener of choice to
  equal 2 T. sugar

In a small saucepan, put brown sugar, cornstarch and cinnamon. Stir until of uniform color. Very slowly add milk, whisking until smooth. Bring mixture to a boil; reduce heat and simmer until slightly thickened. Stir constantly. Remove from heat and add margarine and maple flavoring. Stir in sweetener. Serve warm.
Yield: 3/4 cup or 12 tablespoons

Approximate Per Tablespoon:
Calories: 21
Fat: 0.6 g
Cholesterol: Tr. mg
Carbohydrates: 3 g
Protein: Tr. g
Sodium: 19 mg

Diabetic Exchanges: 1 tablespoon free food; 1/4 cup equals 1 milk

Strawberry Syrup for Pancakes, Waffles or Ice Cream

(Recipe contains approximately 10% fat)

1 c. pure strawberry jam
  with no sugar or pectin added

2 T. water

Put jam and water in a saucepan and melt jam, cooking until mixture comes to a boil. Remove from heat and strain through cheesecloth or fine sieve. Serve over pancakes, waffles or ice cream.
Yield: 3/4 cup

Approximate Per Tablespoon:
Calories: 18
Fat: 0.2 g
Cholesterol: 0.0 mg
Carbohydrates: 4 g
Protein: Tr. g
Sodium: Tr. mg

Diabetic Exchanges: 1/2 fruit

Brunch

Brunch Pizza

(Recipe contains approximately 14% fat)

1 c. flour, whole wheat
    blend, unbleached or
    enriched all-purpose

2 tsp. baking powder
1/4 tsp. salt (opt.)
6 T. skim milk

Blend flour, baking powder and salt. Add milk, tossing with fork to make soft dough. Turn out onto floured surface and roll out. Place on pizza pan, stretching thin and crimping edge.

FILLING:

1 lb. Homestyle turkey
    sausage (see index)
1 c. frozen hash browns,
    thawed
8 slices no-fat American
    cheese, diced

1/4 c. skim milk
Egg substitute to equal
    5 eggs
1/2 tsp. salt (opt.)
1/2 tsp. pepper (less, if
    desired)

Brown sausage and drain off any rendered fat. Spoon crumbled sausage over crust. Top with hash browns, then with cheese. Blend milk, egg substitute, salt and pepper. Beat 2 minute, then pour over meat mixture. Bake in 375° oven for 25 to 30 minutes or until eggs have set and top is lightly browned.
Yield: 6 servings

Approximate Per Serving:
Calories: 340
Fat: 5.2 g
Cholesterol: 68 mg
Carbohydrates: 27 g
Protein: 27 g
Sodium: 979 mg

Diabetic Exchanges: 3 meat; 1 bread; 1 milk

*Instead of using one whole egg, substitute
2 egg whites or 1/4 cup egg substitute.*

Crabmeat Quiche

(Recipe contains approximately 5% fat)

1 (8") baked pie shell,
  lowfat (see index)
Egg substitute to equal
  2 eggs
1 c. "lite" evaporated
  skim milk
1/2 tsp. seasoned salt

1/8 tsp. pepper
8 slices no-fat American
  cheese, diced
1 T. flour
1 (6 1/2 oz.) can crabmeat,
  flaked

In a mixing bowl, put egg substitute, evaporated skim milk, seasoned salt and pepper. Beat for 1 minute with whisk. Combine cheese, flour and crabmeat and sprinkle over bottom of baked shell. Pour egg mixture over top and bake in 325° preheated oven for 45 minutes to 1 hour or until knife inserted in center comes out clean.

Yield: 4 servings

Approximate Per Serving:
Calories: 218
Fat: 1.3 g
Cholesterol: 31 mg
Carbohydrates: 26 g
Protein: 17 g
Sodium: 1,216 mg

Diabetic Exchanges: 1 meat; 1 bread; 1 milk

*When a recipe calls for cheddar cheese and a replacement
will not maintain proper taste, cut the amount of cheese
specified in half and use extra sharp cheddar cheese.*

Crustless Quiche

(Recipe contains approximately 9% fat)

Egg substitute to
  equal 2 eggs
1 1/2 c. flour, whole wheat
  blend, unbleached or
  enriched all-purpose
1 tsp. salt (opt.)
1/8 tsp. pepper
1/4 c. chopped green pepper
2 c. sliced fresh mushrooms
  (can use canned, if desired)

16 slices no-fat American
  cheese, diced
1 can "lite" evaporated
  skim milk, plus enough
  skim milk to make 2 cups
1/4 c. chopped onion
2 c. lean ham, chopped
  (remove all visible fat)

In a large mixing bowl, put all ingredients and whisk until mixture is smooth. Pour into a 9x13-inch baking dish that has been sprayed with cooking oil. Bake in 425° preheated oven for 30 minutes.
Yield: 8 servings

Approximate Per Serving:
Calories: 303
Fat: 3.0 g
Cholesterol: 40 mg
Carbohydrates: 35 g
Protein: 19 g
Sodium: 1,643 mg

Diabetic Exchanges: 2 meat; 1 milk; 1 1/2 bread

*Once an onion has been cut, rub the cut side with
a bit of margarine. It will keep much longer.*

Easy Hash Brown Quiche

(Recipe contains approximately 7% fat)

1 (24 oz.) pkg. shredded
  hash brown potatoes,
  thawed, moisture
  pressed out
Cooking spray
16 slices nonfat American
  cheese, diced
1 c. cooked ham, lean only,
  diced very fine
1/2 c. evaporated skim milk
Egg substitute to equal
  2 eggs
1/2 tsp. seasoned salt
1/8 tsp. pepper

Spray a 9-inch pie plate with cooking oil and press potatoes in dish to make a crust. Spray potatoes with cooking spray. Bake in 450° preheated oven for 25 minutes. Remove from oven and sprinkle cheese and ham over potatoes. Blend milk, egg substitute, seasoned salt and pepper; pour over cheese and ham. Bake at 350° for about 20 minutes, or until firm.
Yield: 6 servings

Approximate Per Serving:
Calories: 241
Fat: 1.9 g
Cholesterol: 2 mg
Carbohydrates: 21 g
Protein: 18 g
Sodium: 1,667 mg

Diabetic Exchanges: 1 bread; 2 meat; 1/2 milk

*For two tablespoons of minced onion, one
teaspoon of onion powder can be substituted.*

Ham and Egg Casserole

(Recipe contains approximately 18% fat)

1 T. tub margarine	6 slices no-fat
3 T. no-fat, no cholesterol	American cheese
mayonnaise	Egg substitute to equal
1 tsp. prepared mustard	4 eggs
12 slices whole wheat	2 c. skim milk
bread, crust removed	1/2 tsp. salt
6 slices thin-sliced ham	1 tsp. paprika

Blend margarine, mayonnaise and mustard. Mix well. Spread on one side of 12 slices of bread. Spray a 9x13-inch glass baking dish with cooking spray and lay 6 slices of bread, buttered-side down, in dish. Top with slice of ham and slice of cheese. Put remaining bread on top of cheese, buttered-side up. Blend egg substitute, milk, salt and paprika. Pour mixture evenly over bread. Put into refrigerator overnight. Bake in 350° preheated oven for 45 to 55 minutes.

Yield: 6 servings

Approximate Per Serving:
Calories: 290
Fat: 5.8 g
Cholesterol: 17 mg
Carbohydrates: 34 g
Protein: 19 g
Sodium: 1,244 mg

Diabetic Exchanges: 1 1/2 bread; 1 meat; 1 milk; 1 fat

If you don't have the fresh herbs a recipe calls for simply substitute with dried ones. Three parts fresh equals one part dried.

Hamburger Quiche

(Recipe contains approximately 19% fat)

1 (9") unbaked, lowfat,
   pie crust (see index)
1/2 lb. ground round
1/2 c. lowfat mayonnaise
1/2 c. skim milk
Egg substitute to equal
   2 eggs

1 T. cornstarch
12 slices no-fat American
   cheese, diced
1/4 c. chopped onion
1/8 tsp. pepper

Brown ground round and drain any rendered fat. Combine mayonnaise, milk, egg substitute and cornstarch, beating until smooth. Stir in meat, diced cheese, onion and pepper. Add salt, if desired. Pour into pastry shell and bake in 350° preheated oven for 35 to 40 minutes or until knife inserted in center comes out clean.

Yield: 6 servings

Approximate Per Serving:
Calories: 261
Fat: 5.5 g
Cholesterol: 32 mg
Carbohydrates: 27 g
Protein: 20 g
Sodium: 825 mg

Diabetic Exchanges: 2 meat; 1 vegetable; 1/2 milk; 1 bread

*To prevent spread of bacteria, clean the wheel of
your can opener often with a sponge dipped in
a solution of hot water and baking soda.*

Holiday No Fry Omelet

(Recipe contains approximately 14% fat)

Egg substitute to equal
8 eggs
1 can evaporated "lite" skim
milk plus enough skim
milk to make 2 cups
1 1/2 c. cubed ham—use
extra lean ham & use
lean only—no visible fat
12 slices no-fat American
cheese, quartered

1/2 c. green bell pepper,
quartered
1/2 c. red bell pepper,
quartered
1 scant tsp. salt (opt.)
2 c. sliced fresh mush-
rooms (can use canned,
if desired)
24 saltine crackers, crushed

Blend together egg substitute and milk, beating for 1 minute. Add ham, cheese, green and red pepper, salt, mushrooms and crackers. Pour into a 9x13-inch baking dish. Bake, uncovered, for 40 to 45 minutes at 325°. Great for when families get together as it can be made up to 2 days in advance.
Yield: 8 servings

Approximate Per Serving:
Calories: 244
Fat: 3.7 g
Cholesterol: 32 mg
Carbohydrates: 18 g
Protein: 16 g
Sodium: 1,442 mg

Diabetic Exchanges: 2 meat; 1 bread; 1 vegetable

If you freeze soft cheese for 15 minutes it will shred easier.

Quick and Easy Do-Ahead Brunch Casserole

(Recipe contains approximately 12% fat)

Egg substitute to equal 6 eggs	1 c. very lean ham cubes, use lean only—no visible fat
1 1/2 c. "lite" skim evaporated milk	2 slices reduced-calorie bread, cubed
1 tsp. dry mustard	8 slices no-fat American cheese, diced
1/2 tsp. salt (opt.)	
1/8 tsp. pepper	

In a mixing bowl, put egg substitute, milk, mustard, salt and pepper. Beat for 1 minute. Add cubed ham and bread cubes. Pour into 8x8-inch baking dish that has been sprayed with cooking spray. Sprinkle cheese over top. Refrigerate overnight. Bake, uncovered, in 325° preheated oven for 45 to 50 minutes or until inserted knife in middle comes out clean.
Yield: 6 servings

Approximate Per Serving:
Calories: 229
Fat: 3.2 g
Cholesterol: 27 mg
Carbohydrates: 17 g
Protein: 16 g
Sodium: 1,199 mg

Diabetic Exchanges: 1 meat; 1 milk; 1/2 bread; 1 fat

Cook dishes in utensils of proper size; don't try to squeeze a 4-cup recipe into a one-quart casserole. And don't use a 4-cup recipe in a 2-quart dish. Use a 1 1/2-quart dish for a 4-cup recipe.

Spanish Omelet, Holiday-Style

(Recipe contains approximately 31% fat)

OMELET:

Egg substitute to equal
  3 eggs
2 T. water

Salt & pepper, to taste
1 tsp. tub margarine

Put egg substitute in bowl and add water and salt and pepper. Whisk to blend. Put margarine in skillet; heat, then add omelet mixture. Shake skillet as eggs cook, to keep omelet from sticking.

FILLING:

1 tsp. tub margarine
1/3 c. green pepper,
  chopped
1/3 c. red bell pepper,
  chopped

1 sm. onion, sliced &
  separated in rings
1 rib celery, chopped
Coarse black pepper

Sauté vegetables in margarine. Pour vegetables over omelet and fold over. Serve immediately.

Yield: 2 servings

Approximate Per Serving:
Calories: 107
Fat: 3.7 g
Cholesterol: 0.0 mg
Carbohydrates: 2 g
Protein: 9 g
Sodium: 439 mg

Diabetic Exchanges: 1/2 vegetable; 1 meat; 1/2 fat

*Small amounts of leftover corn can be
added to pancake batter for variety.*

Tuna Quiche in Rice Crust

(Recipe contains approximately 23% fat)

**Egg substitute to equal
4 eggs**
**2 c. cooked brown rice,
cooked in beef stock
instead of water**
2 T. tub margarine, melted
2 T. finely-chopped onion

**2 (6 1/2 oz.) cans white
tuns, water packed,
drained**
**2 T. finely-chopped green
pepper**
**1/2 tsp. dried marjoram,
crushed**
1 c. skim evaporated milk

Combine egg substitute to equal 1 egg, cooked brown rice, margarine and 1 tablespoon of chopped onion. Press into the bottom of a 10-inch pie plate that has been lightly sprayed with vegetable oil. Put flaked tuna on top of crust. To remaining egg substitute, add milk and remaining onion, green pepper, marjoram and cheese. Pour over tuna. Bake in a 350° preheated oven, uncovered, until knife inserted just off-center comes out clean. Usually about 40 to 45 minutes of baking.
Yield: 8 servings

Approximate Per Serving:
Calories: 152
Fat: 3.9 g
Cholesterol: 13 mg
Carbohydrates: 13 g
Protein: 12 g
Sodium: 94 mg

Diabetic Exchanges: 3/4 bread; 1 1/2 meat

*A leaf of lettuce dropped into the pot absorbs the grease
from the top of soup. Simply remove the lettuce leaf
and throw it away after it has served its purpose.*

Lunch

Soups and Stews

Bean and Turkey Soup
(Recipe contains approximately 7% fat)

1 1/2 c. dried Great
  Northern beans
1 roasted turkey carcass,
  left over from Thanks-
  giving
Leftover pan drippings,
  defatted
1 c. leftover dressing
1 lg. onion, chunked
2 stalks of celery with
  leaves, chunked

3 lg. carrots, chunked
4 qt. water
1 bay leaf
1 tsp. seasoned salt
1/4 tsp. pepper
2 c. leftover turkey,
  chopped
2 lg. carrots, sliced thin
4 med. potatoes, diced

Soak Great Northern beans overnight. The next morning rinse and cover with water. In a large soup kettle, place turkey carcass, pan drippings, onion, celery, carrots, water, bay leaf, seasoned salt and pepper. Bring to a boil, reduce heat and simmer 4 hours. Remove bones and strain stock. Any meat left on bones can be picked off, but don't include in 4 cups of chopped turkey. Put stock back in kettle and add beans. Add more water if needed. Cook over low heat, about 2 hours or until beans are tender. Add turkey, carrots and potatoes; cook another 20 minutes or until vegetables are tender.
Yield: 10 servings

Approximate Per Serving:
Calories: 273
Fat: 2.2 g
Cholesterol: 40 mg
Carbohydrates: 47 g
Protein: 25 g
Sodium: 330 mg

Diabetic Exchanges: 2 bread; 2 vegetable; 1 1/2 meat

Cheese Soup

(Recipe contains approximately 1% fat)

3 c. chicken stock, can
   use canned low-sodium
   chicken broth
1 c. very finely chopped
   celery
1 c. very finely chopped
   onion
2 1/2 c. very finely chopped
   potatoes (or grated
   potatoes)

1 c. shredded carrots
1/2 tsp. salt (opt.)
1/2 tsp. pepper
1 (12 slice) pkg. nonfat
   American cheese,
   quartered
Fresh chopped parsley

Bring broth to a boil and add celery and onion. Cook 20 minutes, then add potatoes, carrots, salt and pepper. Cook another 20 minutes, covered. Add cheese and cook until cheese melts. Serve hot, sprinkled with fresh snipped parsley.

Yield: 8 servings

Approximate Per Serving:
Calories: 145
Fat: 0.1 g
Cholesterol: 15 mg
Carbohydrates: 14 g
Protein: 12 g
Sodium: 1,084 mg

Diabetic Exchange: 1 1/2 meat; 1 bread

*Rub the bottom of soup bowls with a sliced whole
garlic to accent the flavor of navy bean soup.*

Creole Soup

(Recipe contains approximately 10% fat)

1/4 lb. ground pork tenderloin, all visible fat
   removed before grinding
1/4 tsp. chili powder
1 sm. green sweet pepper,
   chopped
1 sm. yellow onion, chopped

1 frozen chicken stock
   cube (see index)
1/4 c. enriched all-purpose
   flour
1 1/2 c. tomatoes, low
   sodium
4 c. chicken stock
1 c. cooked brown rice

Sauté ground pork for 5 minutes. Add chili powder, green pepper, onion and stock cube. Sauté about 5 minutes. Stir in flour, cooking flour for 2 minutes. Add tomatoes and juice, then slowly add stock. Simmer 20 minutes, then add rice and simmer another 5 minutes.

Yield: 8 servings

Approximate Per Serving:
Calories: 112
Fat: 1.3 g
Cholesterol: 6 mg
Carbohydrates: 8 g
Protein: 7 g
Sodium: 381 mg

Diabetic Exchanges: 1 meat; 1 bread

*Freeze defatted broth in ice cube trays - transfer to bags
and use to sauté instead of margarine. Works great!*

Delicious Wild Rice Soup

(Recipe contains approximately 23% fat)

1 T. tub margarine
2 frozen chicken stock cubes (see index)
4 med. fresh mushrooms, chopped fine
2 green onions, chopped fine, use part of green
1/3 c. finely shredded carrot
1/2 c. flour
3 c. chicken stock, can use canned low-sodium chicken broth

2 c. cooked wild rice
1/2 c. minced ham, lean only
1/2 tsp. salt (opt.)
1/4 tsp. white pepper
1 c. "lite" evaporated skim milk
2 T. dry sherry, if desired
Snipped fresh parsley

Melt margarine and frozen stock in large skillet and sauté mushrooms, onions and carrot. Add flour and stir to make a roux, cooking at least 1 to 2 minutes. Remove from stove and slowly whisk in stock, whisking until smooth. Return to stove and bring to a boil, stirring constantly. Boil for 1 minute. Add wild rice, ham and salt and pepper. Blend milk and sherry and stir into mixture. Heat through, but do not boil. Serve hot, garnished with snipped fresh parsley.
Yield: 6 servings

Approximate Per Serving:
Calories: 221
Fat: 5.7 g
Cholesterol: 13 mg
Carbohydrates: 30 g
Protein: 10 g
Sodium: 1,330 mg

Diabetic Exchanges: 1 meat; 1 vegetable; 1 1/2 bread; 1/2 fat

Fat may be quickly eliminated from soup or stew by dropping ice cubes into pot. Stir - remove ice cubes before they melt.

Italian Vegetable Soup

(Recipe contains approximately 29% fat)

3/4 c. stew beef, all visible fat removed; cut into small cubes	2 lg. potatoes, diced small
1 c. onions, diced	1 carrot, sliced thin
6 c. water	1 can green beans, drained
1 green pepper	1/2 tsp. seasoned salt
2 cloves garlic, minced	1/8 tsp. pepper
1 frozen beef stock cube, for sautéing (see index)	2 tsp. basil
	2 (16 oz.) cans tomatoes
	1 c. uncooked eggless noodles

Put beef, onions and water into a large heavy-bottomed pot and simmer for 1 1/2 hours or until beef is tender. Sauté green pepper and garlic in beef stock cube. Add potatoes and carrots and sauté for 10 minutes. Add to beef pot along with green beans, seasoned salt, pepper and basil. Cook 30 minutes. Add tomatoes; bring to a boil and add noodles. Cook until noodles are tender.

Yield: 8 servings

Approximate Per Serving:
Calories: 211
Fat: 6.9 g
Cholesterol: 33 mg
Carbohydrates: 22 g
Protein: 16 g
Sodium: 188 mg

Diabetic Exchanges: 2 meat; 1 bread; 1 vegetable

Thicken soups and stews by putting the onions and celery in the blender for a few seconds before adding.

Mexican Chili (Hot)

(Recipe contains approximately 13% fat)

12 lg. flour tortillas
1 1/2 lb. chicken breast, all
   skin and fat removed,
   chunked
1 med. onion, diced
1 green pepper, chopped
3 cloves garlic, minced
1 to 2 T. crushed hot red
   pepper, depending on
   degree of heat desired
3 T. chili powder

2 tsp. ground cumin
1/2 tsp. dried oregano
1 tsp. dried cilantro (opt.)
1 1/2 tsp. salt (opt.)
2 (16 oz.) cans dark red
   kidney beans, undrained
2 (16 oz.) cans whole
   tomatoes, undrained
1 (8 oz.) can tomato sauce
1 (16 oz.) can whole kernel
   corn, drained

Invert 6 custard cups on cookie sheet and form tortilla around custard cup. Spray lightly with cooking spray and bake in a 375° preheated oven until tortilla cups are crisp, about 15 minutes. Repeat with remaining 6 tortillas. In a large heavy-bottomed skillet, sauté chunked chicken breast. Drain off any rendered fat, then add onion, green pepper, garlic, red chili pepper, chili powder, cumin, oregano, cilantro and salt. Cook, stirring almost constantly, until onion and green pepper are tender. Add beans, tomatoes, tomato sauce and corn. Simmer over low heat for about 45 minutes, breaking up tomatoes when stirring. Serve in tortilla shells.
Yield: 12 servings

Approximate Per Serving:
Calories: 301
Fat: 6.6 g
Cholesterol: 69 mg
Carbohydrates: 24 g
Protein: 36 g
Sodium: 487 mg

Diabetic Exchanges: 3 meat; 2 bread; 2 vegetables

*Beef Stew - About 1/2 hour before done, add 1/2-3/4 cup
red wine. The stew is converted from a "busy day dish"
to a "candlelight entrée." Alcohol cooks away.*

Minestrone

(Recipe contains approximately 5% fat)

1 c. dried kidney beans
6 c. hearty chicken stock, defatted—can use bouillon
2 lg. onion, chopped
2 cloves garlic, crushed
1 carrot, thinly sliced
1 stalk celery, chopped (include leaves)
2 lg. potatoes, diced

1 frozen hearty chicken stock cube, or 2 T. liquid chicken bouillon
Salt & pepper, to taste
2 tsp. basil
2 c. shredded cabbage
2 c. peeled, seeded & chopped tomatoes
1 c. uncooked noodles
1/2 c. frozen peas

Wash beans and soak in 2 cups water overnight. In the morning rinse and put in large pot with chicken stock. Add onions and garlic and simmer 1 hour. Sauté carrots, celery and potatoes in stock; season and add to bean pot. Add salt and pepper, to taste, and basil. Stir in cabbage and chopped tomatoes, stir well and simmer 30 minutes. Add uncooked noodles and frozen peas and cook an additional 15 minutes.
Yield: 12 servings

Approximate Per Serving:
Calories: 129
Fat: 0.7 g
Cholesterol: 0.0 mg
Carbohydrates: 22 g
Protein: 6 g
Sodium: 202 mg

Diabetic Exchanges: 1 bread; 2 vegetable; 1/4 fat

A few drops of lemon juice in the water will whiten boiled potatoes.

Potato Soup with Ribbles

(Recipe contains approximately 3% fat)

6 med. potatoes, peeled
   & diced
1 med. onion, diced
3 c. hearty chicken broth,
   or 4 chicken bouillon
   cubes dissolved in
   3 c. boiling water
1/4 tsp. white pepper

3 c. skim milk
1/3 c. nonfat dry milk
   granules
2 c. flour
1/2 tsp. salt (opt.)
Egg substitute to equal
   1 egg

Put potatoes and onions in a large saucepan and cover with chicken broth. Add 1/4 teaspoon of white pepper and simmer until potatoes are tender. Blend milk granules and milk; add to potato mixture; set aside. Sift flour and salt into egg substitute until fine ribbles are formed by working with fingers. If using salt, put in with flour before adding to egg substitute. Add as many ribbles as needed to thicken soup nicely. Boil 10 minutes. If any ribbles are left they may be kept in a sealed jar for later use.
Yield: 8 servings

Approximate Per Serving:
Calories: 239
Fat: 0.7 g
Cholesterol: 2 mg
Carbohydrates: 44 g
Protein: 10 g
Sodium: 481 mg

Diabetic Exchanges: 2 bread; 1 milk; 1/4 fat

*Add a pinch of basil or oregano to
any recipe that includes tomatoes.*

Salmon Bisque

(Recipe contains approximately 13% fat)

4 c. chicken stock
2 c. nonfat dry milk granules
1 frozen chicken stock cube, for sautéing, or 2 T. cooking stock
1/3 c. onions, finely chopped
1/3 c. green pepper, finely chopped
1/2 c. celery, finely chopped
3 T. flour

1/4 tsp. seasoned salt (opt.)
1/4 tsp. garlic salt or garlic powder
Dash of pepper
1 (7 1/2 oz.) can pink salmon, drained, skin removed & flesh & bones mashed or run through a sieve
2 T. pimentos, chopped

Put stock in a large measuring cup. Add milk granules and stir until dissolved. Set aside. Melt stock cube in a 2-quart saucepan. Sauté onions, green pepper and celery until tender. Stir in flour, seasoned salt, garlic salt and pepper if desired. Brown 1 minute, stirring constantly. Remove from heat and slowly whisk in stock. Return to heat and cook, stirring constantly, until mixture thickens. Do not boil. Stir in salmon and pimento and heat. DO NOT BOIL!
Yield: 4 main course servings

Approximate Per Serving:
Calories: 286
Fat: 4.1 g
Cholesterol: 24 mg
Carbohydrates: 29 g
Protein: 25 g
Sodium: 1,301 mg

Diabetic Exchanges: 2 meat; 1 milk; 2 vegetable; 1/2 bread

A dash of nutmeg does wonders for any soup.

Split Pea and Rice Soup

(Recipe contains approximately 1% fat)

1 c. split peas	1 sm. onion, diced
1 c. brown rice, uncooked	1 frozen beef stock cube,
1/4 tsp. salt (opt.)	for sautéing (see index)
1/8 tsp. pepper	

Cook peas in 2-quart saucepan according to package instructions, adding 1 more cup of water than called for. In a separate saucepan, cook rice according to package instructions. Add salt and pepper. Sauté onion in stock until tender. Add onion and rice to the saucepan containing cooked split peas. Let this mixture simmer about 15 minutes. Add pepper. Serve hot.

Yield: 8 servings

Approximate Per Serving:
Calories: 176
Fat: 0.2 g
Cholesterol: 0.0 mg
Carbohydrates: 35 g
Protein: 8 g
Sodium: 69 mg

Diabetic Exchanges: 2 bread; 1 vegetable

*When out of flour for thickening, use
1/2 to 2/3 tablespoon cornstarch.*

Taco Soup Olé

(Recipe contains approximately 15% fat)

1 lb. ground round
1/2 med. onion, chopped
1 green pepper, chopped
1 clove garlic, minced
1 pkg. taco mix
3/4 c. water
1 can red kidney beans,
  juice included

1 can black beans, juice
  included
1 can whole kernel corn,
  drained
2 cans whole tomatoes,
  chopped (include juice)

Brown ground round, onion, pepper and garlic—do not burn garlic. Add taco seasoning and 3/4 cup water and simmer 15 minutes, stirring occasionally. Pour mixture into soup pot and add remaining ingredients. Simmer 20 minutes.
Yield: 8 servings

Approximate Per Serving:
Calories: 288
Fat: 4.9 g
Cholesterol: 40 mg
Carbohydrates: 42 g
Protein: 26 g
Sodium: 241 mg

Diabetic Exchanges: 2 bread; 2 vegetable; 2 meat

Poultry has one of the most delicate of all food flavors and must be frozen or kept under refrigeration at all times before cooking.

Cock A Doodle Stew with Oatmeal Biscuits

(Recipe contains approximately 24% fat)

2 c. carrots, thinly sliced
3 c. potatoes, peeled &
  diced
1 c. onion, finely chopped
1 c. celery, sliced thin
1 c. frozen peas

1 tsp. salt (opt.)
1/8 tsp. pepper
1 qt. chicken stock
3 c. cooked chicken
  breast, cubed

Put all ingredients in a large pan, except cooked chicken, and simmer until tender. Add cooked chicken to pot when vegetables are tender.

THICKENING:
2 T. flour   1/4 c. water

Mix until smooth and add to chicken and vegetables. Pour into a 9x13-inch baking dish.

BISCUIT TOPPING:
1 c. flour
1/2 tsp. salt (opt.)
1 T. baking powder

1/4 c. tub margarine
1 c. oatmeal
1 c. skim milk

Sift flour, salt and baking powder into a mixing bowl. Cut in margarine until mixture resembles meal. Stir in oats and add milk, tossing with a fork. Turn out on lightly-floured surface and knead 4 or 5 times. Roll out to 1/2-inch thickness. Cut with a 2-inch biscuit cutter. Place biscuits on top of stew and bake in a 425° preheated oven for 12 to 15 minutes or until lightly browned.
Yield: 8 servings

Approximate Per Serving:
Calories: 317
Fat: 8.6 g
Cholesterol: 46 mg
Carbohydrates: 35 g
Protein: 27 g
Sodium: 650 mg

Diabetic Exchanges: 1 bread; 1 vegetable; 1 milk; 2 meat; 1/2 fat

Chicken and Feathery Dumplings

(Recipe contains approximately 17% fat)

4 split chicken breasts, skin & fat left intact	1 potato, chunked
6 c. water	1 tsp. seasoned salt
1 med. onion, quartered	1/4 tsp. garlic powder
1 carrot, chunked	1/8 tsp. pepper

Put all ingredients into a wide-mouthed pot and bring to boil. Simmer 1 hour. Remove chicken. Remove skin and bones and reserve flesh. Put skin and bones back into pot and simmer for another 1 1/2 hours, covered. Cool chicken pot and strain broth, discarding skin, bones and vegetables. Cool, then refrigerate overnight. Next morning defat broth.

When time to serve, add:

2 potatoes, diced fine	1 carrot, sliced thin
1 stalk celery, sliced thin	

Cook vegetables in broth until tender. Add cooked and cubed chicken breast and begin to simmer.

DUMPLINGS:

2 c. enriched all-purpose flour	1/2 tsp. salt
1 T. baking powder	2 T. margarine
	1 1/3 c. skim milk

In large mixing bowl, sift together flour, baking powder and salt. Stir with whisk to blend. Cut in margarine. Gradually add milk as you continue to beat. Beat until mixture is smooth and creamy. Drop by tablespoons onto simmering chicken stew. Cover with tight lid and simmer for 15 to 20 minutes, without removing lid, or until dumplings are fuffy and dry looking. **Yield: 10 servings**

Approximate Per Serving:
Calories: 234
Fat: 4.4 g
Cholesterol: 54 mg
Carbohydrates: 27 g
Protein: 17 g
Sodium: 429 mg

Diabetic Exchanges: 1 bread; 2 meat; 2 vegetable

Sandwiches

Bean Burgers
(These are really good)
(Recipe contains approximately 4% fat)

1 (16 oz.) can dark red
   beans, drained & rinsed
1/4 c. onion, minced
2 T. green pepper, chopped
   very fine
1 T. reduced-calorie
   mayonnaise

1 T. catsup
1 tsp. Dijon mustard (opt.)
1 drop Tabasco sauce
4 English muffins, split
6 slices nonfat American
   cheese, diced

Put beans, onion, green pepper, mayonnaise, catsup, Dijon mustard and Tabasco sauce in blender and process until smooth. Spread mixture over English muffins and heat under broiler or in toaster oven for 3 to 4 minutes or until mixture is bubbly. Sprinkle with cheese and cook another minute or until cheese melts. Serve at once.

Yield: 8 servings

Approximate Per Serving:
Calories: 168
Fat: 0.8 g
Cholesterol: 4 mg
Carbohydrates: 29 g
Protein: 10 g
Sodium: 461 mg

Diabetic Exchanges: 1 bread; 1 milk; 1/2 vegetable

*Make your own hot sauce. Blend: 1 small can hot peppers,
5 cloves garlic and 16 ounces of tomato sauce.*

Canteens

(Recipe contains approximately 18% fat)

1 lb. ground round	2 tsp. dry mustard
1 lb. ground turkey breast	1 tsp. chili powder
1 (8 oz.) can tomato sauce	1 tsp. seasoned salt
1 c. water	1/4 tsp. pepper
1/4 c. vinegar	10 whole wheat reduced-
2 onions, chopped	calorie buns

Mix all ingredients together and simmer in skillet until meat is done and liquid has been absorbed. Put on buns and serve.
Yield: 10 sandwiches

Approximate Per Sandwich:
Calories: 267
Fat: 5.4 g
Cholesterol: 67 mg
Carbohydrates: 18 g
Protein: 29 g
Sodium: 519 mg

Diabetic Exchanges: 1 bread; 1 vegetable; 3 meat

Make your own seasoning salt. Blend: 1 cup salt, 1 tsp. thyme, 1 1/2 tsp. garlic powder, 2 tsp. onion powder, 2 tsp. dry mustard, 2 tsp. curry powder, 2 tsp. paprika, 2 tsp. turmeric, and 1 tsp. sugar.

Deluxe Pattie Melts

(Recipe contains approximately 19% fat)

3/4 lb. ground round	1 lg. onion, sliced thin &
3/4 lb. ground turkey breast	separated into rings
8 crackers, converted to	1 frozen beef stock cube
fine crumbs	1 T. tub margarine
Egg substitute to equal	2 T. no-fat; no-cholesterol
1 egg	mayonnaise
1/2 tsp. seasoned salt	8 slices no-fat American cheese
1/4 tsp. pepper	16 slices rye bread

In a mixing bowl, combine ground round, ground turkey breast, crackers, egg substitute, salt and pepper. Form into 8 patties. Broil or cook on outside barbecue until browned and done. Sauté onions in frozen beef stock cube until done. Blend margarine and mayonnaise and spread over all 16 slices of bread. Put 8 slices in large skillet, butter-side down, and top with meat patty and 1/8 of onions and slice of cheese. Top with slice of bread, butter-side up. Grill until browned. Turn and grill second side.
Yield: 8 servings

Approximate Per Serving:
Calories: 364
Fat: 7.7 g
Cholesterol: 69 mg
Carbohydrates: 33 g
Protein: 37 g
Sodium: 1,089 mg

Diabetic Exchanges: 3 1/2 meat; 1 1/4 bread; 1 milk

*When you prefer not to use white wine in a recipe substitute
an equal amount of apple juice or apple cider.*

French Hamburgers

(Recipe contains approximately 17% fat)

1/2 c. finely-minced fresh onion
1/2 c. dry red wine (can use beef stock)
3/4 lb. ground round
3/4 lb. ground turkey breast
1/2 tsp. salt (opt.)
1/8 tsp. pepper
Egg substitute to equal 1 egg
1 T. flour
10 reduced-calorie whole wheat buns
1 bunch broccoli, broken apart
1/4 c. fat-free Ranch-style dressing

Cook onion in 1 tablespoon red wine until tender, but not browned. Put into mixing bowl and add ground round and ground turkey breast. Add salt, pepper and egg substitute. Form into patties and broil on barbecue or under broiler until done on both sides. In skillet where onions were sautéed pour remaining wine. Whisk in flour, stirring until mixture thickens. Toast buns and put burger on each bun. Spoon some of the wine sauce over each burger. Put onto plate and surround with broccoli flowerets. Drizzle broccoli with salad dressing.
Yield: 10

Approximate Per Hamburger:
Calories: 274
Fat: 5.5 g
Cholesterol: 67 mg
Carbohydrates: 20 g
Protein: 33 g
Sodium: 499 mg

Diabetic Exchanges: 3 meat; 1 bread; 1/2 milk

One-half cup tomato sauce plus 1/2 cup water will substitute for one cup tomato juice.

Grilled Fish on French Bread

(Recipe contains approximately 9% fat)

1 T. soy sauce
2 T. white wine, can use
   chicken stock
1 clove garlic, minced
1/2 tsp. vinegar
2 (6 oz.) flounder fillets,
   halved

8 slices French bread,
   sliced very thin
3 T. no-fat, no-cholesterol
   mayonnaise
1 tsp. dill pickle relish
1/2 tsp. prepared mustard
1 green onion, minced
1/8 tsp. seasoned salt

Blend soy sauce, wine, garlic and vinegar and allow to stand for 30 minutes while flavors marinate. Brush mixture over fish fillets and grill in broiler (or on outside grill), basting often until fish flakes easily. Fish should take about 5 minutes on each side. While fish grills, toast French bread, then spread bread with a mixture of mayonnaise, relish, mustard, onion and seasoned salt. Place fillet on top of bread. If desired, top with lettuce and tomato slice; top with second slice of bread.
Yield: 4 servings

Approximate Per Serving:
Calories: 301
Fat: 2.9 g
Cholesterol: 40 mg
Carbohydrates: 32 g
Protein: 24 g
Sodium: 888 mg

Diabetic Exchanges: 3 meat; 2 bread

*When a recipe calls for cilantro, Chinese parsley or coriander
can be substituted - they are the same thing.*

Jumbo Vienna Sandwich

(Recipe contains approximately 17% fat)

1 lb. turkey sausage	1/4 c. water
(see index)	1/4 tsp. oregano
1/2 lb. ground round	1/4 tsp. rosemary
1 c. chopped onion	1/2 tsp. dried cilantro
1/2 c. chopped green pepper	1 loaf Vienna bread
1 (8 oz.) can tomato sauce	1 (6 oz.) pkg. nonfat
1 (6 oz.) can tomato paste	American cheese slices

Brown sausage and ground round; drain off any rendered fat. Add onions and green pepper and cook 5 minutes. Stir in tomato sauce, tomato paste, water and seasonings. Blend and simmer 15 minutes, stirring occasionally. Cut a lengthwise slice from the top of bread. Scoop out center of bread to form a shell. Place half of cheese in shell. Fill with meat mixture and top with remaining cheese slices. Return top slice to loaf; wrap in foil, tightly. Bake in 400° preheated oven for 6 to 8 minutes. Slice and serve.
Yield: 8 servings

Approximate Per Serving:
Calories: 337
Fat: 6.3 g
Cholesterol: 68 mg
Carbohydrates: 29 g
Protein: 34 g
Sodium: 820 mg

Diabetic Exchanges: 4 meat; 1 1/2 bread

To keep frozen foods from sticking together in bags, freeze on cookie sheets in single layer until firm, then pack in freezer bags.

Grilled Fish on French Bread

(Recipe contains approximately 9% fat)

1 T. soy sauce	8 slices French bread,
2 T. white wine, can use	sliced very thin
chicken stock	3 T. no-fat, no-cholesterol
1 clove garlic, minced	mayonnaise
1/2 tsp. vinegar	1 tsp. dill pickle relish
2 (6 oz.) flounder fillets,	1/2 tsp. prepared mustard
halved	1 green onion, minced
	1/8 tsp. seasoned salt

Blend soy sauce, wine, garlic and vinegar and allow to stand for 30 minutes while flavors marinate. Brush mixture over fish fillets and grill in broiler (or on outside grill), basting often until fish flakes easily. Fish should take about 5 minutes on each side. While fish grills, toast French bread, then spread bread with a mixture of mayonnaise, relish, mustard, onion and seasoned salt. Place fillet on top of bread. If desired, top with lettuce and tomato slice; top with second slice of bread.
Yield: 4 servings

Approximate Per Serving:
Calories: 301
Fat: 2.9 g
Cholesterol: 40 mg
Carbohydrates: 32 g
Protein: 24 g
Sodium: 888 mg

Diabetic Exchanges: 3 meat; 2 bread

When a recipe calls for cilantro, Chinese parsley or coriander can be substituted - they are the same thing.

Jumbo Vienna Sandwich

(Recipe contains approximately 17% fat)

1 lb. turkey sausage	1/4 c. water
(see index)	1/4 tsp. oregano
1/2 lb. ground round	1/4 tsp. rosemary
1 c. chopped onion	1/2 tsp. dried cilantro
1/2 c. chopped green pepper	1 loaf Vienna bread
1 (8 oz.) can tomato sauce	1 (6 oz.) pkg. nonfat
1 (6 oz.) can tomato paste	American cheese slices

Brown sausage and ground round; drain off any rendered fat. Add onions and green pepper and cook 5 minutes. Stir in tomato sauce, tomato paste, water and seasonings. Blend and simmer 15 minutes, stirring occasionally. Cut a lengthwise slice from the top of bread. Scoop out center of bread to form a shell. Place half of cheese in shell. Fill with meat mixture and top with remaining cheese slices. Return top slice to loaf; wrap in foil, tightly. Bake in 400° preheated oven for 6 to 8 minutes. Slice and serve.
Yield: 8 servings

Approximate Per Serving:
Calories: 337
Fat: 6.3 g
Cholesterol: 68 mg
Carbohydrates: 29 g
Protein: 34 g
Sodium: 820 mg

Diabetic Exchanges: 4 meat; 1 1/2 bread

To keep frozen foods from sticking together in bags, freeze on cookie sheets in single layer until firm, then pack in freezer bags.

Maidrites

(Recipe contains approximately 18% fat)

1 lb. ground round	2 tsp. prepared yellow
1 lb. ground turkey breast	mustard
1 sm. onion, diced very fine	2 tsp. chili powder
1 clove garlic, minced	1/2 tsp. dried cilantro
1 tsp. seasoned salt (opt.)	(opt.)
1/4 tsp. pepper	10 reduced-calorie whole
1 (8 oz.) can tomato sauce	wheat buns

In a large skillet, brown ground round, turkey breast, onion, garlic, seasoned salt and pepper. Drain off any rendered fat. Add remaining ingredients except buns and simmer 15 minutes. Use a pastry blender (the type with several wires) to break ground meat into nice, even crumbled consistency. Serve on 10 low-cal hamburger buns.

Yield: 10 sandwiches

Approximate Per Sandwich (including reduced-cal. bun):
Calories: 274
Fat: 5.5 g
Cholesterol: 67 mg
Carbohydrates: 20 g
Protein: 33 g
Sodium: 499 mg

Diabetic Exchanges: 1 bread; 1 vegetable; 3 1/2 meat

*When you burn a pan, use 2 teaspoons cream
of tartar and 1 cup of water and bring to a boil in pan.*

Maid-Rites of Yesteryear
(These taste like the maid-rites you bought 50 years ago)
(Recipe contains approximately 17% fat)

3/4 lb. ground round
3/4 lb. ground turkey breast
1 can low-sodium chicken
   broth
1/4 tsp. pepper

8 reduced-calorie whole
   wheat buns
8 very thin slices of sweet
   onion
24 thin pickle slices

Put ground round and turkey breast in skillet and cook until pink disappears. Add chicken broth and simmer, uncovered, until liquid disappears. Divide meat among 8 buns. Top with onion slice and 3 pickle slices. Serve immediately.
Yield: 8 servings

Approximate Per Serving:
Calories: 261
Fat: 5.0 g
Cholesterol: 64 mg
Carbohydrates: 16 g
Protein: 28 g
Sodium: 599 mg

Diabetic Exchanges: 1 bread; 3 meat; 1 vegetable

*The first function of a good sauce is to
enhance flavor not mask a taste.*

Mermaids

(Recipe contains approximately 9% fat)

6 (6") French rolls
1 (7 oz.) can white tuna
(use the good white tuna
for this)
12 med. shrimp, cooked &
coarsely diced
1/4 c. chopped green pepper
1/4 c. chopped celery
2 green onions, sliced thin
6 pimento stuffed olives,
chopped

6 water chestnuts,
coarsely chopped
1 tsp. Worcestershire
sauce
1 to 2 drops Tabasco sauce
1/2 c. no-fat, no choles-
terol mayonnaise
6 slices no-fat American
cheese, diced coarsely
6 strips of pimento (for
garnish)

Slice off top of rolls and scoop out center of roll. (Scooped out bread can be used for bread crumbs). Put tuna, shrimp, green pepper, celery, onion, olives and water chestnuts in a bowl. Blend Worcestershire sauce and Tabasco sauce into mayonnaise and fold into tuna mixture. Spoon mixture into bread shells, piling up. Sprinkle with cheese. Top with strip of pimento. Place on cookie sheet and bake in 400° preheated oven until bread is crisp, 15 to 20 minutes.
Yield: 6 servings

Approximate Per Serving:
Calories: 230
Fat: 2.2 g
Cholesterol: 39 mg
Carbohydrates: 31 g
Protein: 19 g
Sodium: 643 mg

Diabetic Exchanges: 2 bread; 2 meat

Always refrigerate meat loosely covered as soon as possible.

Mock Pork Tenderloins

(Recipe contains approximately 13% fat)

6 (3 oz.) portions skinless
   turkey breast, pounded
   out to about the size of
   the palm of your hand
Egg substitute to equal
   2 eggs

1 1/2 c. fine cracker
   crumbs, prepared from
   unsalted top crackers
1 1/2 c. chicken stock, can
   use low-sodium canned
   chicken broth
6 reduced-calorie whole
   wheat buns

Remove all fat from turkey breast and pound out. Dredge in egg substitute and roll in cracker crumbs. Put on plate and refrigerate for at least an hour before cooking. This helps the breading to stay on. Put 1/4 cup stock in skillet and heat almost to boiling. Add breaded turkey breast and brown in stock; add more stock, a little at a time. Turn with pancake turner carefully so breading will not come off. When both sides are nicely browned put into 9x13-inch baking dish that has been sprayed with cooking spray. Add a couple of tablespoons of stock, cover with foil and bake in 350° preheated oven for about 30 minutes. Uncover and bake an additional 30 minutes or until breading is crisp. Turn, if desired, to crisp up bottom side
Yield: 6 servings

Approximate Per Serving:
Calories: 323
Fat: 4.8 g
Cholesterol: 71 mg
Carbohydrates: 26 g
Protein: 36 g
Sodium: 668 mg

Diabetic Exchanges: 1 bread; 3 meat; 1 milk

To substitute for one cup ketchup or chili sauce, blend one cup tomato sauce with 1/2 cup sugar and two tablespoons vinegar.

Mushroom Wine Burgers

(Recipe contains approximately 19% fat)

3/4 lb. ground round	1/2 c. beef stock
3/4 lb. ground turkey breast	1/2 c. red dinner wine (can
1/2 c. "lite" evaporated	use stock)
skim milk	1 tsp. Worcestershire
1 T. fresh minced onion	sauce
1 tsp. salt (opt.)	2 T. chopped parsley
1/4 tsp. pepper	1 (4 oz.) can sliced
1 frozen beef stock cube	mushrooms
1 tsp. tub margarine	8 slices French bread
2 T. flour	toasted

In a mixing bowl, combine ground round, ground turkey breast, evaporated milk, onion, salt and pepper. Toss lightly to blend well. Shape into patties. Melt stock cube and margarine in skillet and brown patties, just until both sides are browned. Remove from skillet with slotted spoon and set aside. Add flour to skillet. Stir in bouillon and wine. Cook until mixture bubbles, then add Worcestershire sauce, parsley and mushrooms along with mushroom liquid. Return patties to skillet. Simmer until patties are done. Place a patty on each slice of French bread and spoon sauce over top of patty.

Yield: 8 servings

Approximate Per Serving:
Calories: 293
Fat: 5.5 g
Cholesterol: 64 mg
Carbohydrates: 22 g
Protein: 30 g
Sodium: 558 mg

Diabetic Exchanges: 3 meat; 1 milk; 1/2 bread

Don't have a pizza cutter? Cut pizza with kitchen scissors.

Pineapple Hamburgers
(These are very good)
(Recipe contains approximate 16% fat)

3/4 lb. ground round
3/4 lb. ground turkey
1/4 c. ketchup
2 tsp. yellow mustard
1 T. brown sugar

1 tsp. Worcestershire
　sauce
2 T. pineapple juice
8 slices pineapple
8 reduced-calorie buns,
　toasted

In a mixing bowl, put ground round, ground turkey breast, ketchup, mustard, brown sugar, Worcestershire sauce and pineapple juice. Blend well. Form into 6 patties. Broil 5 to 8 minutes on each side. The last 3 minutes of broiling time on second side, place a pineapple slice on burger. Place broiled burger on bun and serve.

Yield: 8 servings

Approximate Per Serving:
Calories: 279
Fat: 5.1 g
Cholesterol: 63 mg
Carbohydrates: 24 g
Protein: 31 g
Sodium: 271: mg

Diabetic Exchanges: 3 meat; 1 bread; 1 milk

*Instead of purchasing a costly gourmet "mushroom brush,"
try an inexpensive soft toothbrush. Works great!*

Pizza Cups

(Recipe contains approximately 19% fat)

1/2 lb. ground round	1/4 tsp. sweet basil
1/2 lb. ground turkey breast	1/8 tsp. garlic powder
1 (6 oz.) can tomato paste	6 slices whole wheat bread,
1 tsp. Italian seasoning	cut into 12 rounds to fit
1/2 tsp. salt (opt.)	muffin tins
1/4 c. finely-chopped onion	1/2 c. part-skim mozzarella
1/4 c. finely-chopped green	cheese, shredded
pepper	

Brown ground round and ground turkey breast. Drain off all rendered fat (there really should not be any). Add tomato paste, Italian seasoning and salt. Blend. Remove from stove and add onion, green pepper, basil and garlic powder. Blend well. Spray a 12-cup muffin tin with cooking spray. Put a round of bread in bottom and spray bread lightly. Divide meat mixture among 12 muffin cups, then top with cheese. Bake in 400° oven for 12 minutes or until golden brown.
Yield: 12 pizza cups

Approximate Per Pizza:
Calories: 117
Fat: 2.5 g
Cholesterol: 28 mg
Carbohydrates: 7 g
Protein: 14 g
Sodium: 188 mg

Diabetic Exchanges: 1 1/2 meat; 1/2 bread

Use a pancake turner to slide sandwiches into sandwich bags.
This keeps sandwiches with soft fillings together.

Pizza on English Muffin

(Recipe contains approximately 15% fat)

1/2 lb. ground round, browned & all rendered fat removed
1/4 c. chopped onion
1/4 c. chopped green pepper
1/2 tsp. salt
6 English muffins, split
2 T. no-fat, no-cholesterol mayonnaise
1 (8 oz.) can tomato sauce
1 tsp. oregano
6 sm. mushrooms, sliced; or 1 (4 oz.) can sliced mushrooms
2 oz. lowfat, part skim mozzarella cheese
3 slices no-fat American cheese, diced

To browned meat, add onion, green pepper and salt. Stir to blend well. Spread mayonnaise thinly over split English muffins and place on large baking sheet. Mix tomato sauce and oregano and spread on English muffin halves, allowing about 1 tablespoon for each muffin half. Add meat mixture, top with sliced mushrooms. Mix mozzarella and diced American cheese and sprinkle over top of muffins. Bake in 350° preheated oven for about 15 minutes or until cheese melts and muffins start to brown.
Yield: 12 individual pizzas

Approximate Per Pizza:
Calories: 134
Fat: 2.2 g
Cholesterol: 16 mg
Carbohydrates: 17 g
Protein: 10 g
Sodium: 566 mg

Diabetic Exchanges (2 muffin pizza halves per serving):
1 bread; 1 meat

Slice English muffins in half before frezing. This saves work later and they thaw more quickly.

Quick Pizza Melt

(Recipe contains approximately 19% fat)

6 English muffins, split
1 (6 oz.) can tomato sauce
1/2 tsp. oregano
1/4 tsp. basil
1/4 tsp. garlic powder

6 very thin (1/2 oz.) slices
  Canadian bacon
2 oz. reduced-fat, part-
  skim mozzarella cheese

Blend tomato sauce, oregano, basil and garlic powder and spread on English muffins. Top with a thin slice of Canadian bacon and sprinkle with cheese. Put in toaster oven for 3 to 5 minutes.

Yield: 6 servings

Approximate Per Serving:
Calories: 223
Fat: 4.7 g
Cholesterol: 19 mg
Carbohydrates: 31 g
Protein: 14 g
Sodium: 1,031 mg

Diabetic Exchanges: 1 1/4 bread; 1/2 meat; 1 milk; 1/2 fat

Sloppy Joes

(Recipe contains approximately 17% fat)

1/2 lb. ground turkey breast
1/2 lb. ground round
1/2 c. chopped celery
1/2 c. chopped onion
1/4 c. finely-chopped
  green pepper (opt.)

1/2 tsp. seasoned salt
1/8 tsp. pepper
1 (8 oz.) can tomato sauce
6 reduced-calorie whole
  wheat hamburger buns

In a skillet sauté turkey breast, ground round, celery, onion and green pepper. When browned drain any rendered fat and return to stove. Add salt, pepper and tomato sauce. Simmer about 10 to 15 minutes. Spoon onto hamburger buns, allowing about 1/2 cup meat mixture per bun.

Yield: 6 servings

Approximate Per Serving:
Calories: 239
Fat: 4.6 g
Cholesterol: 56 mg
Carbohydrates: 18 g
Protein: 29 g
Sodium: 664 mg

Diabetic Exchanges: 3 meat; 1/2 vegetable; 1 bread

Stroganoff on French Bread

(Recipe contains approximately 17% fat)

1 lb. ground round
1 c. dry-style cottage
  cheese, lowfat
1 T. lemon juice
1/4 tsp. garlic powder
1/2 tsp. seasoned salt
  (opt.)
1 tsp. Worcestershire
  sauce
1/4 c. chopped green onion,
  including green tops

1 loaf French bread,
  unsliced
Cooking spray (use
  good grade)
2 tomatoes, sliced thin
1 green pepper, cut in
  thin rings
10 slices no-fat American
  cheese

In a skillet, cook ground round until pink disappears. Drain off any rendered fat. In a blender, process cottage cheese, lemon juice, garlic powder, seasoned salt and Worcestershire sauce. Blend until smooth. Add green onion and blend. Add to meat mixture, heating through, but not boiling. Cut French loaf in half lengthwise and place cut-side-up on cookie sheet. Spray bread with vegetable spray and put under broiler for 3 to 5 minutes or until lightly toasted. Remove from oven and spread half of mixture on each side of bread. Top with tomato slices, then green pepper. Lay cheese slices on top of green pepper. Broil 2 to 3 minutes longer. Cut in slices and serve.
Yield: 8 servings

Approximate Per Serving:
Calories: 345
Fat: 6.7 g
Cholesterol: 48 mg
Carbohydrates: 37 g
Protein: 32 g
Sodium: 1,023 mg

Diabetic Exchanges: 1 1/2 bread; 1 vegetable; 3 meat; 1 milk

*Use muffin tins sprayed with vegetable oil as
molds when baking stuffed peppers.*

Taco Bean Burgers
(Delicious)
(Recipe contains approximately 5% fat)

1 (16 oz.) can red kidney
  beans, drained & mashed
1 (16 oz.) can Great
  Northern beans, drained
  (reserve juice) & mashed
1/4 c. onion, minced

2 T. green pepper, chopped
  very fine
1 frozen beef stock cube
  (see index)
1 pkg. dry taco mix
4 English muffins, split
4 slices cheese, diced

Put onion and green pepper in skillet with stock cube and sauté until vegetables are soft. Add mashed beans and stir in juice. Add taco mix and simmer for about 15 minutes or until most of liquid has been absorbed. Water can be added during cooking, if needed. Divide mixture among 8 muffin halves. Sprinkle with cheese. Bake in toaster oven 10 to 15 minutes or until heated through.
Yield: 8 servings

Approximate Per Muffin Half:
Calories: 220
Fat: 1.2 g
Cholesterol: 3 mg
Carbohydrates: 37 g
Protein: 11 g
Sodium: 415 mg

Diabetic Exchanges: 1 bread; 1 milk; 2 vegetable; 1/4 fat

Chill lowfat cheese to grate it easier.

Tacos

(Recipe contains approximately 27% fat)

1/2 lb. ground turkey breast	1 c. tomatoes, diced
1/2 lb. ground round	1/2 c. chopped onion
1 pkg. taco seasoning mix	1/2 c. chopped green
3/4 c. water	pepper
12 taco shells	6 slices no-fat American
1 c. shredded lettuce	cheese, sliced

Over medium heat, cook ground turkey breast and ground round. When meat is browned, drain off any rendered fat (there really should not be any). Add taco seasoning mix and water. Simmer 10 to 15 minutes or until thickened. Warm taco shells in oven according to package directions. On each taco shell spoon 3 tablespoonfuls of meat mixture and top with lettuce, tomatoes, onion, green pepper and cheese. Fold.
Yield: 12 tacos

Approximate Per Taco:
Calories: 254
Fat: 7.6 g
Cholesterol: 31 mg
Carbohydrates: 24 g
Protein: 17 g
Sodium: 245 mg

Diabetic Exchanges (2 tacos per serving): 1 meat; 1 bread; 1 fat; 1 milk

Store cottage cheese cartons upside down.
The cottage cheese will keep twice as long.

Sweet Hamburger Relish

(Recipe contains approximately 15% fat)

4 c. ground cucumber,
    peeled
1 lg. onion
1 lg. green pepper
1/2 lg. red pepper
2 T. salt or salt substitute
1 c. vinegar

1/2 tsp. mustard seed
1/2 tsp. celery seeds
1/2 tsp. parsley flakes
1/2 tsp. turmeric
24 pkt. Equal sweetener,
    or sweetener of choice to
    equal 1 cup sugar

Grind cucumbers, onion, green pepper and red pepper. Stir in salt. Put in refrigerator overnight. Next day, drain and set aside. In a saucepan, put vinegar, mustard seeds, celery seeds, parsley flakes and turmeric. Bring to a boil and boil for 10 minutes. Remove from heat and add ground vegetables. Cook for 20 minutes. Remove from heat. Add sugar replacement. Put mixture in refrigerator for 24 hours. Drain if too much liquid accumulates. Pack in scalded jars; seal.
Yield: 2 1/2 pints

Approximate Per Tablespoon:
Calories: 6
Fat: 0.3 g
Cholesterol: 0.0 mg
Carbohydrates: 1 g
Protein: Tr. g
Sodium: 61 mg

Diabetic Exchanges: Free food in very limited amounts

When buying cucumbers, choose long slender green ones.
Cucumbers with yellow on them are undesirable.

Vegetable-Oven Burgers

(Recipe contains approximately 18% fat)

1 lb. loaf frozen bread
    dough, low fat, thawed
1 lb. ground round
1 sm. head cabbage,
    shredded

1 carrot, shredded
1 lg. onion, chopped fine
1/2 tsp. seasoned salt
1/8 tsp. pepper

Put ground round in skillet and brown. Add cabbage, carrot and onion; cook until tender. Stir in seasoned salt and pepper. Pour mixture in strainer and strain, pushing down on mixture to remove any excess fat and liquid. Divide dough into 8 pieces. Roll each piece into 6-inch circle. Place 1/8 of meat mixture in center of circle. Bring bread up over meat and pinch together to form a ball-like shape. Place on baking sheet, seam-side down. Allow to rise 20 minutes. Bake in 350° preheated oven for 20 minutes or until light brown. Remove from oven and place on serving platter covered with white linen napkin (these sometimes ooze a little). Serve immediately.
Yield: 8 servings

Approximate Per Serving:
Calories: 269
Fat: 5.5 g
Cholesterol: 40 mg
Carbohydrates: 30 g
Protein: 23 g
Sodium: 352 mg

Diabetic Exchanges: 1 1/2 bread; 2 meat; 2 vegetable

*When buying peas and lima beans select pods
that are well-filled but not bulging.*

Vegetable-Pasta Patties

(Recipe contains approximately 7% fat)

1 c. cooked macaroni,
chopped fine
Egg substitute to equal
2 eggs
4 slices no-fat American
cheese, diced
1 c. red kidney beans,
chopped fine
1/4 c. finely-shredded
carrots

1 green onion, chopped
fine
1/4 c. enriched all-purpose
flour
1 T. skim milk
1/4 tsp. salt
1/4 tsp. garlic powder
1 tsp. canola oil

In a large mixing bowl, put macaroni, egg substitute, cheese, beans, carrots and onion. Blend well. Add flour, milk, salt and garlic powder; blend. Form into 4 patties. Put oil in skillet and heat. Brown patties in skillet over medium heat until nicely browned on each side.
Yield: 6 servings

Approximate Per Serving:
Calories: 145
Fat. 1.2 g
Cholesterol: 3 mg
Carbohydrates: 21 g
Protein: 10 g
Sodium: 4.3 mg

Diabetic Exchanges: 1 bread; 1 vegetable; 1 meat

*To rid cutting board of onion, garlic or fish smell, cut a
lime in half and rub the surface with cut side of lime.*

Potatoe Entrées

Broccoli Stuffed Potatoes
(Recipe contains approximately 2% fat)

3 lg. unpeeled baking
  potatoes
1 c. fresh broccoli flowerets,
  chopped (can use frozen)

1/2 c. commercial reduced-
  calorie Italian dressing
  (oil-free is best)

Bake potato in 400° oven for 1 hour or until done.* Cool slightly. Cut potato in half lengthwise and scoop out pulp leaving shell to serve as bowl. Mash scooped out potato and set aside, keeping warm. Steam broccoli or boil in small amount of water until crisp-tender, 3 to 5 minutes. Add steamed broccoli to potato and toss lightly. Stuff mixture into potato shells. Drizzle with Italian dressing. If desired, add a little salt and pepper.
Yield: 6 servings

Approximate Per Serving:
Calories: 76
Fat: 0.2 g
Cholesterol: 0.0 mg
Carbohydrates: 17 g
Protein: 3 g
Sodium: 200 mg

Diabetic Exchanges: 1 bread

*If a little salt is rubbed into skin before baking the potato, shell will be much stronger. This should not be done if potato skin is to be consumed.

*One fresh clove of garlic can be replaced with
1 tsp. garlic salt or 1/8 tsp. garlic powder.*

Cheese and Chili Pepper Stuffed Potato

(Recipe contains approximately 9% fat)

4 lg. baking potatoes
1/4 c. skim milk
1/2 tsp. salt (opt.)
Dash of pepper
2 oz. shredded part-skim
    Cheddar cheese

8 slices no-fat American
    cheese, diced
2 T. canned, chopped green
    chilies (more if desired)
2 egg whites

Bake potatoes in 400° oven for 1 hour or until done. Cut potatoes in half lengthwise and put potato pulp in bowl, leaving shells. Add milk, salt and pepper; beat until smooth with no lumps. Stir in Cheddar cheese, American cheese and green chilies. Blend well. Set aside.

Beat egg whites at high speed until soft peaks form. Fold into potato mixture. Fill shells; place on cookie sheet. Bake in 375° preheated oven for 20 to 25 minutes.

Yield: 8 servings

Approximate Per Serving:
Calories: 136
Fat: 1.3 g
Cholesterol: 9 mg
Carbohydrates: 19 g
Protein: 10 g
Sodium: 508 mg

Diabetic Exchange: 1 meat; 1 bread; 1/4 milk

*Three-fourths cup tomato paste plus one cup of
water will substitute for 2 cups tomato sauce.*

Chicken Filled Potatoes

(Recipe contains approximately 11% fat)

4 lg. baking potatoes	2 green onions, sliced thin
2 cans white meat of chicken, drained	2 T. chopped green pepper
	1/2 tsp. seasoned salt
3 slices no-fat American cheese, diced	1/8 tsp. pepper
	1/4 c. no-fat, no cholesterol mayonnaise
1 c. frozen peas	

Bake potatoes in 400° oven for 1 hour or until done. Split potatoes lengthwise and scoop out pulp. Mash potatoes slightly with fork. Add cheese, peas, onions, green pepper, and toss to blend. Put seasoned salt and pepper in mayonnaise and pour over potato mixture. Toss to blend. Fill shells; place on cookie sheet and put back into oven (350°) for 10 to 20 minutes.

Yield: 8 servings

Approximate Per Serving:
Calories: 127
Fat: 1.6 g
Cholesterol: 2 mg
Carbohydrates: 19 g
Protein: 8
Sodium: 518 mg

Diabetic Exchanges: 1 meat; 1 bread; 1 vegetable

One eighth to one fourth teaspoon garlic powder equals one clove garlic.

Chili Stuffed Potatoes

(Recipe contains approximately 14% fat)

4 lg. baking potatoes
1/2 lb. ground turkey breast
1/2 lb. ground round
1/4 c. chopped onions
1/4 c. chopped green
   pepper
1 clove garlic, minced
1 c. seeded, chopped
   tomatoes (no juice,
   low-sodium)

1 c. dark red kidney beans,
   drained
1/2 c. tomato sauce
1/4 c. water
2 to 3 tsp. chili powder
1/2 tsp. ground cumin
1/2 tsp. seasoned salt
Dash of pepper

Bake potatoes in a 400° preheated oven for 1 hour or until tender. Brown ground turkey and ground round with onions, green pepper and garlic. Add remaining ingredients, except potato, and simmer for 5 to 10 minutes. Cut potatoes in half lengthwise and fluff potato pulp with a fork. Top with chili mixture.

Yield: 8 servings

Approximate Per Serving:
Calories: 199
Fat: 3.0 g
Cholesterol: 42 mg
Carbohydrates: 22 g
Protein: 22 g
Sodium: 133 mg

Diabetic Exchanges: 2 1/2 meat; 1 bread; 1 vegetable

One cup uncooked macaroni equals 2 1/2 cups cooked.

Shrimp Stuffed Potatoes

(Recipe contains approximately 4% fat)

4 lg. potatoes
1 frozen chicken stock
   cube, thawed
2 green onions, sliced
1/4 c. chopped green
   pepper
1 (16 oz.) pkg. cooked,
   frozen shrimp, thawed

1/4 c. no-fat, no choles-
   terol mayonnaise
1/2 tsp. seasoned salt
1/8 tsp. pepper
8 slices no-fat American
   cheese, diced
1/4 c. chopped parsley,
   can use dried

Bake potatoes in a 400° preheated oven for 1 hour or until done. Put stock cube in skillet and melt. Sauté onion and green pepper. Add shrimp and sauté another minute. Split potatoes lengthwise and put pulp in bowl, being sure to leave skins in tact. Fluff potatoes and add shrimp mixture. Add mayonnaise, salt and pepper. Add half of cheese. Fill potato shells and sprinkle tops with remaining cheese and parsley. Place on baking sheet and broil under broiler for 2 minutes or until cheese melts.
Yield: 8 servings

Approximate Per Serving:
Calories: 179
Fat: 0.8 g
Cholesterol: 92 mg
Carbohydrates: 19 g
Protein: 21 g
Sodium: 743 mg

Diabetic Exchanges: 1 bread; 2 meat; 1 vegetable

One medium onion equals 1/2 cup chopped.

Taco Stuffed Potatoes

(Recipe contains approximately 11% fat)

4 lg. baking potatoes	3/4 c. water
1/2 lb. turkey breast	1 can dark red kidney
1/2 lb. ground round	beans, drained
1/4 c. chopped onion	1 tomato, seeded &
1/4 c. chopped green	chopped
pepper	1 c. shredded lettuce
1 pkg. taco seasoning	4 slices no-fat American
mix	cheese, diced

Bake potatoes in 400° oven for 1 hour or until done. Cut potatoes in half lengthwise. Mash pulp slightly, leaving in shell. Sprinkle with a little salt and pepper, if desired. In a skillet, brown turkey breast, ground round, onion and green pepper. Drain off any rendered fat. Add taco mix and water. Stir well and simmer 10 to 15 minutes. Add red beans and heat through. Top potatoes with this mixture. Garnish with tomato, lettuce and cheese.
Yield: 8 servings

Approximate Per Serving:
Calories: 254
Fat: 3.2 g
Cholesterol: 45 mg
Carbohydrates: 27 g
Protein: 26 g
Sodium: 263 mg

Diabetic Exchanges: 3 meat; 1 1/2 bread; 1 vegetable

Save your next empty salt box to store homemade bread crumbs.
Fill with funnel and shake out of spout as needed.

Lunch Entrees

Busy Day Casserole

(Recipe contains approximately 17% fat)

6 med. red potatoes,
  peeled & sliced thin
1 lb. ground round (ground
  meat must be very lean)

1 med. onion, sliced very
  thin
1 can red kidney beans,
  drained
1 can tomato soup

Put thin sliced potatoes in 7 1/2 x 11-inch shallow baking dish that has been sprayed with cooking spray. Crumble ground round evenly over potatoes and top with onion slices. Sprinkle beans over top, then spread undiluted tomato soup over top of casserole. Cover and bake 1 hour and 30 minutes or until potatoes are done, in a 375° preheated oven.
Yield: 8 servings

Approximately Per Serving:
Calories: 246
Fat: 4.6 g
Cholesterol: 40 mg
Carbohydrates: 28 g
Protein: 22 g
Sodium: 286 mg

Diabetic Exchanges: 2 bread; 2 meat

Poultry is truly a cosmopolitan food. There are unlimited ways in which it can be prepared. Acquaint yourself with some of them.

Chicken Patties with Cranberry Sauce

(Recipe contains approximately 15% fat)

2 c. cooked chicken, diced fine
Egg substitute to equal
   2 eggs
2 c. fresh bread crumbs,
   use reduced-calorie bread

2 T. fresh onion, minced
1 tsp. tub margarine, melted
1 frozen stock cube,
   melted (see index)
1 c. whole cranberry sauce

In a mixing bowl, put chicken, egg substitute, crumbs and onion. Form into 4 patties. Place on broiler tray and broil. Mix margarine and stock cube; brush patties as they brown. Stir canned cranberry sauce and serve with patties.

Yields: 4 servings

Approximate Per Serving:
Calories: 312
Fat: 5.1 g
Cholesterol: 60 mg
Carbohydrates: 41 g
Protein: 25 g
Sodium: 251 mg

Diabetic Exchanges: 2 meat; 2 bread; 1 milk

A teaspoon of dry mustard can be replaced with a tablespoon of prepared mustard.

Crispy Italian Chicken Breasts

(Recipe contains approximately 23% fat)

6 (3 oz.) skinless, boneless
  chicken breast fillets
1/2 c. oil-free Italian salad
  dressing

1/2 tsp. salt (opt.)
1/4 tsp. pepper
1 1/2 c. cornflake crumbs

Mix oil-free Italian salad dressing, salt and pepper. Marinate chicken breast fillets in mixture for at least 1 hour, turning several times. Remove chicken from marinade and coat with cornflake crumbs, pressing firmly to make crumbs stick. Place on a cooking sheet that has been sprayed with cooking spray. Bake, uncovered, in a 400° preheated oven for about 35 minutes or until chicken is golden brown.
Yield: 6 servings

Approximate Per Serving:
Calories: 178
Fat: 4.6 g
Cholesterol: 66 mg
Carbohydrates: 5 g
Protein: 22 g
Sodium: 390 mg

Diabetic Exchanges: 3 meat; 1/4 bread

*Wrap onions individually in foil to keep them
from becoming soft or sprouting.*

Easiest Ever Goulash

(Recipe contains approximately 12% fat)

1/2 lb. ground round	1/2 tsp. seasoned salt
1/2 lb. ground turkey breast	1/2 tsp. garlic powder
2 c. tomato juice	1/4 tsp. pepper
1 c. water	1 tsp. chili powder
2 c. macaroni, uncooked	1 (8 oz.) can tomato sauce
1 T. sugar	

Mix ground round and turkey together and put in deep skillet. Brown; drain off any rendered fat. Add remaining ingredients. Bring to boil; boil 10 to 15 minutes or until macaroni is done. Stir occasionally while cooking.
Yield: 6 servings

Approximate Per Serving:
Calories: 324
Fat: 4.3 g
Cholesterol: 56 mg
Carbohydrates: 41 g
Protein: 30 g
Sodium: 1,152 mg

Diabetic Exchanges: 3 meat; 2 bread; 1 milk

When extra counter space is needed, pull out a cabinet drawer and place a pastry board or tray across it.

One cup uncooked noodles equals one cooked.

Ham and Asparagus Bake

(Recipe contains approximately 22% fat)

2/3 c. "lite" evaporated skim milk	1/4 c. finely-chopped onion
2 c. cubed, cooked ham, lean only	2 med. fresh mushrooms, diced
2 c. cooked brown rice	1 (10 oz.) pkg. frozen asparagus spears
8 slices nonfat American cheese, diced	1/2 c. corn flakes
1 recipe cream soup substitute, prepared (see index)	Cooking spray

Add enough water to evaporated milk to make 3/4 cup. In a mixing bowl, combine ham, rice, cheese, soup substitute and onion. Stir in chopped mushrooms. Put asparagus spears in mixing bowl and cover with boiling water to enable separation. Drain and set aside. Put half of ham mixture into 7x11-inch baking dish that has been sprayed with cooking spray. Top with asparagus spears, then add remaining layer of ham mixture. Crush corn flakes and sprinkle over top. Spray with cooking spray. Bake in 375° preheated oven for 25 to 50 minutes or until heated through and lightly browned.

Yield: 4 servings

Approximate Per Serving:
Calories: 252
Fat: 6.2 g
Cholesterol: 30 mg
Carbohydrates: 24 g
Protein: 13 g
Sodium: 994 mg

Diabetic Exchanges: 1 meat; 1 milk; 1 bread; 1 fat

*To keep skewers from scattering throughout the drawer,
store them in plastic toothbrush containers.*

Lowfat Ham, Cheese and Macaroni

(Recipe contains approximately 9% fat)

3 c. cooked macaroni
1 tsp. tub margarine
2 c. skim milk
1/2 tsp. seasoned salt
1/8 tsp. pepper

1/2 c. ham, cut into very small cubes (use lean only)
1 (12 slice) pkg. no-fat American cheese, diced
Egg substitute to equal 3 eggs

Stir margarine in hot drained macaroni to coat. Add remaining ingredients and pour into baking dish that has been sprayed with cooking spray. Bake in 325° preheated oven for 1 hour. Allow to stand 10 minutes before serving.
Yield: 6 servings

Approximate Per Serving:
Calories: 250
Fat: 2.4 g
Cholesterol: 21 mg
Carbohydrates: 32 g
Protein: 18 g
Sodium: 1,269 mg

Diabetic Exchanges: 1 1/2 bread; 1 milk; 1 meat; 1/2 fat

If a lemon is a little dried up, put it in boiling water for five minutes. It will yield more juice.

Luncheon Salmon Salad

(Recipe contains approximately 18% fat)

1 sm. can salmon, drained
  (reserve 1 T. liquid)
1 c. cooked brown rice
1/2 c. celery chopped
1/2 c. green pepper,
  chopped
2 green onions, chopped

1 T. dill relish
1/2 tsp. seasoned salt
  (opt.)
1/3 c. no-fat, no choles-
  terol mayonnaise
1 T. salmon liquid
1 tsp. lemon juice

Remove skin from salmon. Flake salmon meat and mash salmon bones. Blend together. Put salmon in mixing bowl and add rice, celery, green pepper, onions and dill relish. Toss to blend. Blend seasoned salt, mayonnaise, salmon liquid and lemon juice. Pour over salmon mixture and blend. Chill. Serve on saltines.

Yield: 6 servings

Approximate Per Serving With Six Saltine Crackers:
Calories: 110
Fat: 2.2 g
Cholesterol: 11 mg
Carbohydrates: 13 g
Protein: 7 g
Sodium: 495 mg

Diabetic Exchanges: 1 meat; 1/2 bread; 1 vegetable

*All meat is more tender and juicy if
cooked at lower temperatures.*

Mining Town Pasties
(This was a popular food in the
mining towns of yesteryear)
(Recipe contains approximately 17% fat)

1 loaf whole wheat (or
   white) frozen bread dough,
   thawed
1 lb. ground round
3 lg. red potatoes, peeled
   & diced

1 onion, chopped fine
1 carrot, grated
1 tsp. salt (opt.)
1/4 tsp. pepper

In a mixing bowl, blend ground round, potatoes, onion, carrot, salt and pepper. Divide dough into sixths and roll into circles. Divide mixture among 6 bread circles, mounding mixture on 1/2 of circle and leaving a half-inch border. Moisten border and fold circle of bread over meat mixture, pinching to seal. After sealing, press down on edge of half circle with fork to make decorative pattern. Place on baking sheet that has been lightly sprayed with cooking spray. Prick the top with fork and bake in 375° preheated oven for 45 minutes or until nicely browned.
Yield: 6 servings

Approximate Per Serving:
Calories: 396
Fat: 7.3 g
Cholesterol: 53 mg
Carbohydrates: 48 g
Protein: 32 g
Sodium: 639 mg

Diabetic Exchanges: 2 bread; 1 milk; 1 vegetable; 2 meat; 1/2 fat

If a cracked dish is boiled for 45 minutes in sweet milk, the crack will be so welded together that it will hardly be visible and will be so strong it will stand the same usage as before.

Old-Fashioned Goulash From Yesteryear

(Recipe contains approximately 18% fat)

1 lb. ground round
1 onion, chopped
1 (16 oz.) can tomatoes
1 (16 oz.) can cream-style
  corn
1 (16 oz.) can red kidney
  beans
1/2 tsp. salt (opt.)
1/8 tsp. pepper

Brown ground round and onion until pink disappears from meat. Drain off any rendered fat. Add remaining ingredients; blend. Simmer 20 to 30 minutes.
Yield: 6 servings

Approximate Per Serving:
Calories: 300
Fat: 6.0 g
Cholesterol: 53 mg
Carbohydrates: 34 g
Protein: 28 g
Sodium: 244 mg

Diabetic Exchanges: 2 bread; 1 vegetable; 2 1/2 meat

Oven Baked Chicken Hash

(Recipe contains approximately 13% fat)

2 c. diced, peeled, boiled
  potatoes
2 c. cooked & cubed chicken
  breast, skin & fat removed
1 c. evaporated skim milk
1 T. grated onion
1 tsp. salt (opt.)
1/4 tsp. pepper

Combine all ingredients and pour into a 9x9-inch baking dish that has been sprayed with cooking spray. Bake 20 minutes or until bubbling hot.
Yield: 4 servings

Approximate Per Serving:
Calories: 199
Fat: 2.9 g
Cholesterol: 62 mg
Carbohydrates: 19 g
Protein: 27 g
Sodium: 615 mg

Diabetic Exchanges: 1/2 bread; 2 meat; 1 milk

Turkey Porcupines

(Recipe contains approximately 11% fat)

1 med. onion, chopped
   fine
1/2 green pepper, chopped
   fine
1 frozen chicken stock
   cube, for sautéing
   (see index)
1/2 c. uncooked brown rice

1/2 tsp. salt (opt.)
1/8 tsp. pepper
Egg substitute to equal
   1 egg
2 c. leftover cooked turkey
   breast, ground
1 can tomato soup

Sauté onion and green pepper in stock. Add rice and toss around to coat. Remove from stove and pour into a mixing bowl. Add salt, pepper and egg substitute. Blend well, then add ground turkey breast. Form into 12 balls and place in a shallow casserole that has been sprayed with vegetable oil. Pour tomato soup over turkey balls and bake in a 350° preheated oven for 1 1/2 hours, basting 2 or 3 times during cooking.
Yield: 6 servings

Approximate Per Serving:
Calories: 190
Fat: 2.3 g
Cholesterol: 37 mg
Carbohydrates: 21 g
Protein: 18 g
Sodium: 756 mg

Diabetic Exchanges: 1 bread; 1 vegetable; 2 meat

Notes & Recipes

Ethnic
Foods

Ethnic Food

Learning to Prepare Your Own Ethnic Food

Ethnic foods are becoming more and more popular. Italian, Chinese and Mexican restaurants can be found all over the country. Many people, when they want a good ethnic meal, dine out at an ethnic restaurant. However, this is not necessary. Whether it be Italian, Chinese or Mexican food that is desired, it can all be prepared very successfully in the home. Another nice thing about preparing it yourself is the control you gain over the ingredients used. Try some of the ethnic food in this chapter. You'll be surprised how much fun they are to prepare.

A little vinegar rubbed on meat will help to tenderize the meat.

Chinese, Italian & Mexican

Chinese

Chinese Chicken
(Recipe contains approximately 17% fat)

1 1/2 lb. boneless, skinless
  chicken breasts, all
  visible fat removed
1 tsp. ginger
2 tsp. sugar
1 T. cornstarch
3 T. water
3 T. reduced-sodium soy
  sauce

1/3 c. cooking sherry (can
  use chicken stock)
1 T. canola oil
2 (6 oz.) pkg. Chinese pea
  pods
1 can water chestnuts,
  sliced (opt.)
4 c. cooked brown rice

Cut chicken breasts into 1/2-inch cubes; set aside. In a bowl, put ginger, sugar and cornstarch. Blend water, soy sauce and cooking sherry; add to cornstarch mixture, blending until smooth. Set aside. Heat oil in wok or iron skillet. Add chicken and cook until done (this only takes a few minutes). Add soy mixture and cook until mixture thickens. Add pea pods and water chestnuts; cook until heated through. Serve over 1/2 cup brown rice.
Yield: 8 servings

Approximate Per Serving:
Calories: 309
Fat: 6.0 g
Cholesterol: 58 mg
Carbohydrates: 32 g
Protein: 28 g
Sodium: 317 mg

Diabetic Exchanges: 3 meat; 2 bread; 1 vegetable

Chinese Pepper Steak

(Recipe contains approximately 23% fat)

1 lb. round steak, slightly
   frozen & sliced across
   the grain into very thin
   slices
1 T. cornstarch
1/4 tsp. fresh ground ginger
1/4 c. low-sodium soy sauce
1 T. canola oil

3 med. green peppers, cut
   into strips
1 sm. onion, chopped fine
1 clove garlic, minced
1/2 c. water
2 lg. tomatoes, cut into
   wedges
2 c. cooked brown rice

In a small bowl, combine cornstarch and ginger. Add soy sauce and stir to blend. Put thin-sliced meat into mixing bowl and mix well with fingers to coat meat well. Over medium heat, heat oil in wok or heavy iron skillet. Add beef to hot oil and stir until meat is brown. Remove beef from wok with slotted spoon. Reduce heat and add peppers, onion, garlic and water. Cook 5 minutes, then return meat to pan and add tomatoes. Heat through. Serve over 1/2 cup brown rice per serving.
Yield: 4 servings

Approximately Per Serving Over Rice:
Calories 287
Fat: 7.2 g
Cholesterol: 60 mg
Carbohydrates: 15 g
Protein: 29 g
Sodium: 770 mg

Diabetic Exchanges: 3 meat; 1 vegetable; 1 milk

*Ginger: To use fresh, clean carefully scraping the skin
before using. Then chop, mince, slice or grate as needed.*

Chop Suey

(Recipe contains approximately 21% fat)

1/2 lb. ground round
1/2 lb. ground turkey breast
1/2 med. onion, chopped
2 stalks celery, chopped
1/2 tsp. salt (opt.)
1/2 tsp. pepper
1 c. hot water

1 can fancy mixed Chinese
   vegetables (can use
   bean sprouts)
1/2 c. cold water
2 T. cornstarch
2 tsp. low-sodium soy
   sauce
1 tsp. sugar
2 c. cooked brown rice

Brown ground round and turkey in skillet until pink disappears. Drain any rendered fat. Add onion and celery and cook 3 to 4 minutes. Add salt and pepper. Add hot water, Chinese vegetables, and cook until warmed through. Combine water and cornstarch, stirring until smooth. Add soy sauce and sugar and stir until sugar partially dissolves. Pour mixture over skillet mixture and simmer 30 to 40 minutes. Serve over brown rice.
Yield: 6 servings

Approximate Per Serving Over 1/2 Cup Brown Rice:
Calories: 154
Fat: 3.6 g
Cholesterol: 56 mg
Carbohydrates: 5 g
Protein: 24 g
Sodium: 314 mg

Diabetic Exchanges: 3 meat; 1 vegetable

*Once you have enjoyed broiled fish you will
wonder why you liked it so well fried.*

Oriental Chicken Salad

(Recipe contains approximately 18% fat)

2 c. cooked chicken
  breast, diced (skin &
  fat removed)
1/4 c. reduced-sodium soy
  sauce
1 tsp. sugar or equivalent
  sweetener

1 T. canola oil
2 1/2 c. cooked brown rice
1 c. chopped celery
1/2 c. sliced green onions
1/4 c. finely-chopped green
  pepper
1 can Chinese vegetables

Put chicken breasts in mixing bowl. Blend soy sauce, sugar and oil. Pour over chicken, tossing to coat. Refrigerate for 1 hour while chicken marinates. Add remaining ingredients and chill until time to serve.
Yield: 4 servings

Approximate Per Serving:
Calories: 332
Fat: 6.6 g
Cholesterol: 60 mg
Carbohydrates: 41 g
Protein: 27 g
Sodium: 729 mg

Diabetic Exchanges: 1 1/2 bread; 1 vegetable; 1 milk; 2 meat

To quickly loosen burned food in a casserole dish, add boiling water to which a tablespoon of soda has been dissolved.

Oriental Pork Fried Rice

(Recipe contains approximately 21% fat)

1 frozen chicken stock
  cube (see index)
1 tsp. canola oil
1/2 c. chopped onion
1 clove garlic, minced
1/2 lb. pork tenderloin, all
  visible fat removed &
  cut into very small pieces
1 c. chopped green onion
  (use part of green)

4 c. cooked brown rice
1/3 c. low-sodium soy
  sauce
1 tsp. sugar
1 tsp. chopped fresh ginger
  (can use 1/2 tsp. ground
  ginger)
Egg substitute to equal 2
  eggs, scrambled &
  chopped up fine

Melt stock cube and add oil. Stir to blend. Sauté onion, garlic and pork until tenderloin is done. This just takes a few minutes. Add green onion and rice and cook another 5 minutes. Blend soy sauce, sugar and ginger; stir into rice mixture. Add scrambled egg substitute, lifting and turning to distribute evenly.
Yield: 6 servings

Approximate Per Serving:
Calories: 307
Fat: 7.2 g
Cholesterol: 33 mg
Carbohydrates: 38 g
Protein: 19 g
Sodium: 637 mg

Diabetic Exchanges: 1 1/2 meat; 2 bread; 1 vegetable; 1 fat

One bunch celery equals 4 1/2 cups chopped.

Shrimp Egg Foo Yong

(Recipe contains approximately 22% fat)

Egg substitute to equal
6 eggs
1/2 tsp. salt
1/2 c. cooked shrimp,
diced
1/4 c. finely-chopped
celery

1 c. bean sprouts
1/4 c. finely-chopped
water chestnuts
4 med., fresh mushrooms,
sliced thin
2 tsp. canola oil

SAUCE:
1 T. cornstarch
1 tsp. low-sodium soy
sauce

1/2 c. beef broth

Prepare egg substitute and add salt, shrimp, celery, beans sprouts, water chestnuts and mushrooms. Heat 1/2 teaspoon oil in skillet and add one-fourth of mixture. Cook over medium heat, browning on both sides. Repeat procedure, using 1/2 teaspoon oil for each batch. Prepare sauce by putting beef broth, soy sauce and cornstarch in pan. Stir until smooth, then cook over medium heat until sauce thickens. Serve over hot egg foo yong.
Yield: 4 servings

Approximate Per Serving:
Calories: 172
Fat: 4.2 g
Cholesterol: 46 mg
Carbohydrates: 6 g
Protein: 14 g
Sodium: 648 mg

Diabetic Exchanges: 2 meat; 1 vegetable; 1 fat

One cup uncooked rice equals 3 cups cooked.

Italian

Cheesy Manicotti

(Recipe contains approximately 21% fat)

1/2 lb. ground round	1 (28 oz.) can tomatoes,
1/2 lb. ground turkey breast	cut into pieces
1 med. onion, chopped	1/2 c. fresh parsley, chopped fine
1/4 med. green pepper,	1/2 tsp. oregano (more
chopped fine	if desired)
1 clove garlic, minced	1/2 tsp. basil
1 (12 oz.) can tomato paste	1/2 tsp. seasoned salt
1 (8 oz.) can tomato sauce	1/4 tsp. pepper

Brown ground round, turkey breast, onion, green pepper and garlic until pink disappears from meat. Pour off any rendered grease. Add remaining ingredients and simmer for 30 minutes over low heat.

CHEESE FILLING:

1 (16 oz.) ctn. ricotta cheese	1/2 c. grated Parmesan cheese
4 oz. mozzarella cheese,	Egg substitute to equal 2 eggs
shredded	2 T. fresh parsley, chopped fine
6 slices no-fat American	1/4 tsp. pepper
cheese, diced	16 uncooked manicotti shells

Blend ricotta, mozzarella, American and Parmesan cheeses. Add egg substitute, parsley and pepper. Blend well. Fill uncooked manicotti shells, using small spatula, knife or little finger to push filling into shell. Pour half of sauce into 9x13-inch baking dish and lay shells on top of filling. Pour remaining sauce over shells.

To Bake in Oven: Cover with foil and bake in 350° oven for about 1 hour. Baste several times during cooking.

To Bake in Microwave: Cover with plastic wrap and bake on HIGH power for 10 minutes. Turn shells, baste, cover and microwave on 70% power for about 15 minutes. Allow to stand 15 minutes before serving.

Yield: 8 servings

Approximate Per Serving:
Calories: 287
Fat: 6.8 g
Cholesterol: 56 mg
Carbohydrates: 24 g
Protein: 30 g
Sodium: 702 mg

Diabetic Exchanges: 1 bread; 3 meat; 1 vegetable; 1/2 milk

Easy Cannelloni

(Recipe contains approximately 30% fat)

1/2 lb. ground round
1/4 c. chopped green
    pepper
1/4 c. chopped onion
1/4 c. Parmesan cheese
Egg substitute to equal
    to 1 egg
1 tsp. Italian seasoning
1/2 tsp. garlic salt or
    garlic powder

8 manicotti shells,
    uncooked
1 (16 oz.) can tomatoes
    with juice
1 (8 oz.) can tomato sauce
1/4 c. water
1 (4 oz.) pkg. lowfat part
    skim mozzarella cheese
6 slices nonfat American
    cheese, diced

Brown meat, green pepper and onion. Stir in 1/4 cup Parmesan cheese, egg substitute and seasoning. Blend well. Fill manicotti shells and place in large shallow baking dish that has been sprayed with vegetable oil. Blend chopped tomatoes and juice, tomato sauce and water. Pour over manicotti shells. Cover and bake in 350° oven for 1 hour. Top with mozzarella and American cheese. Bake until cheese melts and is bubbly.

Yield: 4 servings

Approximate Per Serving:
Calories: 185
Fat: 6.1 g
Cholesterol: 29 mg
Carbohydrates: 18 g
Protein: 16 g
Sodium: 317 mg

Diabetic Exchanges: 2 meat; 1 bread; 1/2 vegetable

Eight ounces uncooked spaghetti equals 4 cups cooked.

Italian Fricasseed Chicken

(Recipe contains approximately 28% fat)

1 T. canola oil
1/2 c. all-purpose enriched
   flour
1/2 tsp. black pepper
1/2 tsp. salt (opt.)
4 (4 oz.) boneless, skinless
   chicken breast fillets,
   all fat removed
2/3 c. dry white wine (can
   use chicken stock)

1 sm. onion, sliced thin
   & separated into rings
1 green pepper, cut into
   thin strips
1 med. carrot, sliced very
   thin
1/2 stalk celery, cut into
   thin strips
1 clove garlic, minced
2/3 c. Italian tomatoes,
   chopped (include juice)

Heat oil in skillet over medium heat. Blend flour, pepper and salt. Dredge chicken fillets in flour and brown in hot oil, cooking until browned on both sides. Remove chicken from skillet, and keep warm. Drain any rendered fat. Turn heat to high and add wine. Boil until wine has reduced to half. Turn heat down to medium and add onion rings. Cook about 5 minutes, stirring twice. Return chicken breasts to skillet. Add remaining ingredients to skillet and cook 30 to 35 minutes, turning several times during cooking period. Remove chicken to serving platter and pour sauce over chicken.
Yield: 4 servings

Approximate Per Serving:
Calories: 155
Fat: 4.9 g
Cholesterol: 17 mg
Carbohydrates: 13 g
Protein: 19 g
Sodium: 338 mg

Diabetic Exchanges: 3 meat; 2 vegetable

An easy way to open the end of a box that instructs to "Press here":
Use a beverage can opener. Saves fingernails.

Lasagna—Lowfat

(Recipe contains approximately 23% fat)

1/2 lb. ground round
1 lb. ground turkey breast
1/2 med. onion
1 (28 oz.) can whole
  tomatoes
1 (12 oz.) can tomato paste
1 tsp. garlic salt
1 tsp. garlic powder
1 1/2 tsp. oregano
1 tsp. basil

1 (12 oz.) pkg. lasagna
  noodles, cooked per
  pkg. directions
2 c. lowfat cream-style
  cottage cheese
1/4 c. Parmesan cheese
8 oz. mozzarella cheese,
  shredded
1 (8 oz.) pkg. no-fat
  American cheese slices,
  diced

In a large skillet, brown ground round, turkey and onion. Drain off any rendered fat. Cut up tomatoes and add tomatoes and juice to meat along with tomato paste, garlic salt and powder, oregano and basil. Heat to boiling, turn down heat and simmer for 30 minutes. Blend cottage cheese and Parmesan cheese.

Put 1/3 of sauce in bottom of 9x13-inch baking dish and top with half of noodles, 1/2 of cottage cheese mixture, half of mozzarella cheese and American cheese. Repeat layers. Bake in 350° oven, uncovered, for 45 minutes. Allow to stand 15 minutes before cutting.

Yield: 8 servings

Approximate Per Serving:
Calories: 336
Fat: 8.6 g
Cholesterol: 60 mg
Carbohydrates: 16 g
Protein: 30 g
Sodium: 543 mg

Diabetic Exchanges: 3 meat; 1/2 bread; 1/2 milk; 1 fat; 1 vegetable

*When a screw-top jar won't open, simply wrap a few
rubber bands around the lid to make a firm grip.*

Spaghetti Bake

(Recipe contains approximately 19% fat)

1/2 lb. ground round	1 tsp. salt (opt.)
1 lb. ground turkey breast	1 tsp. oregano
1 med. onion, chopped	1/4 tsp. cilantro
1 clove garlic, minced	1 tsp. basil
1 (28 oz.) can Italian	1 (8 oz.) pkg. spaghetti,
tomatoes, chopped up	broken into 2" pieces &
1 (15 oz.) can tomato sauce	cooked per package
1 (3 oz.) can sliced mush-	directions
rooms	1 (4 oz.) pkg. mozzarella
2 tsp. sugar	cheese, grated

Brown ground beef, turkey breast, onion and garlic until pink disappears from meat. Drain off all rendered fat. Add tomatoes, tomato sauce, mushrooms, sugar, salt, oregano, cilantro and basil. Simmer 30 minutes, uncovered. Add cooked spaghetti and blend well. Put half of spaghetti mixture into a 9x13-inch baking dish that has been sprayed with vegetable oil. Add half of mozzarella cheese. Layer remaining spaghetti mixture and top with remaining cheese. Bake in a 350° preheated oven for 30 minutes.
Yield: 6 servings

Approximate Per Serving:
Calories: 288
Fat: 6.2 g
Cholesterol: 50 mg
Carbohydrates: 24 g
Protein: 27 g
Sodium: 597 mg

Diabetic Exchanges: 3 meat; 2 vegetable; 1 bread

Keep a package of pipe cleaners handy in the kitchen.
They are great to close opened bags of food.

Mexican

Burritos in a Hurry

(Recipe contains approximately 11% fat)

1/2 lb. ground round
1/2 lb. turkey breast
1 onion, chopped fine
2 c. homestyle refried
  beans (see index)
1 (4 oz.) can green
  chilies, chopped

1 (16 oz.) jar picante
  sauce
1 pkg. of 10 flour tortillas
16 slices no-fat American
  cheese, diced

In a skillet, over medium heat brown ground round, ground turkey breast and onion. Drain off any rendered fat and add refried beans, chilies and picante sauce. Stir to blend and heat until warm. Put 1/3 cup of mixture on each tortilla; top with 1/10 of cheese and fold over envelope style. Place in a 9x13-inch glass dish, seam-side down. Cover with Saran Wrap and microwave 8 minutes on medium (level 6) until cheese melts.
Yield: 10 servings

Approximate Per Serving:
Calories: 306
Fat: 3.9 g
Cholesterol: 42 mg
Carbohydrates: 39 g
Protein: 30 g
Sodium: 1,036 mg

Diabetic Exchanges: 3 meat; 2 bread; 2 vegetable

*A lump of sugar added to olive oil will
prevent it from turning rancid.*

Chicken Enchiladas

(Recipe contains approximately 20% fat)

1 (16 oz.) can whole
   tomatoes
1 (4 oz.) can green chilies
1/2 tsp. salt (opt.)
1 c. "yogurt cheese"
   (see index)
1 scant tsp. cornstarch
2 c. cooked chicken,
   finely diced

1/2 c. ricotta cheese
1/4 c. finely-chopped
   onion
1/2 tsp. dried cilantro
1/2 tsp. salt (opt.)
Vegetable spray
12 (6") corn tortillas
6 slices no-fat American
   cheese, diced

Pour undrained tomatoes into blender and add drained chilies. Add salt and process until smooth. Pour out into mixing bowl and stir in "yogurt cheese", with cornstarch blended in, just until mixed. Set aside. Combine chicken, ricotta cheese, onion, cilantro and salt. Spray tortillas with vegetable spray lightly on both sides. Spoon 1/12 of chicken mixture onto each tortilla. Roll up and place seam-side-down in a shallow baking dish. Pour tomato mixture over tortillas; cover with foil and bake at 350° in a preheated oven for 30 minutes. Remove foil and sprinkle diced cheese over top. Put in oven until cheese melts.

Yield: 6 servings

Approximate Per Serving:
Calories: 251
Fat: 5.6 g
Cholesterol: 54 mg
Carbohydrates: 26 g
Protein: 26 g
Sodium: 956 mg

Diabetic Exchanges: 2 meat; 1 bread; 1 milk

Fish should be poached; never, never boiled.

Chili Relleno Casserole

(Recipe contains approximately 9% fat)

2/3 c. uncooked brown
   rice, cooked per pkg.
   directions
1 (8 oz.) can tomato sauce
1/4 c. green onions, sliced
1/2 tsp. garlic powder
1/2 tsp. cilantro seasoning
   (opt.)

1 tsp. oregano
2 c. homestyle refried
   beans (see index)
2 (4 oz.) cans diced green
   chilies, drained
6 slices not-fat American
   cheese, diced

Combine tomato sauce, onion, garlic powder, cilantro seasoning and oregano. Set aside. Blend refried beans and rice. Spread half of this mixture on bottom of a 1 1/2-quart casserole that has been sprayed with vegetable oil. Top with chilies, then diced cheese. Add remaining bean/rice mixture and top with seasoned tomato sauce. Bake in 350° preheated oven for 30 minutes.

Yield: 6 servings

Approximate Per Serving:
**Calories: 146
Fat: 1.4 g
Cholesterol: 5 mg
Carbohydrates: 22 g
Protein: 13 g
Sodium: 729 mg**

Diabetic Exchanges: 1 meat; 1 bread; 1 vegetable; 1/4 milk

Use canned fish often, especially fish canned in water. Not only is it economical, but it will produce many good dishes.

Corn Bread Olé

(Recipe contains approximately 30% fat)

1 c. cornmeal
1 c. enriched all-purpose
    flour
1 tsp. baking powder
Egg substitute to equal
    1 egg
1 c. skim milk
3 T. canola oil

10 oz. whole kernel corn,
    drained
1/4 c. green onions,
    chopped
4 oz. jalapeño peppers,
    drained & sliced
1 (4 oz.) jar pimentos,
    drained & chopped
1/2 tsp. salt

Put all ingredients in a mixing bowl and blend until just moistened—do not beat. Pour into 9x9-inch pan that has been sprayed with vegetable oil and bake for 30 to 35 minutes.
Yield: 9 (3x3-inch) servings

Approximate Per Serving:
Calories: 179
Fat: 5.7 g
Cholesterol: Tr. mg
Carbohydrates: 25 g
Protein: 5 g
Sodium: 162 mg

Diabetic Exchanges: 1 bread; 1/2 milk; 1 fat; 1 vegetable

Save on household cleansers. Make your own; it's easy, safe and cheap.

Crab Enchiladas

(Recipe contains approximately 20% fat)

1 T. tub margarine
1 chicken stock cube
   (frozen), for sautéing
1 c. chopped onion
1/2 c. chopped green
   pepper
1 clove garlic, minced
1/2 c. flour
1 can chicken broth
2 (4 oz.) cans green
   chilies, chopped
1 c. "yogurt cheese"
   (see index)
1 tsp. cornstarch
8 slices nonfat American
   cheese
1/4 tsp. salt (opt.)
1/4 tsp. pepper
Dash Tabasco sauce
2 cans crabmeat, sorted
   & flaked
8 (10") flour tortillas

In a large skillet, melt margarine and stock cube. Add onion, green pepper and garlic, and sauté until tender. Stir in flour, cooking for about 1 minute, then slowly add broth, whisking until smooth. Add green chilies and cook until thick and bubbly, stirring constantly. Remove from heat and cool 3 minutes. Blend "yogurt cheese" and cornstarch and add along with half of cheese. Add salt, pepper and Tabasco sauce. Carefully fold in flaked crabmeat so as not to break up too much. Dip tortillas into mixture, then fill each tortilla with mixture and roll up. Place in shallow casserole, that has been sprayed with cooking spray, seam-side down. Sprinkle remaining cheese over enchiladas. Bake in 350° preheated oven for about 30 minutes or until cheese is bubbly.

Yield: 10 enchiladas

Approximate Per Enchilada:
Calories: 254
Fat: 5.7 g
Cholesterol: 31 mg
Carbohydrates: 38 g
Protein: 17 g
Sodium: 1,271 mg

Diabetic Exchanges: 2 bread; 1 milk; 1 meat

Easy Taco Salad

(Recipe contains approximately 13% fat)

1/2 lb. ground round	3 tomatoes, diced
1/2 lb. ground turkey breast	1 onion, diced
1 (8 oz.) can tomato sauce	1 (12-slice) pkg. no-fat
2 pkg. taco seasoning	American cheese, diced
1 head lettuce	

Brown ground round and turkey breast. Add tomato sauce and 1 package taco seasoning. Season until liquid cooks off and is absorbed. In a large mixing bowl, tear up lettuce and put in bowl along with tomatoes, onion and diced cheese. Pour meat mixture over lettuce mixture. Blend and serve immediately. Serve with taco chips. To make taco chips, cut tortillas in 6 pie-shaped pieces. Lightly spray with cooking spray and sprinkle with dry taco seasoning. Bake in 400° oven for 10 minutes or until crisp.
Yield: 6 servings

Approximate Per Serving:
Calories: 347
Fat: 5.0 g
Cholesterol: 61 mg
Carbohydrates: 40 g
Protein: 34 g
Sodium: 1,107 mg

Diabetic Exchanges: 2 bread; 1 vegetable; 3 meat

Round toothpicks make good skewers
for closing stuffed turkey or chicken.

Enchilada Casserole

(Recipe contains approximately 21% fat)

1/4 c. chopped onion
1/2 c. chopped green pepper
1 frozen beef stock cube
1 lb. ground round
1 T. flour
1 c. skim milk
6 slices no-fat American
    cheese

1 (4 oz.) jar pimentos,
    drained & chopped
1/3 c. evaporated milk
1 (4 oz.) can chopped
    green chilies
1 c. whole tomatoes,
    drained
12 (6") corn tortillas
1/4 c. shredded Monterey
    Jack cheese

Sauté onion and pepper in frozen stock cube. Stir in ground round and cook until pink disappears. Drain off any rendered fat. Set aside. In a medium saucepan, put flour and gradually add milk until smooth. Add American cheese, pimentos, milk, green chilies and tomatoes. Cook until thickened and cheese melts, stirring constantly; set aside. In a 2-quart deep casserole tear tortillas (3 at a time torn into pieces). Add meat mixture, then top with cheese sauce. Top with shredded Monterey Jack cheese. Bake 20 minutes. Allow to stand a few minutes before serving.

Yield: 6 servings

Approximate Per Serving:
Calories: 415
Fat: 9.7 g
Cholesterol: 65 mg
Carbohydrates: 47 g
Protein: 39 g
Sodium: 574 mg

Diabetic Exchanges: 3 meat; 2 bread; 1 vegetable; 1 milk

*Chill candles in the refrigerator for 24 hours before using;
they will burn evenly and will not drip.*

Macaroni Taco Casserole

(Recipe contains approximately 11% fat)

2 c. uncooked macaroni,
  cooked per directions
1 lb. ground round
1 pkg. dry taco seasoning
  mix
1 (16 oz.) can tomato sauce
1 (15 oz.) can dark red
  kidney beans, drained,
  rinsed & drained

1/4 c. skim milk
8 slices no-fat American
  cheese, shredded
1 c. shredded lettuce
1 med. tomato, diced
Taco sauce

In a large skillet, brown meat and pour off any rendered fat. Add taco seasoning, tomato sauce and beans. Simmer, uncovered, 5 minutes; set aside. Stir milk and cheese into hot macaroni, blending well until cheese melts. In a 9x13-inch casserole, put half of macaroni; 1/2 of meat. Repeat layers. Bake in 375° preheated oven for 20 to 25 minutes. Top with lettuce, tomatoes and taco sauce.

Yield: 8 servings

Approximate Per Serving:
Calories: 372
Fat: 4.5 g
Cholesterol: 40 mg
Carbohydrates: 38 g
Protein: 35 g
Sodium: 843 mg

Diabetic Exchanges: 1 bread; 2 milk; 2 meat

Scouring Powder - Dampened salt on cloth or brush. Use salt to clean coffee pot. Works good and does not leave a bitter taste.

Mexicali Chicken and Rice

(Recipe contains approximately 16% fat)

1 lb. boned chicken breasts (skin removed & cut in strips)
1 frozen chicken stock cube, for sautéing (see index)
1 tsp. olive oil
2 c. chicken broth, can use low-sodium canned broth
1 (8 oz.) can tomato sauce
1 pkg. dry taco seasoning
1 (12 oz.) can corn, drained
1 med. green pepper, cut in small strips
1 1/2 c. brown rice, cooked per pkg. directions
6 slices no-fat American cheese, diced
10 corn tortillas, cut into pie shapes, sprayed with cooking spray & baked until crisp

Sauté chicken in stock and oil until opaque. Add broth, tomato sauce, and taco seasoning. Bring to boil and simmer, covered, for 5 minutes. Add corn and green pepper; blend. Add cooked rice. Stir until heated through. Serve sprinkled with cheese and with tortilla chips.

Yield: 6 servings

Approximate Per Serving:
Calories: 326
Fat: 5.9 g
Cholesterol: 41 mg
Carbohydrates: 40 g
Protein: 26 g
Sodium: 1,037 mg

Diabetic Exchanges: 2 bread; 2 meat; 1 vegetable; 1/2 milk

Cleaning Windows - Mix 1/2 cup kerosene or vinegar with a quart of warm water.

Mexicali Rice Casserole

(Recipe contains approximately 15% fat)

1 lb. ground round	1 c. uncooked brown rice
1/4 tsp. seasoned salt (opt.)	1 (8 oz.) can tomato sauce
1/4 tsp. pepper	1 1/2 c. water
1 sm. green onion, chopped fine	4 slices no-fat American cheese, diced
1 sm. green pepper, chopped fine	1 med. green pepper, sliced in rings
1 pkg. taco seasoning	

Brown ground round, salt, pepper, onion and green pepper. Drain off any rendered fat. Stir in taco seasoning. Remove from stove and set aside. In a 9x13-inch pan sprayed with cooking spray, sprinkle uncooked rice and top with browned ground round. Pour tomato sauce and water over top. Bake in 375° oven, covered, for 60 minutes or until rice is tender. Add more water, if needed. Remove from oven and top with green pepper rings and sprinkle with cheese. Bake another 15 minutes or until cheese is melted. **Yield: 6 servings**

Approximate Per Serving:
Calories: 315
Fat: 5.4 g
Cholesterol: 57 mg
Carbohydrates: 32 g
Protein: 29 g
Sodium: 657 mg

Diabetic Exchanges: 3 meat; 2 bread

Rub fish down with lemon or lime before cooking.
Gives them a nice fresh taste.

Mexican Lasagna

(Recipe contains approximately 22% fat)

1/2 lb. ground round
1/2 lb. ground turkey breast
1 med. onion, chopped
1/4 c. finely-chopped green
    pepper
1 pkg. corn tortillas
1/2 tsp. garlic salt or
    powder
1 (16 oz.) can tomato
    sauce

10 extra-large ripe olives,
    chopped
1 c. dry curd cottage
    cheese
1 c. sour cream substitute
    for hot dishes (see
    index)
1 (4 oz.) can green chilies
1 (8-slice) pkg. no-fat
    American cheese,
    quartered

Sauté ground round, ground turkey breast, onion and green pepper in skillet. Drain off any rendered fat (should not be much). Set aside. With kitchen scissors, cut tortillas in very small pieces; spray with vegetable oil and bake in oven on baking sheet until crisp, stirring occasionally.

Combine garlic salt, tomato sauce and chopped olives; set aside. Blend cottage cheese, sour cream substitute and chilies. Spray a 2 1/2-quart casserole with vegetable oil. Put half of tortilla chips on bottom of dish and top with half of meat mixture, half of tomato mixture and half of cheese. Repeat layers. Bake in 350° preheated oven for 30 to 35 minutes.

Yield: 8 servings

Approximate Per Serving:
Calories: 301
Fat: 7.5 g
Cholesterol: 73 mg
Carbohydrates: 30 g
Protein: 31 g
Sodium: 892 mg

Diabetic Exchanges: 3 meat; 1 bread; 1 milk

*A large roast will carve more easily if allowed
to stand 15 to 30 minutes before carving.*

Mexican Roll-Ups
(Recipe contains approximately 13% fat)

1 lb. turkey sausage
  (see index)
4 green onions, chopped
1/2 c. chopped green
  pepper
1 (4 oz.) can chilies
1 clove garlic, minced

1 pkg. taco mix
3/4 c. water
1 can red kidney beans,
  drained, rinsed &
  mashed
6 slices American no-fat
  cheese, diced
12 flour tortillas (soft)

Brown turkey sausage, onions and green pepper. Add chilies and garlic and cook another 2 minutes. Add taco mix and water and cook at a simmer for 12 to 15 minutes or until most of water is absorbed. Stir in mashed beans, stirring until mixture is well blended. Divide mixture among 12 tortillas, putting in center of tortilla and spreading to the edge of tortilla. Sprinkle with cheese and roll up tightly. Place in 9x13-inch baking dish that has been sprayed with vegetable oil. Cover and bake at 350° for 15 to 20 minutes.
Yield: 12 servings

Approximate Per Serving:
Calories: 239
Fat: 3.5 g
Cholesterol: 33 mg
Carbohydrates: 32 g
Protein: 20 g
Sodium: 364 mg

Diabetic Exchanges: 2 bread; 1/2 vegetable; 2 meat

Try waxing your ash trays. Ashes won't cling odors won't linger and they can be wiped clean with a paper towel.

Mexican-Style Chicken Fricassee

(Recipe contains approximately 29% fat)

8 (3 oz.) skinless, boneless
   chicken breast fillets
1/2 c. cornmeal
1/2 tsp. seasoned salt
1/4 tsp. pepper
2 tsp. canola oil
1 tsp. tub margarine
1 lg. onion, chopped
3 cloves garlic, minced
2 T. chili powder

1 tsp. ground coriander
1/2 tsp. ground cumin
1 (16 oz.) can peeled,
   seeded & chopped
   canned tomatoes
   (use juice)
4 c. chicken stock, can use
   low-sodium canned
   chicken broth
20 stuffed green olives,
   chopped

Blend cornmeal, seasoned salt and pepper; dust chicken breast fillets with mixture. In a large skillet, melt oil and margarine and brown chicken breasts on both sides. Remove chicken from skillet with a slotted spoon. Put onion and garlic in skillet and sauté until onions are soft. Be careful not to burn garlic. Add chili powder, coriander and cumin to onions; stir to blend. Return chicken to skillet, turning to coat both sides of fillets with mixture. Add tomatoes and juice, stirring to blend. Return chicken to skillet, turning to coat both sides of fillets with mixture. Add tomatoes and juice, stirring to blend. Cover and simmer for 15 minutes. Add chicken broth; bring to boil and simmer for 1 hour or until chicken is tender. With a slotted spoon, transfer chicken to heated platter. Turn up heat and reduce liquid in skillet by one-fourth. Pour into large strainer and strain into a bowl, pressing on vegetables with the back of a spoon to recover all of the liquid. Return to skillet and add chopped olives. Simmer for 5 minutes. Pour over chicken and serve.

Yield: 8 servings

Approximate Per Serving:
Calories: 249
Fat: 8.1 g
Cholesterol: 68 mg
Carbohydrates: 11 g
Protein: 30 g
Sodium: 918 mg

Diabetic Exchanges: 3 meat; 1 milk

Taco Salad for a Crowd

(Recipe contains approximately 11% fat)

1 lb. ground round
1 lb. ground turkey breast
1 sm. onion, chopped fine
1/2 sm. green pepper,
   chopped fine
1 clove garlic, minced
2 pkg. dry taco seasoning
1 c. water
2 cans dark red kidney
   beans, drained & rinsed
8 slices no-fat American
   cheese, diced

1 recipe of taco-flavored
   Oven Tortilla Chips
   (see index), broken
   into small pieces
2 sm. heads lettuce,
   chopped
3 fresh tomatoes, seeded
   & chopped
2 btl. low-cal Ranch-style
   dressing

In a large skillet, brown ground round, ground turkey breast, onion, green pepper and garlic. Drain off any rendered fat. Add taco seasoning, blend well. Add water and simmer 15 minutes. Add kidney beans and heat through. In a very large mixing bowl, put meat mixture and add cheese, taco-flavored tortilla chips, lettuce, tomatoes and salad dressing. Blend very well and serve immediately.

Yield: 12 servings

Approximate Per Serving:
Calories: 381
Fat: 4.8 g
Cholesterol: 59 mg
Carbohydrates: 36 g
Protein: 34 g
Sodium: 938 mg

Diabetic Exchanges: 3 meat; 2 bread; 1 vegetable; 1/2 milk

Use muffin tins to make large ice cubes for use in punch bowl.
And instead of water, use some of the punch.

Mock Sangria

(Recipe contains no fat)

2 (40 oz.) btl. unsweetened
white grape juice, chilled
2 (32 oz.) btl. low-calorie
cran-apple juice, chilled

1 c. lime juice, chilled
1 (33.8 oz.) btl. sugar-free
club soda, chilled

Blend white grape juice and cran-apple juice. Fill a 1-quart metal bowl or 3 ice cube trays with mixture. Freeze. Return remaining mixture to refrigerator. When ready to serve, put large ice form (or ice cubes) in punch bowl. Add chilled fruit juices and club soda. Blend and serve.
Yield: 20 servings

Approximate Per Serving:
Calories: 88
Fat: 0.0 g
Cholesterol: 0.0 mg
Carbohydrates: 20 g
Protein: 0.0 g
Sodium: 3 mg

Diabetic Exchanges: 2 fruit

Notes & Recipes

Special
Entrées

Special Entrées

With this book due to be released in November, I thought it would be nice to include some holiday entrées. Entrées that are a little more special than most everyday food.

The ones I have chosen are not difficult to prepare, but go to the table with a look of elegance.

Wine has been used in some of them. If you prefer, chicken or beef stock can be substituted. However, it should be remembered that the alcohol in wine cooks off immediately, making the dish a good offering even for children. It's the special taste the wine emits that makes the dish stand out.

So, for the holidays if you are looking for something special, give one of the recipes in this chapter a try.

For a great energy saver, when you're near the end of the baking time, turn the oven off and keep the door closed. The heat will stay the same long enough to finish baking and you'll save all that energy.

Apricot Stuffed Pork Tenderloin with Vegetables

(Recipe contains approximately 35% fat)

1 (16 oz.) pkg. dried apricots
1 (2 1/2 lb.) pork tenderloin, all visible fat removed (this will shrink to allow about 8 (3 1/2 oz.) servings)
1 lg. Granny Smith apple
1 frozen chicken stock cube (see index)
1/2 tsp. seasoned salt (opt.)
1/8 tsp. pepper
3/4 c. chicken stock (can use 1/2 c. chicken stock) & 1/4 c. white wine mixed
8 med. potatoes (if possible, use new potatoes & leave skin on)
4 lg. carrots, scraped & cut into large sticks (or use 24 baby carrots)

Put apricots in bowl and cover with water. Allow to soak overnight. Split tenderloin down center without cutting loin in two, to make a pocket for fruit. Drain apricots and set aside in mixing bowl. Peel and slice apple. Stuff apricots and apples in pocket. Close pocket and tie securely at 3-inch intervals. Melt stock in skillet and brown tenderloin on both sides. Using an iron skillet with tight lid, add stock to skillet. Set shallow rack inside skillet and place loin on rack. Sprinkle with salt and pepper. Place potatoes and carrots around roast on rack. Cover and bake in 350° preheated oven for 1 hour or until loin is tender, basting several times with stock-wine mixture. Remove from skillet, untie string and slice.
Yield: 8 servings

Approximate Per Serving:
Calories: 307
Fat: 11.9 g
Cholesterol: 75 mg
Carbohydrates: 26 g
Protein: 31 g
Sodium: 281 mg

Diabetic Exchanges: 3 meat; 1 vegetable; 1 fruit; 1 bread

Broiled Leg of Lamb

(Recipe contains approximately 39% fat)

6 to 7 lb. leg of lamb, boned,
  trimmed of all visible fat
  & butterflied
1 onion, sliced paper-thin
2 sm. garlic cloves, minced
3 T. fresh lemon juice
3 bay leaves

2 T. chopped fresh parsley
1 tsp. oregano
1/2 tsp. fresh ground
  pepper
1 T. soy sauce
2/3 c. white wine or chicken
  stock

Combine all ingredients, except lamb. Spread lamb out in shallow pan and pour marinade over it. Refrigerate for 24 hours, turning every 6 to 8 hours. Remove from refrigerator and allow to come to room temperature. Transfer lamb to broiling pan. Broil meat 4 to 6 inches from heat for 15 minutes. Brush with marinade, turn and brush top side. Broil 12 minutes longer. Carve against grain in 1/4-inch slices. Heat marinade and serve on side with meat.
Yield: 10 servings

Approximate Per Serving:
Calories: 195
Fat: 8.5 g
Cholesterol: 84 mg
Carbohydrates: 2 g
Protein: 23 g
Sodium: 113 mg

Diabetic Exchanges: 3 meat; 1/2 vegetable

*Put vegetables in water after the water boils - not before -
to be sure to preserve all the vegetable's vitamins.*

Crown Roast of Pork with Vegetables

(Recipe contains approximately 40% fat)

1 crown roast (12 chops) about 3 oz. of lean on each chop	24 sm. baby carrots, boiled until almost tender
24 sm. potatoes, scraped lightly to clean, if necessary, boiled	24 sm. mushrooms
	1 frozen chicken stock cube (see index)
	1 tsp. tub margarine

Have butcher prepare a 12-chop crown roast. Place roast on rack in baking pan and cover raw bones with foil to prevent burning. Roast, uncovered, in a 400° preheated oven for 1 to 1 1/2 hours or until tender and nicely browned. Remove from oven and remove foil; put on frills. If you have no paper frills, make some from foil. In a heavy-bottomed skillet, boil potatoes and carrots until almost tender. Drain well. Put frozen stock cube and margarine in skillet and melt. Add potatoes and carrots; toss until lightly browned and done. Add mushrooms and toss about for about 3 to 4 minutes. Put around roast with parsley garnish. Serve immediately.
Yield: 12 servings

Approximate Per Serving:
Calories: 276
Fat: 12.2 g
Cholesterol: 75 mg
Carbohydrates: 9 g
Protein: 28 g
Sodium: 74 mg

Diabetic Exchanges: 3 meat; 2 vegetable; 1 fat

For a quick thickener for gravies, add some instant potatoes to the gravy. Just remember to count the extra calories in the gravy from the instant potatoes.

Chicken Breast Bordeaux

(Recipe contains approximately 21% fat)

6 boneless, skinless 3 oz.
chicken breast pieces,
all visible fat removed
1/2 c. all-purpose enriched
flour
1/2 tsp. seasoned salt
1/8 tsp. pepper
1/4 tsp. dried oregano
1/2 tsp. dried cilantro

1 frozen chicken stock
cube plus 1 tsp.
margarine (see index)
2 tsp. brown sugar
1 c. canned tomatoes,
cut up, juice included
1 c. chicken broth
1 c. red Burgundy
1 c. fresh mushrooms,
sliced
2 tsp. tub margarine

Blend flour, salt, pepper, oregano and cilantro. Pound chicken breast with a mallet until uniform in size, but not too thin. Melt stock cube and 1 teaspoon margarine in skillet. Dredge chicken in flour mixture and brown in stock and margarine. Brown both sides, then remove from pan. Stir flour into pan liquid and blend to make a smooth paste. Cook 1 or 2 minutes to brown flour. Add brown sugar, tomatoes and juice, plus extra 2 tablespoons of water if needed. Add chicken broth. Heat to boiling, stirring constantly. Reduce heat and simmer 5 minutes. Add wine and cook until thickened. Sauté mushrooms in 2 teaspoons of margarine. Arrange chicken in 9x13-inch baking dish that has been sprayed with vegetable oil. Top with sautéed mushroom slices and pour tomato sauce over chicken. Cover and bake in 325° preheated oven for 30 minutes. Uncover and bake 10 to 15 minutes or until chicken has browned slightly and liquid has cooked down some.
Yield: 6 servings

Approximate Per Serving:
Calories: 275
Fat: 6.4 g
Cholesterol: 66 mg
Carbohydrates: 16 g
Protein: 31 g
Sodium: 394 mg

Diabetic Exchanges: 3 meat; 1 vegetable; 1/2 bread; 1/2 milk

Chicken Breasts Wellington

(Recipe contains approximately 14% fat)

6 frozen rolls (uncooked
  bread dough)
1 (6 oz.) box long-grain
  & wild rice
6 (3 oz.) pieces boneless,
  skinless chicken

2 T. white wine (can use
  chicken stock)
6 oz. red currant jelly
1/2 tsp. Dijon-style
  mustard
1 T. orange juice

Thaw dough for rolls and allow to rise. Punch down and allow to rest for 10 minutes. Meanwhile, cook rice according to package directions and allow to cool. Roll out dough into a thin 8-inch circle. Place 1 chicken breast in center and top with 1/6 of rice. Bring sides up around chicken and rice and pinch together. Repeat with remaining ingredients. Place, seam-side down, in a 9x13-inch baking dish and refrigerate overnight.

Bake in 375° preheated oven for 35 to 45 minutes. Cover lightly with aluminum foil once bread dough has browned to liking. Combine remaining ingredients in saucepan and heat over low heat. Serve with chicken.
Yield: 6 servings

Approximate Per Serving:
Calories: 428
Fat: 6.7 g
Cholesterol: 66 mg
Carbohydrates: 57 g
Protein: 35 g
Sodium: 773 mg

Diabetic Exchanges: 2 bread; 3 meat; 1 1/2 fruit; 1 milk

*Thaw fish in milk. The milk draws out the frozen
taste and provides a fresh-caught flavor.*

Delicious Ham En Milk

(Recipe contains approximately 29% fat)

1 center-cut ham slice
  (1 1/2 lb., lean only),
  all visible fat removed
1 tsp. dry mustard

3 T. brown sugar
1 T. vinegar
Skim milk to just cover
  ham slice

In a small mixing bowl, combine dry mustard and brown sugar. Stir in vinegar to make a smooth paste. Spread evenly over ham slice and place in baking dish that has been sprayed with cooking spray. Add milk to just cover ham and bake in a 325° preheated oven for 1 hour.
Yield: 6 servings

Approximate Per Serving:
Calories: 217
Fat: 6.9 g
Cholesterol: 89 mg
Carbohydrates: 7 g
Protein: 29 g
Sodium: 1,536 mg

Diabetic Exchanges: 1 milk; 3 meat

The fishy smell can be removed from hands by washing them in a blend of vinegar and water or salt and water.

Dr. Bob's Deluxe Salmon Patties

(Recipe contains approximately 37% fat)

To reduce fat use pink salmon, however red is better for special entrées.

1 (16 oz.) can red salmon, drained, skin removed, flaked; bones mashed
20 saltine crackers with unsalted tops, crushed very fine
1/4 c. very finely minced fresh onion
1/4 c. very finely minced green pepper
1/4 tsp. dried cilantro (or coriander) (opt.)
1/2 tsp. seasoned salt
1/4 tsp. garlic powder
Egg substitute to equal 2 eggs
1/8 tsp. pepper
1/8 tsp. basil
1 T. canola oil
6 lemon slices

In a mixing bowl, put flaked, skinless salmon and mashed bones. Add cracker crumbs, onion and green pepper, cilantro, seasoned salt, garlic powder, egg substitute, pepper and basil. Blend well. Mixture should be of even texture and somewhat dry. If too dry to form patties, add a teaspoon or 2 of skim milk. Form salmon mixture into 6 patties. Heat oil in heavy-bottomed skillet and brown patties on both sides. Serve immediately with lemon slices.

Yield: 6 servings

Approximate Per Serving:
Calories: 218
Fat: 8.9 g
Cholesterol: 28 mg
Carbohydrates: 10 g
Protein: 19 g
Sodium: 712 mg

Diabetic Exchanges: 1/2 bread; 2 meat; 1/2 milk; 1/2 fat

Wear rubber gloves to transfer a turkey from roasting pan to platter.

Duck A L'Orange

(Recipe contains approximately 29% fat)

A skinned duck contains only 45 calories; 2.3 grams of fat and 21 milligrams of cholesterol per ounce of meat.

1 (5 to 6 lb.) domestic duck, skinned with all visible fat removed	1 c. chicken stock, can use canned chicken broth
1/2 tsp. salt (opt.)	Juice of 4 med. oranges
1/8 tsp. pepper	Juice of 1 sm. lemon
1 c. dry white wine	1/4 c. brandy (can use chicken stock)
1 T. sugar	1 lg. orange, separated into segments
1 T. vinegar	1 bunch of watercress

Skin duck completely. This is accomplished by starting at the breast portion of bird and sliding hand under skin and slowly working skin from body. For legs and wings score with a sharp knife and use fingers to work skin away from flesh. Remove any other visible fat. Rub salt and pepper all over the bird. Place in roasting pan on a rack and roast for 15 minutes in 400° preheated oven. Reduce heat to 350° and roast about 2 hours for 5-pound bird; 2 hours 20 minutes for 6-pound bird or until bird is tender. Baste every 15 minutes with white wine to keep skinned bird moist.

In a saucepan, put sugar and vinegar. Stir while mixture caramelizes. Remove duck from pan and keep warm. Drain off rendered juices and put into deffating cup. Defat and add to the mixture of orange juice, lemon juice and brandy. Add the caramelized mixture and cook slowly for 10 minutes. Cut in half vertically so each half has equal portion of breast. Now cut 2 halves in two down center. There are now four pieces of breast; 2 pieces contain a leg; 2 pieces contain a wing. Put duck pieces back on platter, putting together to make a whole duck (can use picks to hold, if desired). Pour sauce over duck and sprinkle with julienne strips of orange rind. Garnish with orange segments and watercress. Makes a very attractive dish.

Yield: 4 (3-ounce) servings

Approximate Per Serving:
Calories: 255
Fat: 8.1 g
Cholesterol: 64 mg
Carbohydrates: 16 g
Protein: 20 g
Sodium: 689 mg

Diabetic Exchanges: 3 meat; 1 vegetable; 1 fruit; 1 fat

Easy Chicken Divan

(Recipe contains approximately 18% fat)

6 (3 oz.) boneless chicken breasts, skin & all fat removed
1 pkg. frozen broccoli; or about 1 lb. fresh
1 c. white sauce (see index)
6 slices no-fat American cheese

In a 9x13-inch baking dish, sprayed with cooking spray, arrange chicken breasts. Put broccoli around chicken breasts and pour white sauce over chicken and broccoli. Top chicken breasts with slice of cheese. Bake in a 350° preheated oven, covered, for 40 to 50 minutes or until tender. Uncover for 10 to 15 minutes to allow casserole to brown.
Yield: 6 servings

Approximate Per Serving:
Calories: 235
Fat: 4.6 g
Cholesterol: 71 mg
Carbohydrates: 6 g
Protein: 34 g
Sodium: 491 mg

Diabetic Exchanges: 3 1/2 meat; 1/2 milk

Always prepare and marinate meats in a non-reactive container such as glass, ceramic or stainless steel.

Favorite Round Roast in Wine Sauce

(Recipe contains approximately 33% fat)

1 (4 lb.) round roast
1/2 c. beef stock
1/2 c. Burgundy wine

1/4 c. soy sauce
1 clove garlic, minced

Put roast in roaster (I use a deep iron skillet) on a rack or wire trivet placed in the bottom. Pour a couple of tablespoons of baste over roast and roast in 350° oven for about 3 hours or until tender. With a baster, baste roast often during cooking, to keep moist and add flavor to meat. Remove from oven when done and allow to cool 10 minutes before slicing. Defat drippings and make gravy using 1 tablespoon of flour for each cup juice.
Yield: 8 to 12 servings, depending on size of roast

Approximate Per 3-Ounce Serving of Cooked Meat:
Calories: 156
Fat: 5.7 g
Cholesterol: 60 mg
Carbohydrates: 0.0 g
Protein: 26 g
Sodium: 54 mg

Diabetic Exchanges: 3 meat

*Marinades can become a sauce for cooked meat if
the marinade has been heated to boiling temperature.*

Florentine Chicken En Phyllo Dough

(Recipe contains approximately 24% fat)

1 med. onion, finely
   chopped
1 frozen chicken stock
   cube (see index)
2 (10 oz.) pkg. frozen,
   chopped spinach, thawed
   & squeezed dry
1 lb. ricotta cheese
Egg substitute to equal
   1 egg
6 slices no-fat American
   cheese, diced
1 tsp. basil

1/2 tsp. cilantro
1 tsp. Italian seasoning
1/4 c. reduced-calorie
   mayonnaise
1/2 tsp. seasoned salt
1/8 tsp. pepper
8 (3 oz.) boned & skinned
   chicken breast fillets
Vegetable spray
2 T. tub margarine
1/3 c. fresh grated
   Parmesan cheese
16 sheets phyllo dough

Sauté onion in melted stock cube until soft. Pour into mixing bowl and add spinach, ricotta cheese, egg substitute, diced American cheese, basil, cilantro, Italian seasoning, mayonnaise, salt and pepper. Blend. Place 2 sheets of phyllo dough together and spread out. Spray top surface with cooking spray and place a piece of boned chicken about 3 inches from bottom of dough. Top with 1/8 of spinach filling. Fold bottom of dough up and over chicken; fold both sides over chicken, folding dough entire length of phyllo sheet. Roll package up like a jellyroll. Place seam-side-down in baking sheet, with filling on top of roll. Repeat with remaining chicken. Brush top of roll with melted margarine. Sprinkle with Parmesan cheese. Bake in 375° preheated oven for 25 minutes.

Yield: 8 servings

Approximate Per Serving:
Calories: 514
Fat: 13.5 g
Cholesterol: 91 mg
Carbohydrates: 37 g
Protein: 41 g
Sodium: 1,110 mg

Diabetic Exchanges: 4 meat; 1 bread; 1 milk; 2 vegetable; 2 fat

Mushroom Filled Meatloaf

(Recipe contains approximately 23% fat)

1 lg. onion, chopped coarsely	1 tsp. seasoned salt
1/2 c. finely-chopped celery	1/4 tsp. pepper
1 frozen beef stock cube, thawed	1/2 c. "light" sour cream
	1 lb. ground turkey breast
1 tsp. tube margarine	1 lb. ground round
1 lb. sm. fresh mushrooms, sliced	1/4 c. skim milk
	Egg substitute to equal 2 eggs
3/4 c. tomato sauce	1/2 c. oatmeal
1 c. soft bread crumbs	

Sauté onions and celery in frozen beef stock and margarine. Remove half of mixture and set aside. To mixture remaining in skillet, add mushrooms and sauté for about 3 minutes. Add 1/2 cup tomato sauce and simmer 10 minutes. Remove from heat and add bread crumbs, 1/2 teaspoon seasoned salt and 1/8 teaspoon pepper. Stir in sour cream and set aside. In second mixing bowl, put reserved sautéed vegetables, ground turkey breast, ground round, milk, egg substitute, oatmeal and remaining tomato sauce. Blend. If a little dry, add a little more milk. Pat mixture into a loaf pan that has been sprayed with cooking oil. Scoop out a trench in center of meatloaf, leaving about an inch shell around pan. Fill with mushroom mixture and pat meat over filling, covering entire trench. If desired, spread a little tomato sauce over top. Bake in 450° preheated oven for 20 minutes. Reduce heat to 350° and bake an additional 40 minutes or until done.

Yield: 10 servings

Approximate Per Serving:
Calories: 195
Fat: 5.0 g
Cholesterol: 56 mg
Carbohydrates: 8 g
Protein: 27 g
Sodium: 375 mg

Diabetic Exchanges: 3 meat; 1/2 vegetable; 1/2 bread

Scallops Mornay

(Recipe contains approximately 20% fat)

1 c. dry white wine (can
   use chicken stock)
1/2 tsp. salt (opt.)
1/8 tsp. white pepper
1/4 c. water
1 lb. fresh or frozen
   scallops
1 c. sliced fresh mushrooms
1 T. tub margarine

1/4 c. chopped onion
3 T. flour (scant)
1 c. skim milk
1/4 c. shredded Swiss
   cheese
6 slices no-fat American
   cheese, diced
2 T. fresh parsley, snipped

In a saucepan, combine wine, salt, pepper and water. Bring mixture to a boil and add scallops and mushrooms. Boil for 5 to 6 minutes or until scallops are tender (DO NOT OVERCOOK). With a slotted spoon, remove scallops and mushrooms; set aside. Reduce liquid to 1/2 cup by boiling for 15 to 20 minutes, uncovered.

In a small saucepan, put margarine and cook onions until tender. Stir in flour and blend until smooth. Add 1/2 cup scallop liquid and milk. Cook, stirring constantly, until thickened. Stir in cheeses and cook until melted. Remove from heat and add scallops and mushrooms. Pour into a 2-quart casserole that has been sprayed with cooking spray. Bake, uncovered, in 350° preheated oven for 15 to 20 minutes. Sprinkle parsley over top and serve.

Yield: 6 servings

Approximate Per Serving:
Calories: 233
Fat: 5.3 g
Cholesterol: 54 mg
Carbohydrates: 9 g
Protein: 27 g
Sodium: 1,001 mg

Diabetic Exchange: 3 meat; 1 milk

Scallop Stir-Fry

(Recipe contains approximately 21% fat)

1 lb. frozen scallops
1 T. olive oil
3 cloves garlic, minced
1 c. coarsely-diced celery
  cabbage
1 c. coarsely-chopped
  broccoli

1 c. silced fresh mush-
  rooms
1 pkg. frozen sugar snap
  peas
1/2 c. teriyaki sauce
2 T. flour
3 c. cooked brown rice

Heat 1 tablespoon oil in wok or heavy-bottomed pan (iron skillet is good). Add scallops, garlic and chopped celery cabbage and stir-fry 2 minutes. Add broccoli, mushrooms and sugar snap peas and stir-fry 3 minutes. Add teriyaki sauce and flour. Stir-fry until scallops are done (DO NOT OVER-COOK). Serve over brown rice.

Yield: 6 servings

Approximate Per Serving Using 1/2 Cup Brown Rice:
Calories: 141
Fat: 3.3 g
Cholesterol: 40 mg
Carbohydrates: 7 g
Protein: 20 g
Sodium: 233 mg

Diabetic Exchanges: 3 meat; 1/2 bread

One fourth cup unpopped corn equals 5 cups popped corn.

Seafood Jambalaya

(Recipe contains approximately 8% fat)

1 frozen chicken stock
  cube, melted for sautéing
  (see index)
2 lg. yellow onions, chopped
2 cloves garlic, minced
2 (28 oz.) cans Italian plum
  tomatoes, drained
  (reserve 1/2 c. juice)
2 1/2 c. chicken broth,
  can use low-sodium,
  canned chicken broth
1 med. green bell pepper,
  seeded & chopped

1/2 tsp. dried thyme,
  crumbled
1/2 tsp. dried red pepper,
  flakes, crushed
1 bay leaf
1/4 tsp. sweet basil
1 tsp. seasoned salt (opt.)
1/4 tsp. pepper
2 c. uncooked brown rice
1 lb. lg. shrimp, peeled
  & deveined (fresh or
  frozen)
1 lb. scallops, fresh or
  fresh or frozen

Melt frozen chicken stock cube in heavy iron skillet or heavy-bottomed skillet over low heat. Add onions and garlic and sauté, stirring constantly, until onions are soft, about 3 minutes, BE CAREFUL NOT TO BURN GARLIC. Add tomatoes and reserved juice along with broth, bell pepper, thyme, pepper flakes, bay leaf, sweet basil, seasoned salt and pepper. Blend, then stir in rice. Cover and simmer about 45 minutes. Add more water, if needed. Add shrimp and scallops to rice mixture and cook until seafood is just opaque, 2 to 3 minutes. DO NOT OVERCOOK SEAFOOD. Serve immediately.

Yield: 10 servings

Approximate Per Serving:
Calories: 254
Fat: 2.2 g
Cholesterol: 76 mg
Carbohydrates: 34 g
Protein: 22 g
Sodium: 635 mg

Diabetic Exchanges: 3 meat; 1 bread; 1 vegetable

Shrimp and Scallops Bobby Dean

(Recipe contains approximately 9% fat)

1 tsp. canola oil
1 frozen chicken stock cube
1 med. onion, chopped
2 fresh tomatoes, peeled
   & chopped or 1 can
   canned, drained
1 sm. green pepper, sliced
   very thin
2 cloves garlic, minced
1 lb. fresh or frozen shrimp,
   shelled & deveined

3/4 lb. fresh or frozen sea
   scallops
1/2 tsp. seasoned salt
1/8 tsp. black pepper
1 to 2 drops Tabasco
   sauce, if desired
1/4 c. dry white wine (can
   use bouillon)
3 c. cooked brown rice,
   prepared with chicken
   stock instead of water

Melt oil and frozen stock cube and sauté onions until soft. Add tomatoes, green pepper and garlic. Cook over medium heat for about 5 minutes, stirring constantly to prevent garlic from burning. Add shrimp and scallops, cooking over medium-high heat for 2 minutes, stirring constantly. Add salt and pepper along with Tabasco and stir to blend. Pour in wine and cook 1 minute to allow alcohol to burn off. Serve over rice.

Yield: 6 servings

Approximate Per Serving:
Calories: 234
Fat: 2.3 g
Cholesterol: 110 mg
Carbohydrates: 24 g
Protein: 27 g
Sodium: 338 mg

Diabetic Exchanges: 3 meat; 1/2 bread; 1 vegetable: 1 fruit

One slice bread equals 1/2 cup crumbs.

Shrimp Gumbo, Cajun-Style

(Recipe contains approximately 13% fat)

2 frozen chicken stock
   cubes (see index)
1 T. canola oil
1/3 c. browned flour (see
   index)
2 c. hearty chicken stock
   or 1 can low-sodium
   chicken broth (13 oz.)
1 (8 oz.) can tomato sauce
2 lg. onions, chopped fine
2 c. celery, chopped
1 lg. green pepper, chopped
1 (10 oz.) pkg. frozen, cut
   okra

1/4 c. chopped fresh parsley (or 2 T. dried parsley)
3 med. bay leaves
2 T. Worcestershire sauce
1 T. thyme
1 tsp. dried cilantro
2 tsp. garlic salt
2 tsp. pepper
2 tsp. Cajun seasoning
2 lb. med. shrimp, peeled
   & deveined
2 cans crabmeat, drained
   & sorted
6 c. cooked brown rice

Put frozen stock cube and canola oil in skillet and melt. Add flour and blend well. Stir in chicken stock, whisking until smooth. Whisk in tomato sauce. Add remaining ingredients except shrimp, crabmeat and rice. Simmer for 1 hour; if sauce becomes too thick, add water. Add shrimp, crabmeat and rice. Simmer 15 minutes. Remove bay leaves and serve.
Yield: 12 servings

Approximate Per Serving:
Calories: 242
Fat: 3.4 g
Cholesterol: 104 mg
Carbohydrates: 34 g
Protein: 17 g
Sodium: 879 mg

Diabetic Exchanges: 2 meat; 2 bread; 1 vegetable

Oven mits are great when rearranging foods in the freezer.

Teriyaki Salmon Steaks

(Recipe contains approximately 27% fat)

1 c. white wine (can use
  chicken stock)
1/4 c. low-sodium soy
  sauce
2 cloves garlic, minced

2 tsp. ground ginger
1/2 tsp. oregano
Pepper, to taste
6 salmon steaks, about
  4 oz. each

Combine wine, soy sauce, garlic cloves, ginger, oregano and pepper in a 9x13-inch shallow baking dish. Put salmon steaks in marinade; cover and refrigerate 6 hours or overnight. Bake steaks in a 350° preheated oven for 30 to 35 minutes in the marinade. Watch closely as these should not be overcooked. Fish is done when meat flakes easily. Pour off marinade and serve on platter; spread with a clean white napkin.
Yield: 6 servings

Approximate Per Serving:
Calories: 211
Fat: 6.4 g
Cholesterol: 80 mg
Carbohydrates: 0.0 g
Protein: 28 g
Sodium: 381 mg

Diabetic Exchanges: 4 meat

Before washing meat grinder, run a piece of bread through it.

Turkey O Beautiful

(Recipe contains approximately 22% fat)

1 turkey of desired size or	1 1/2 tsp. salt (opt.)
1 whole turkey breast	1/2 tsp. pepper
5 c. stock prepared from	1 1/2 c. onions
giblets & defatted, can	1 c. minced celery
use low-sodium, canned	2 tsp. tub margarine
chicken broth	Egg substitute to equal
8 c. day-old bread, crusts	2 eggs
removed & cubed	1/2 c. white wine
4 c. day-old corn bread,	1/2 tsp. seasoned salt
crumbled	1 clove garlic minced
1/4 c. minced parsley	1 tsp. lemon juice
3 T. sage	Cooking spray

Put cubed bread and crumbled cornbread in a large mixing bowl. Add parsley, sage, salt and pepper. Toss to blend. In a skillet, put 1/4 cup broth and 2 teaspoons tub margarine. Add onion and celery and sauté for about 5 minutes or until vegetables are soft. Pour into mixing bowl with bread. Add egg substitute and enough broth to moisten dressing. Wash turkey and pat dry with paper towels. Sprinkle cavity and skin very lightly with salt and pepper. Loosely spoon part of dressing into cavity. Do not pack tightly. Sew up openings and truss turkey tightly. Blend 1/4 cup broth, wine, seasoned salt, garlic and lemon juice. Set aside to use as baste. Spray turkey with cooking spray. Put a rack in a roasting pan and position turkey on its side. Roast in 425° preheated oven for 15 minutes. Turn turkey to other side and roast for 15 minutes. Reduce heat to 325° and turn turkey breast-side up on rack. Spray a piece of cheesecloth with cooking spray and spread it out over turkey. Roast turkey the amount of time indicated on package or insert a meat thermometer in meaty part of thigh and roast until thermometer registers 180°. Baste turkey every 20 minutes. If turkey is not properly browned, remove the cheesecloth the last part of baking. Put leftover dressing in shallow pan and bake until nicely browned, about 30 minutes.

GRAVY: Remove drippings from pan and defat broth. Put 2 tablespoons defatted broth in saucepan and add 1 tablespoon tub margarine. Stir in 3 tablespoons flour and cook for 2 minutes to cook flour. Slowly whisk in 2 to 3 cups defatted broth until gravy is of the right consistency.

Continued on following page

Continued from preceding page

Approximate Per 3-Ounce Serving White Meat (without skin and 2 tablespoons gravy plus 1/2 cup per serving dressing):
Calories: 257
Fat: 6.2 g
Cholesterol: 66 mg
Carbohydrates: 6 g
Protein: 27 g
Sodium: 402 mg

Diabetic Exchanges: 1/2 bread; 4 meat

(This turkey takes a little more time and attention than a foil-wrapped turkey, but it is worth every extra minute spent on it.)

Notes & Recipes

Vegetables

Vegetables

We all know how to boil or steam vegetables or prepare them in their standard forms. However, it is the special vegetable recipes that most cooks seek out—a new way to prepare vegetables for Sunday dinner or when company is on hand.

In the vegetable chapter, I have endeavored to take some of the fat out of preparing special vegetables. However, it should be noted that these are special vegetable recipes to be used on special occasions. For the most part, prepare vegetables without the extra calories by steaming or boiling.

Reserve these recipes for company and special occasions. You don't have to give up the special vegetable dishes, just don't consume them on a daily basis.

Cheesy Asparagus
(Recipe contains approximately 4% fat)

2 bunches fresh asparagus or 2 jars long stemmed asparagus
1 tsp. salt (opt.)

1 c. chicken stock or canned, low-sodium chicken stock
1 T. browned flour (see index)
12 slices no-fat American cheese, quartered

Boil asparagus in enough water to cover with salt added, if desired. While asparagus cooks, put flour into small saucepan and gradually add stock, whisking until smooth. Put on stove and cook until thick, stirring constantly. Add cheese and cook until cheese melts. When asparagus is tender, remove from pan with tongs onto hot serving platter. Pour cheese sauce over asparagus and serve immediately.
Yield: 8 servings

Approximate Per Serving:
Calories: 101
Fat: 0.5 g
Cholesterol: 8 mg
Carbohydrates: 10 g
Protein: 11 g
Sodium: 880 mg

Diabetic Exchanges: 2 vegetable; 1 meat

Scalloped Cabbage

(Recipe contains approximately 10% fat)

1 med. head cabbage,
   coarsely shredded
8 slices no-fat American
   cheese, shredded

2 c. saltine cracker
   crumbs, use unsalted
   topped crackers
1 (13 oz.) can evaporated
   milk

Cook cabbage until tender. Drain. Put half of cabbage in bottom of a 2-quart casserole that has been sprayed with vegetable oil. Top with half of cheese and half of crumbs. Repeat layers, reserving crumb layer. Pour milk over casserole and top with crumbs. Spray crumbs with cooking spray and bake in 350° oven for 30 to 40 minutes.

Yield: 8 servings

Approximate Per Serving:
Calories: 156
Fat: 1.8 g
Cholesterol: 7 mg
Carbohydrates: 20 g
Protein: 9 g
Sodium: 654 mg

Diabetic Exchanges: 1 bread; 1 vegetable: 1 meat

*A wooden pick or two inserted through a cabbage
wedge will hold the leaves together during cooking.*

Carrots Supreme

(Recipe contains approximately 3% fat)

1 lb. carrots, sliced	1/4 tsp. salt (opt.)
1/4 c. reduced-calorie	Dash of pepper
mayonnaise	6 saltine crackers,
4 tsp. chopped onion	crushed
1 T. prepared horseradish	6 slices no-fat American
	cheese, diced

Cook carrots in boiling water until crisp-tender, about 10 minutes. Drain and place in 1-quart casserole that has been sprayed with vegetable oil. Blend mayonnaise, onion, horseradish, salt and pepper. Mix with carrots. Sprinkle carrots with cracker crumbs and top with slices of cheese. Bake, uncovered, in 350° preheated oven for 45 minutes. If cheese browns too quickly, cover with foil.

Yield: 6 servings

Approximate Per Serving:
Calories: 86
Fat: 0.3 g
Cholesterol: 5 mg
Carbohydrates: 9 g
Protein: 8 g
Sodium: 699 mg

Diabetic Exchanges: 1 vegetable; 1 meat

If vegetables are scorched, set the pot in a pan of cold water and allow to stand for 15 to 30 minutes. Do not scrape the bottom of the pan.

Broccoli and Corn Casserole

(Recipe contains approximately 12% fat)

1 can cream-style corn
Egg substitute to equal
   1 egg
1 T. grated fresh onion
1 pkg. frozen broccoli,
   cooked per pkg.
   directions

1 1/2 c. seasoned crou-
   tons, crushed fine
   (see index)
8 slices no-fat American
   cheese, diced
2 tsp. tub margarine
Cooking spray

In a mixing bowl, put corn, egg substitute, onion, broccoli, 1 cup crouton crumbs and cheese. Stir to blend well. Pour into a 1 1/2-quart casserole that has been sprayed with vegetable oil. Dot with margarine and top with 1/2 cup crumbs. Spray the crumbs with cooking spray and bake in a 350° preheated oven for 1 hour or until bubbly and crumbs have browned.
Yield: 8 servings

Approximate Per Serving:
Calories: 133
Fat: 1.8 g
Cholesterol: 5 mg
Carbohydrates: 21 g
Protein: 8 g
Sodium: 656 mg

Diabetic Exchanges: 1 bread; 1 vegetable; 1/2 meat

*Dampen a paper towel and brush downward on
cob of corn; every strand of silk will come off.*

Easy Scalloped Corn
(The cinnamon gives this corn a special taste)
(Recipe contains approximately 4% fat)

2 cans cream-style corn,
  low sodium
1 can Mexican corn (with
  green & red peppers)
1 1/2 c. saltine cracker
  crumbs, use unsalted tops

1 tsp. sugar
1 T. tub margarine
1/2 tsp. salt (opt.)
1/8 tsp. white pepper
1 tsp. cinnamon

Put all ingredients in mixing bowl and stir until well blended. Pour into a 2-quart baking dish that has been sprayed with vegetable oil. Bake in 350° preheated oven for 30 to 45 minutes or until golden brown.
Yield: 12 servings

Approximate Per Serving:
Calories: 131
Fat: 2.2 g
Cholesterol: 2 mg
Carbohydrates: 29 g
Protein: 3 g
Sodium: 207 mg

Diabetic Exchanges: 1 bread; 2 vegetable; 1/2 fat

If on a sodium-restricted diet, make your own salt substitute by blending: 1 tsp. chili powder, 1 T. garlic powder, 2 tsp. onion powder, 2 tsp. dry mustard, 2 tsp. curry powder, 2 tsp. paprika, 2 tsp. turmeric and 1 tsp. sugar.

Holiday Corn Casserole

(Recipe contains approximately 24% fat)

1 can cream-style corn
1 can whole kernel corn,
   drained
3 T. tub margarine
1 1/2 c. "yogurt cheese"
   (see index)
1 tsp. cornstarch

Egg substitute to equal
   2 eggs
1 box Jiffy corn muffin mix
8 slices nonfat American
   cheese, diced
1/2 tsp. seasoned salt (opt.)
1/4 tsp. pepper

Put cream-style and whole kernel corn in mixing bowl and add margarine. Blend "yogurt cheese" and cornstarch and add to corn. Add remaining ingredients. Blend well and pour into 2-quart casserole that has been sprayed with vegetable oil. Bake in 350° preheated oven for 45 minutes.
Yield: 12 servings

Approximate Per Serving:
Calories: 222
Fat: 5.8 g
Cholesterol: 5 mg
Carbohydrates: 34 g
Protein: 8 g
Sodium: 833 mg

Diabetic Exchanges: 2 bread; 1/2 meat; 1 vegetable

*A little vinegar used in dish water will help
to remove grease from dishes.*

California Casserole

(Recipe contains approximately 3% fat)

1 (20 oz.) pkg. California-style mixed vegetables	1/2 tsp. dried cilantro
1 can sliced water chestnuts, drained	1/4 tsp. pepper
1 c. skim milk	12 slices nonfat American cheese, diced
2 T. flour	4 med. fresh mushrooms, diced
1 tsp. seasoned salt	1 c. seasoned croutons, crushed (see index)
1/2 tsp. garlic powder	

Put California mix and water chestnuts in a mixing bowl and set aside. Put milk in saucepan and whisk in flour. Add seasoned salt, garlic powder, cilantro and pepper. Cook over medium heat, stirring constantly, until mixture thickens. Add cheese and mushrooms; cook until cheese melts. Pour over vegetable mixture and blend well. Pour into baking dish that has been sprayed with vegetable oil and top with crushed croutons. Bake in 350° preheated oven for 45 minutes.

Yield: 8 servings

Approximate Per Serving:
Calories: 122
Fat: 0.4 g
Cholesterol: 8 mg
Carbohydrates: 14 g
Protein: 10 g
Sodium: 947 mg

Diabetic Exchanges: 1 meat; 3/4 bread; 1/2 vegetable

*When buying snap beans go for the ones
with small seeds in the pods.*

Company Green Beans

(Recipe contains approximately 10% fat)

2 oz. ham, diced (lean only)
1 med. onion, chopped
1/2 med. green pepper,
   chopped (opt.)
1 (8 oz.) can tomato sauce
2 tsp. brown sugar
1 tsp. dry mustard

1/2 tsp. chili powder
Salt & pepper, to taste
1 (4 oz.) can sliced mushrooms, drained
2 cans whole green beans,
   drained

Put ham, onion and green pepper in skillet; add 1 teaspoon water and sauté. Add tomato sauce, sugar, dry mustard, chili powder and salt and pepper to taste. Fold in mushrooms and green beans. Pour into casserole that has been sprayed with vegetable oil and bake in 350° preheated oven, covered, for 45 minutes.

This recipe works well to prepare the day before baking.

Yield: 8 servings

Approximate Per Serving:
Calories: 47
Fat: 0.5 g
Cholesterol: 6 mg
Carbohydrates: 6 g
Protein: 5 g
Sodium: 387 mg

Diabetic Exchanges: 1 vegetable; 1/2 meat

*A touch of sugar to any sweet vegetable
will enhance its flavor.*

Green Beans with a Zing

(Recipe contains approximately 20% fat)

1/4 c. chopped onion
1 tsp. tub margarine
1 1/2 tsp. flour
1/4 c. water
1 1/2 tsp. vinegar
1/8 tsp. dill weed

1/2 tsp. salt (opt.)
Dash of pepper
1/4 c. "light" sour cream
1 (10 oz.) pkg. frozen,
   cut green beans, cooked
   in 1/2 c. water

In a saucepan, cook onion in margarine until tender. Stir in flour, cooking for a minute to brown flour. Add water, vinegar and dill; cook, stirring constantly until bubbly. Add salt and pepper; blend well. Stir in sour cream. When well blended, add cooked green beans. Heat through. DO NOT BOIL.

Yield: 4 servings

Approximate Per Serving:
Calories: 59
Fat: 1.3 g
Cholesterol: Tr. mg
Carbohydrates: 6 g
Protein: 2 g
Sodium: 308 mg

Diabetic Exchanges: 1/2 vegetable; 1/2 bread

*When a recipe calls for a 10-cup baking dish, use: a
9 x 9 x 2-inch square pan; an 11 3/4 x 7 1/2 x 1 3/4-inch
baking pan or a 15 x 10 x 1-inch jelly roll pan.*

Holiday Green Beans

(Recipe contains approximately 5% fat)

3 green onions, sliced thin
(include some of green
top)
1 tsp. tub margarine
1 T. flour
1/2 tsp. seasoned salt (opt.)
1/2 tsp. paprika
1/2 tsp. Worcestershire
sauce
1/4 tsp. dry mustard

1 (13 oz.) can evaporated
milk
2 cans French-style green
beans, drained
12 slices no-fat American
cheese
1/2 c. saltine cracker
crumbs, crushed (use
unsalted topped
crackers)

Sauté onions in margarine. Stir in flour, salt, paprika and Worcestershire sauce. Add dry mustard, blending well. Remove from heat and gradually stir in evaporated milk. Return to heat and stir until mixture bubbles. Remove from heat and add green beans and cheese; blend. Pour into 1 1/2-quart casserole that has been sprayed with cooking spray. Top with cracker crumbs. Spray crumbs with cooking spray. Bake in a 350° pre-heated oven for about 30 minutes or until bubbly and cracker crumbs have browned.

Yield: 8 servings

Approximate Per Serving:
Calories: 152
Fat: 0.9 g
Cholesterol: 11 mg
Carbohydrates: 19 g
Protein: 11 g
Sodium: 1,046 mg

Diabetic Exchanges: 1/2 milk; 1 vegetable; 1/2 bread; 1/2 meat

Use an egg slicer to cut cooked or canned potatoes,
beets, fresh mushrooms or peeled cucumber sections.

Oriental Green Beans

(Recipe contains approximately 19% fat)

1 lb. fresh green beans or
  2 (10 oz.) pkg. frozen
  green beans
1 tsp. canola oil
1 tsp. minced ginger root
1 clove garlic, minced
2 T. water

1 T. low-sodium soy sauce
1 tsp. cornstarch
1/2 tsp. brown sugar
1/2 tsp. crushed dried red
  peppers
1/4 tsp. salt (opt.)
Dash of pepper

Steam fresh green beans about 5 minutes or cook frozen green beans according to package directions. Drain. Blanch in very cold water and drain again. Spray a large nonstick skillet with cooking spray and add canola oil. Over medium heat, heat until hot, then add ginger root and garlic. Cook 30 to 40 seconds, then add green beans and sauté 6 minutes. Blend water, soy sauce, cornstarch, brown sugar, crushed red peppers, salt and pepper. Blend until smooth, then add to bean mixture. Cook, stirring constantly until heated through.

Yield: 8 servings

Approximate Per Serving:
Calories: 33
Fat: 0.7 g
Cholesterol: 0.0 mg
Carbohydrates: 6 g
Protein: 1 g
Sodium: 220 mg

Diabetic Exchanges: 1 vegetable

To prevent fishing for cooked ears of corn in boiling water, put them in a French-fry basket before lowering them into the water.

Peas Oriental

(Recipe contains approximately 6% fat)

2 (10 oz.) pkg. frozen peas
1 can sliced water chest-
nuts, drained
1/2 c. chicken stock

1 pkg. reduced-calorie dry
Ranch dressing mix
Cooking spray

Combine peas, water chestnuts, stock and dressing mix. Blend well. Pour into small casserole that has been sprayed with cooking spray. Spray top with cooking spray; cover with aluminum foil and bake in 325° preheated oven for 15 to 20 minutes.
Yield: 8 servings

Approximate Per Serving:
Calories: 80
Fat: 0.5 g
Cholesterol: 0.0 mg
Carbohydrates: 13 g
Protein: 5 g
Sodium: 50 mg

Diabetic Exchanges: 1/2 bread; 1 vegetable

Sautéed Onion Rings

(Recipe contains approximately 20% fat)

3 med. onions
1 tsp. canola oil
1 frozen beef stock cube

1/4 tsp. salt (opt.)
Dash of pepper

Slice onions very thinly and separate into rings. Put oil and stock cube in skillet and melt. Add onions, salt and pepper, and toss to coat. Cook over medium heat for about 10 minutes or until onions are crisp and lightly browned. Serve immediately.
Yield: 4 (1/2 cup) servings

Approximate Per Serving:
Calories: 55
Fat: 1.2 g
Cholesterol: 0.0 mg
Carbohydrates: 9 g
Protein: 2 g
Sodium: 146 mg

Diabetic Exchanges: 2 vegetable; 1/4 fat

Easy Scalloped Tomatoes

(Recipe contains approximately 6% fat)

1 (16 oz.) can tomatoes
1 green onion, sliced thin
   (use green top also)
1 T. green pepper, minced
3 T. finely-chopped celery
3 T. flour
2 T. sugar

1/2 tsp. salt (opt.)
1/4 tsp. pepper
1/2 c. crumbs prepared
   from seasoned croutons
   (see index)
Cooking spray

Combine tomatoes, onion, green pepper and celery. Blend flour, sugar, salt and pepper; stir into tomato mixture. Pour into a small casserole that has been sprayed with vegetable oil. Sprinkle crouton crumbs over top and spray with vegetable oil. Bake, uncovered, in 350° oven for 45 minutes.
Yield: 6 servings

Approximate Per Serving:
**Calories: 57
Fat: 0.4 g
Cholesterol: 0.0 mg
Carbohydrates: 12 g
Protein: 1 g
Sodium: 280 mg**

Diabetic Exchanges: 1/2 bread; 1 vegetable

Tomatoes Provencale

(Recipe contains approximately 8% fat)

4 med.-sized tomatoes
1/4 tsp. salt
Dash of pepper

1 frozen chicken stock cube
1/2 c. fresh white bread crumbs
1 clove garlic, minced

Cut tomatoes in half and season cut surface with salt and pepper. In a skillet, melt stock cube and add crumbs. Add minced garlic and a little pepper, if desired. Divide mixture among tomato halves and put under moderate broiler until crumbs are golden brown.
Yield: 4 servings

Approximate Per Serving:
**Calories: 53
Fat: 0.5 g
Cholesterol: 0.0 mg
Carbohydrates: 11 g
Protein: 2 g
Sodium: 290 mg**

Diabetic Exchanges: 1/2 bread; 1/2 vegetable

Potatoes

Boiling Potatoes

About everyone believes they can boil a potato, but can they boil one for maximum taste? Most people put the potatoes in water, bring the water to a boil, cover and simmer until the potatoes are done, sometimes overdone. The potatoes are then drained and prepared. This will not net the best boiled potatoes.

Potatoes need to dry out, to shed some of the water they picked up as they boiled covered with water. Getting rid of excess water in the potato can be done in two ways.

First, the potato can be boiled to within about 5 minutes of doneness. It should then be drained, put back on the stove, a clean kitchen towel crumpled down over the potatoes and the lid put back on. The potatoes should then be allowed to steam over a very low heat for about 5 minutes.

If preferred, the potatoes can be drained, then put into a colander, a towel crumpled over them and a lid placed on top, and put over a pan of boiling water for 5 to 10 minutes. Either way the process should be continued until the potato takes a dry look. You will then have a very delicious tasting potato. And trust me—if properly done, the potatoes will not burn and will have a superior taste.

To make your kitchen appliances shine like new apply car wax and polish. The results are unbelievable.

Cheesy Potatoes

(Recipe contains approximately 4% fat)

8 med. red potatoes,
   washed & sliced thin
12 slices nonfat American
   cheese, diced

2 c. "yogurt cheese" (see index)
2 scant tsp. cornstarch
1/2 tsp. garlic salt
1/4 tsp. pepper

Blend "yogurt cheese", cornstarch, garlic salt and pepper, then alternate layers of potato slices, cheese and sour cream. Bake, covered, in 350° preheated oven for 1 1/2 hours. If desired, cover can be removed the last 15 minutes of baking.
Yield: 8 servings

Approximate Per Serving:
Calories: 205
Fat: 1.0 g
Cholesterol: 14 mg
Carbohydrates: 29 g
Protein: 10 g
Sodium: 1,039 mg

Diabetic Exchanges: 2 bread; 1 meat

Creamy Skillet Potatoes

(Recipe contains approximately 10% fat)

8 med. red potatoes,
   boiled in skin
3/4 c. beef or chicken
   stock, can use low-
   sodium canned broth

1/4 tsp. salt (opt.)
1/8 tsp. pepper
Dash of nutmeg
2 tsp. tub margarine
1/2 c. skim milk

Peel boiled potatoes and slice thin. Layer in large skillet; pour stock over potatoes and sprinkle with salt, pepper and a dash of nutmeg. Dot with margarine; bring to boil and cook, uncovered, for 5 minutes. Add milk and simmer potatoes, covered, until soft—allowing sauce to thicken and become creamy.
Yield: 8 servings

Approximate Per Serving:
Calories: 97
Fat: 1.1 g
Cholesterol: Tr. mg
Carbohydrates: 18 g
Protein: 4 g
Sodium: 402 mg

Diabetic Exchanges: 1 bread; 1/4 milk; 1/4 fat

Delicious Scalloped Potatoes

(Recipe contains approximately 1% fat)

3 lg. red potatoes, peeled
  & thinly sliced
1 qt. water
6 ice cubes
1 frozen chicken stock
  cube
1 tsp. tub margarine
2 T. flour
2 c. skim milk, scalded
  (heated to almost boiling)

1/3 tsp. dry mustard
1/3 tsp. paprika
1/2 tsp. salt (opt.)
1/8 tsp. pepper
1 med. onion, very thinly
  sliced
3 slices no-fat American
  cheese, quartered

Into water put ice cubes and soak thinly sliced potatoes for 30 minutes. In a saucepan, put frozen chicken stock cube and margarine; melt and add flour. Stirring constantly, cook for 3 minutes to cook flour. Very, very slowly add scalded milk, stirring with whisk. Add mustard, paprika, salt and pepper. Remove potatoes from water and pat dry. In a 1 1/2-quart casserole that has been sprayed with vegetable oil, layer half of potatoes; top with thin onion slices and pour half of sauce over potatoes and onions. Repeat layers. Top with cheese. Cover with foil and bake in a 375° pre-heated oven for 45 minutes. Remove foil and put cheese on top. Bake another 45 minutes, covered. Remove cover the last 20 minutes of baking.
Yield: 6 servings

Approximate Per Serving:
Calories: 134
Fat: 0.1 g
Cholesterol: 4 mg
Carbohydrates: 23 g
Protein: 7 g
Sodium 456 mg

Diabetic Exchanges: 1 bread; 1/2 milk; 1 vegetable

Delmonico Potatoes

(Recipe contains approximately 2% fat)

9 med.-size red potatoes,
boiled in jacket until firm
1 tsp. dry mustard
1 c. evaporated skim milk
12 slices nonfat American cheese
1 tsp. salt (opt.)
1 c. skim milk
Dash of white pepper
Dash of nutmeg

Cool potatoes and peel. Grate fine into 1 1/2-quart baking dish that has been sprayed with vegetable oil. With hands push potatoes out of pile so they are even in dish, but do not stir grated potatoes. In a saucepan, put remaining ingredients and heat over medium heat until cheese melts and mixture is smooth. Pour over grated potatoes. Bake in 325° preheated oven for 1 hour or until done.
Yield: 10 servings

Approximate Per Serving:
Calories:154
Fat: 0.3 g
Cholesterol: 7 mg
Carbohydrates: 24 g
Protein: 23 g
Sodium: 765 mg

Diabetic Exchange: 2 bread

Dilly Potatoes

(Recipe contains approximately 5% fat)

8 sm. new potatoes, boiled
1/2 c. plain lowfat yogurt
1 T. prepared horseradish
Dash of salt
1/8 tsp. dried dill weed
1 green onion, chopped
fine (include green)

Scrub potatoes and boil until done. Cut each potato in half; set aside. Blend yogurt, horseradish, salt and dill weed. Spread mixture over each potato half and place on serving platter. Sprinkle with chives. Serve.
Yield: 4 servings

Approximate Per Serving:
Calories: 103
Fat: 0.6 g
Cholesterol: 2 mg
Carbohydrates: 19 g
Protein: 4 g
Sodium: 99 mg

Diabetic Exchanges: 1 bread; 1/4 milk

Jalapeño Potatoes

(Recipe contains approximately 7% fat)

6 med. red potatoes, boiled in jackets	2 tsp. tub margarine
1 sm. green pepper, cut in very, very fine slivers	1 c. skim milk
1 sm. can pimento, drained & chopped	1 (12-slice) pkg. no-fat American cheese, diced
1 T. flour	1 (4 oz.) can green chilies, chopped

Peel and slice potatoes. Spray an 8x8-inch baking dish with cooking spray and layer potatoes, green pepper and pimentos. In a saucepan, mix flour and margarine to make a roux. Gradually add milk, whisking until smooth. Cook sauce just until it comes to a boil (DO NOT BOIL); add cheese and stir until cheese melts. Add green chilies and pour sauce over potatoes. Bake in 350° oven for 45 minutes to 1 hour.
Yield: 6 servings

Approximate Per Serving:
Calories: 206
Fat: 1.5 g
Cholesterol: 17 mg
Carbohydrates: 29 g
Protein: 14 g
Sodium: 917 mg

Diabetic Exchanges: 1 bread; 1 milk; 1/2 meat; 1 vegetable

Coat a rubber drainboard tray with a light film of polishing wax to prevent rapid staining and make for easy cleaning.

Lowfat Western Fries

(Recipe contains approximately 1% fat)

6 med. baking potatoes
(be sure skin is new
& edible)
2 T. barbecue sauce

1 tsp. A-1 steak sauce
1 tsp. sodium-free
seasoned salt
Pepper, to taste

Boil potatoes in skins until crisp-tender. Remove from water and cool. Refrigerate for at least 2 hours. Cut potato in 4 to 6 wedges, depending on size desired. Put aluminum foil on cookie sheet and spray with cooking spray. Place potato wedges on cookie sheet, skin-side down, and brush with mixture of barbecue sauce and A-1 steak sauce. Sprinkle with seasoned salt and pepper. Bake at 400° oven for 25 to 30 minutes or until potatoes are nicely browned. Turn once during cooking.
Yield: 6 servings

Approximate Per Serving:
Calories: 82
Fat: 0.1 g
Cholesterol: 0.0 mg
Carbohydrates: 18 g
Protein: 2 g
Sodium: 62 mg

Diabetic Exchanges: 1 1/4 bread

When a recipe calls for a 12-cup baking dish or over, use: a 13 1/2 x 8 x 2-inch glass baking pan; a 13 x 9 x 2-inch metal baking pan or a 14 x 10 1/2 x 2 1/2-inch roasting pan.

Oven-Fried Potatoes

(Recipe contains approximately 19% fat)

4 lg. baking potatoes,
boiled in skins & chilled
in refrigerator

Cooking spray
Salt & pepper, to taste

Remove skins and slice potatoes into 1/2-inch thick rounds. Put a piece of aluminum foil on baking sheet and spray lightly with cooking spray. Lay out potato rounds and lightly spray tops of potatoes. Sprinkle with salt and pepper as desired and bake, uncovered, in 425° preheated oven for 25 to 30 minutes. Turn once while cooking.

VARIATIONS:

Taco Fried Potatoes: Sprinkle with a little dry taco mix instead of salt.

Barbecued Fried Potatoes: Brush with barbecue sauce on top and again after turning.

Parmesan Fried Potatoes: Sprinkle potatoes with 1 tablespoon grated Parmesan cheese.

Onion Fried Potatoes: Sprinkle potatoes with onion powder before cooking.

Garlic Fried Potatoes: Sprinkle with garlic powder before cooking.

Yield: 6 servings

Approximate Per Serving:
Calories: 79
Fat. 1.7 g
Cholesterol: 0.0 mg
Carbohydrates: 17 g
Protein: 2 g
Sodium: 3 mg

Diabetic Exchanges: 1 bread; 1/4 fat

A pinch of salt added to a recipe calling for sugar, will bring out enough of the natural sweetness in the food to replace 1/4 cup sugar called for.

Parmesan Oven Fries

(Recipe contains approximately 12% fat)

Cooking spray (good grade)
6 med. red potatoes,
   unpeeled & quartered
1/4 c. flour

1/4 c. grated Parmesan
   cheese
1/2 tsp. salt (opt.)
1/4 tsp. pepper

Spray potatoes with cooking spray. Blend flour, Parmesan cheese, salt and pepper; put in plastic bag. Shake sprayed potatoes in bag mixture and put in 9x13-inch baking dish that has been sprayed with vegetable oil. Bake in 375° preheated oven for 1 hour, turning every 15 minutes.

Yield: 6 servings

Approximate Per Serving:
Calories: 112
Fat: 1.5 g
Cholesterol: 3 mg
Carbohydrates: 20 g
Protein: 4 g
Sodium: 78 mg

Diabetic Exchanges: 1 1/2 bread; 1/4 fat

Pat's Deviled Potatoes

(Recipe contains approximately 18% fat)

6 med. red potatoes, peeled
   & cut in large dice
1 T. tub margarine
1 tsp. prepared mustard of choice

1 tsp. vinegar
1/4 tsp. salt
1/8 tsp. white pepper

Boil potatoes until almost done. Drain and put back on stove. Stuff towel in pan and cover with lid for 3 to 5 minutes or until potatoes dry out. While potatoes finish cooking, put margarine in saucepan and add mustard, vinegar, salt and pepper. Cook 2 or 3 minutes. Add potatoes to pan and shake pan until potatoes are all coated. Avoid stirring, as this has a tendency to break potatoes and make them mushy.

Yield: 6 servings

Approximate Per Serving:
Calories: 94
Fat: 1.9 g
Cholesterol: 0.0 mg
Carbohydrates: 16 g
Protein: 2 g
Sodium: 109 mg

Diabetic Exchanges: 1 bread; 1/2 fat

Potato-Broccoli Bake

(Recipe contains approximately 5% fat)

6 med. potatoes, peeled
  & diced
1 tsp. tub margarine
1 tsp. salt
Dash of pepper
1/3 c. skim milk

1 (10 oz.) pkg. frozen,
  chopped broccoli, cook-
  ed per pkg. directions
6 slices no-fat American
  cheese, diced

Cook potatoes; drain and mash with margarine, salt, pepper and milk. Fold broccoli into mashed potatoes. Put into a casserole that has been sprayed with cooking spray. Top with cheese and bake in 350° preheated oven for 15 minutes or until cheese melts.

Yield: 10 servings

Approximate Per Serving:
Calories: 87
Fat: 0.5 g
Cholesterol: 3 mg
Carbohydrates: 14 g
Protein: 5 g
Sodium: 490 mg

Diabetic Exchanges: 1 bread; 1/2 meat

Potato Dumplings

(Recipe contains approximately 5% fat)

4 sm. red potatoes, peeled,
  diced & mashed
Egg substitute to equal
  3 eggs

1/2 c. flour
Dash of salt & pepper
1 1/2 qt. beef broth, can
  use canned

Put cooked potatoes and egg substitute in mixing bowl and beat until smooth. Add flour and salt and pepper, continue beating until smooth. Bring broth to a boil and drop the dumpling batter by tablespoonfuls. Boil for about 5 minutes or until dumplings rise to surface.

Yield: 8 servings

Approximate Per Serving:
Calories: 103
Fat: 0.6 g
Cholesterol: 0.0 mg
Carbohydrates: 16 g
Protein: 6 g
Sodium: 623 mg

Diabetic Exchanges: 1 bread; 1/2 meat

Potato Pie Crust

(Recipe contains approximately 5% fat)

3 lg. red potatoes, peeled
   diced & boiled (see index
   for directions on boiling)
1/4 tsp. salt
1/8 tsp. white pepper

1 T. skim milk
1/4 tsp. basil
Egg substitute to
   equal 1 egg
1 egg white

Cook potatoes, drain and put back on stove for a few seconds to dry out. Add salt, pepper, skim milk, basil and egg substitute. Whip until potatoes are light and fluffy. Spoon into pie plate that has been sprayed with cooking spray and spread over pie plate with back of spoon to form a crust. Brush with egg white that has been slightly beaten. Put into 350° preheated oven and bake 10 to 15 minutes or until crust is lightly browned.
Yield: 8 servings

Approximate Per Serving:
Calories 55
Fat: 0.3 g
Cholesterol: Tr. mg
Carbohydrates: 10 g
Protein: 3 g
Sodium: 90 g

Diabetic Exchanges: 2 vegetable

*A pinch of ginger sprinkled in a cup of hot tea
will sometimes ease a stomach ache.*

Potato-Rice Balls

(Recipe contains approximately 8% fat)

These can be made ahead to point of baking. Will keep in the refrigerator for 5 to 6 days.

1/2 med. onion, diced	2 T. Worcestershire sauce
1 lg. stalk celery, diced	2 T. barbecue sauce
1 frozen chicken stock	1/2 c. soft bread crumbs
cube, for sautéing	1/8 tsp. pepper
1 1/2 c. mashed potatoes	2 T. fresh snipped parsley
1 c. cooked brown rice	or 1 T. dried parsley

Sauté onion and celery in chicken stock until tender. Put into mixing bowl and add remaining ingredients. Form mixture into 12 (1 1/2-inch) balls and place on baking sheet that has been sprayed with vegetable oil. Bake in oven for 20 to 25 minutes or until lightly browned.

If baking after being in refrigerator, allow an extra 5 to 10 minutes.

Yield: 12 servings

Approximate Per Serving:
Calories: 56
Fat: 0.5 g
Cholesterol: Tr. mg
Carbohydrates: 12 g
Protein: 1 g
Sodium: 169 mg

Diabetic Exchanges: 3/4 bread

*A watering can with a small spout works
great for filling ice cube trays.*

Potato Skins

(Recipe contains approximate 23% fat)

4 lg. new baking potatoes
   with tender skins
Cooking spray
1/2 tsp. garlic salt
1 tsp. paprika

1/4 tsp. pepper
1/2 c. lowfat "light" sour
   cream
2 T. green onion, minced

Scrub potatoes well and prick with fork. Bake in 450° preheated oven for about 1 hour or until done. Put baked potatoes on rack to cool to the touch. Cut potatoes in half lengthwise. Scoop out pulp (it can be reserved for another use), leaving about 1/8-inch shell. Cut each shell into 4 strips. Place on baking sheet and spray lightly with cooking spray. Sprinkle with a mixture of garlic salt, paprika and pepper. Bake in 425° preheated oven for about 15 minutes or until crisp.

Combine sour cream and onion. When skins come out of oven, spread with sour cream mixture and serve at once.

Yield: 32 appetizers

Approximate Per Skin:
Calories: 20
Fat: 0.5 g
Cholesterol: 0.0 mg
Carbohydrates: 3
Protein: 1 g
Sodium: 39 mg

Diabetic Exchanges: 1 vegetable

These can also be served as the potato course at a meal. Allow 4 skins per person.

Yield: 8 servings

Approximate Per Serving:
Calories: 80
Fat: 2.0 g
Cholesterol: 0.0 mg
Carbohydrates: 10 g
Protein: 2 g
Sodium: 157 mg

Diabetic Exchanges: 1 vegetable; 1/2 milk; 1/4 fat

Pure and Simple Scalloped Potatoes

(Recipe contains approximately 2% fat)

6 med. red potatoes, sliced
very thin (use 1 potato
per number of person
being served)

Evaporated "lite" skim milk
Salt & pepper, to taste

In a shallow casserole, sprayed with cooking spray, layer sliced potatoes; adding salt and pepper, if desired. Slightly cover with milk. Bake in 350° oven, covered, for 1 hour and 30 minutes to 2 hours. Uncover the last 20 minutes of cooking, for browned top.
Yield: 6 servings

Approximate Per Serving:
Calories: 109
Fat: 0.3 g
Cholesterol: 2 mg
Carbohydrates: 21 g
Protein: 5 g
Sodium: 26 mg

Diabetic Exchanges: 1 bread; 1/2 milk

*Add a little milk to the water when cooking
cauliflower and it will remain white.*

Zesty Mashed Potatoes

(Recipe contains approximately 24% fat)
(These have enough flavor—they really don't need gravy)

2 lb. red potatoes, peeled & chunked	1/2 tsp. seasoned salt
	1/8 tsp. white pepper
1 c. nonfat plain yogurt	1/4 tsp. baking powder
1 T. tub margarine	2 green onions, minced
1/2 tsp. garlic powder	(include part of green)

In a medium saucepan, cover potatoes with water and boil 15 minutes. Remove from stove and drain. Stuff a clean, crumpled kitchen towel down over potatoes, cover and return to stove for 5 minutes or until potatoes are tender. Potatoes should now have a dry look. If they are not dried, cook another minute or two with towel and cover. Remove from stove and pour into mixing bowl; add yogurt, margarine, garlic powder, seasoned salt, white pepper and baking powder. Beat with an electric mixer until fluffy. Add green onions and stir into potatoes with spoon until well distributed. Serve immediately.
Yield: 6 servings

Approximate Per Serving:
Calories: 103
Fat: 2.7 g
Cholesterol: 2 mg
Carbohydrates: 16 g
Protein: 4 g
Sodium: 231 mg

Diabetic Exchanges: 1 bread; 1/4 milk

*Fresh tomatoes keep longer if stored
in the refrigerator with stems down.*

Sweet Potato and Apple Scallop

(Recipe contains approximately 13% fat)

8 med. sweet potatoes,
   cooked, peeled & sliced
   1/2" thick
4 med. tart apples, cored
   & cut into rings

1/4 c. brown sugar, firmly
   packed
1/2 c. mini marshmallows
1 tsp. salt (opt.)
1 T. tub margarine

Spray a 2-quart casserole with vegetable oil and arrange layers of sweet potatoes, apples, brown sugar and marshmallows. Sprinkle with salt, if desired, and dot with margarine. Cover and bake in a moderate 350° oven for 50 minutes.

Yield: 8 servings

Approximate Per Serving:

Calories: 119
Fat. 1.7 g
Cholesterol: 0.0 mg

Carbohydrates: 40 g
Protein: 2 g
Sodium: 190 mg

Diabetic Exchanges: 2 bread; 1 fruit

Thumbprint Sweet Potatoes

(Recipe contains approximately 29% fat)

2 c. cooked sweet
   potatoes, mashed
Egg substitute to equal
   1 egg
2 tsp. grated orange peel
1 T. brown sugar

1/2 tsp. salt
1/4 c. very finely chopped
   pecans
1 T. tub margarine, melted
2/3 c. whole cranberry
   sauce

Combine sweet potatoes, egg substitute, orange peel, brown sugar and salt. Whip until smooth. Form into balls using a heaping tablespoonful of mixture. Roll balls lightly in nuts and place on a baking sheet that has been sprayed with vegetable oil.

Place thumb in center of ball and push to make a well. Drizzle with margarine and bake in 425° preheated oven for 20 minutes or until nicely browned. Remove from oven and place on serving platter. Place a spoonful of cranberry sauce in center of each thumbprint. If you wish to make them look like Christmas, place a piece of green maraschino cherry in center of cranberry sauce.

Yield: 12 servings

Approximate Per Serving:

Calories: 84
Fat: 2.7 g
Cholesterol: 0.0 mg

Carbohydrates: 11 g
Proetin 1 g
Sodium: 123 mg

Diabetic Exchanges: 1 bread; 1/2 fat

Steamed Rice

If you have a problem with rice being light and fluffy, try cooking it using the steaming method. In a saucepan, bring to a boil 2 quarts of water or stock. Sprinkle 3/4 cup brown rice into water and simmer over medium-high heat for 25 minutes. Drain the rice in a large colander or strainer and rinse with water. Place the colander over a pan of boiling water, covered with a tea towel and lid, for 30 to 40 minutes or until it is dry. Makes about 2 cups cooked rice.

Notes & Recipes

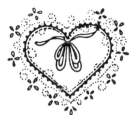

Salads

Salads

Taking the Fat and Sugar Out of Salads

When we think of salad we think of eating something that is good for us. Nothing could be further from the truth. Many, many salads are filled with fat and sugar and even cholesterol.

In this chapter the fat has been greatly reduced and the sugar content has been next to removed completely. And the good part about it is the fact that nobody will be the wiser. That is because the salads still taste good. We are living in a world where the manufacturers have gone to great lengths to remove the cholesterol and most of the fat in salad dressings while maintaining a good degree of taste.

There is also a mayonnaise on the market that contains no fat and no cholesterol. I don't think it quite stacks up to other mayonnaise, but hey— we can't have it all. I solve this by adding other ingredients to the "free" mayonnaise. In the chapter you will find a number of recipes designed to enhance the taste of "free" mayonnaise. Never consider a salad as a low fat and low sugar food. Make sure you know there is no hidden fat lurking in that salad.

When preparing flavored gelatin, add gelatin to boiling water instead of boiling water to Jello. It requires less stirring.

Vegetable Salads

Cooked Vegetable Salad

(Recipe contains approximately 11% fat)

2 lg. red potatoes, peeled, diced & cooked
2 med. carrots, sliced med. thin & cooked
1 (10 oz.) pkg. frozen green beans, cooked per pkg. directions
1 (10 oz.) pkg. frozen peas, cooked per pkg. directions
1 cucumber, peeled, seeded & diced
2 stalks celery, diced
1 sm. onion, minced
1/2 c. nonfat, no-cholesterol mayonnaise
1/2 c. sour cream, "light" style
1 T. lemon juice
1/2 tsp. seasoned salt (opt.)
1/4 tsp. garlic powder (opt.)
1/8 tsp. pepper

Drain cooked vegetables very well and put into large mixing bowl. Add cucumber, celery and onion. Combine mayonnaise, sour cream, lemon juice, seasoned salt, garlic powder and pepper. Blend well and pour over vegetables. Toss gently. Chill.
Yield: 6 servings

Approximate Per Serving:
Calories: 120
Fat: 1.4 g
Cholesterol: 0.0 mg
Carbohydrates: 21 g
Protein: 6 g
Sodium: 436 mg

Diabetic Exchanges: 1 bread; 1 vegetable; 1/2 meat

Carrot and Pineapple Salad

(Recipe contains approximately 2% fat)

1 pkg. sugar-free orange-
   flavored gelatin
1 c. boiling water
1 c. cool water

2 c. shredded carrots
1 sm. can unsweetened
   crushed pineapple,
   drained

Dissolve gelatin in boiling water and stir in cool water. Refrigerate until mixture begins to thicken. Add shredded carrots and crushed pineapple. Pour into serving dish (or dishes) and chill until firm.

Yield: 6 servings

Approximate Per Serving:
Calories: 45
Fat: 0.1 g
Cholesterol: 0.0 mg
Carbohydrates: 4 g
Protein: 2 g
Sodium: 6 mg

Diabetic Exchanges: 1 vegetable; 1/2 fruit

Coleslaw—Sugar-Free

(Recipe contains approximately 11% fat)

12 c. shredded cabbage
1 1/2 c. shredded carrots
1/2 c. chopped green peppers
1/4 c. finely-chopped onion
1/4 c. reduced-calorie mayonnaise
1/4 c. plain lowfat yogurt

1/4 c. vinegar
1 T. celery seed
1 tsp. seasoned salt (opt.)
1 tsp. garlic powder
8 pkt. Equal sweetener, or equivalent sweetener of choice

In a very large mixing bowl, put cabbage, carrots, green pepper and onion. Blend well. In a small mixing bowl, put mayonnaise, yogurt, vinegar, celery seed, seasoned salt, garlic salt and sweetener. Blend well, then pour over vegetables. Blend and refrigerate. Recipe may be halved.

Yield: 12 servings

Approximate Per Serving:
Calories: 55
Fat: 0.7 g
Cholesterol: Tr. mg
Carbohydrates: 10 g
Protein: 3 g
Sodium: 103 mg

Diabetic Exchanges: 2 vegetable

Corn and Cabbage Slaw

(Recipe contains approximately 17% fat)

2 c. shredded red cabbage	1 c. halved salad tomatoes
1 can whole kernel corn, drained	1/4 green pepper, chopped fine
2 oz. part-skim mozzarella cheese	1/2 tsp. salt (opt.)
1/2 c. diced radishes	1/8 tsp. pepper
1/2 c. diced apple	1/2 c. "free" Ranch-style dressing

In a large mixing bowl, put cabbage, corn, cheese, radishes, apple, tomatoes and green pepper. Blend salt, pepper and Ranch dressing; pour over mixture. Toss to blend. Chill at least 3 hours.

Yield: 8 servings

Approximate Per Serving:
Calories: 89
Fat: 1.7 g
Cholesterol: 4 mg
Carbohydrates: 17 g
Protein: 4 g
Sodium: 466 mg

Diabetic Exchanges: 1/2 bread; 2 vegetable; 1/4 fat

To easily remove the white membrane from oranges - for fancy desserts or salads - soak them in boiling water for five minutes before peeling the orange.

Deluxe Mushroom and Artichoke Salad

(Recipe contains approximately 7% fat)

2 pkg. frozen artichoke
    hearts
2 lb. sm. mushrooms, sliced
    (these must be fresh
    mushrooms)
1 1/2 c. water
1 c. cider vinegar

1/2 c. "free" Italian
    dressing
1 clove garlic, halved
1 tsp. salt (opt.)
1/2 tsp. peppercorns
1/2 tsp. basil
1/2 tsp. oregano

Cook artichoke hearts per package directions. Drain and set aside. Clean and slice mushrooms in thirds. Put mushrooms and artichokes in large bowl with tight lid. Combine remaining ingredients and pour over vegetables. Refrigerate overnight. To serve, pour off liquid and put salad in serving dish.

Yield: 8 servings

Approximate Per Serving:
Calories: 51
Fat: 0.4 g
Cholesterol: 0.0 mg
Carbohydrates: 7 g
Protein: 1 g
Sodium: 558 mg

Diabetic Exchanges: 2 vegetable

*When storing lettuce in the refrigerator, put
half a lemon with it to keep it fresh.*

Hominy-Vegetable Salad

(Recipe contains approximately 2% fat)

1 can white hominy, drained	1/2 med. onion, diced
1 can whole kernel corn, drained	1/4 c. chopped green pepper
10 cherry tomatoes, halved	10 ripe olives, sliced
1 stalk celery, sliced thin	1/2 tsp. seasoned salt
	1/4 tsp. pepper
	1/4 c. "Free" Italian dressing

In a large mixing bowl, put hominy, corn, tomatoes, celery, onion, green pepper, olives, salt and pepper. Toss gently. Add dressing and toss. Chill before serving.

Yield: 10 servings

Approximate Per Serving:
Calories: 90
Fat: 1.6 g
Cholesterol: 0.0 mg
Carbohydrates: 17 g
Protein: 2 g
Sodium: 371 mg

Diabetic Exchanges: 3/4 bread; 1 vegetable; 1/4 fat

Always use fresh ingredients for salads.
Stale vegetables or fruits makes for a dull salad.

Hot Potato Salad

(Recipe contains approximately 19% fat)

5 med. potatoes, peeled,
   diced & boiled
4 slices Canadian Bacon,
   1 oz. slices, diced
1/4 c. vinegar
1/4 c. water
Egg substitute to equal
   1 egg

1/2 tsp. salt
1/4 tsp. pepper
1 pkt. Equal sweetener
   or sweetener equivalent
   to 2 tsp. sugar
1/2 c. chopped onion
1/4 c. green pepper (opt.)
1/2 c. celery

Put cooked potatoes in bowl. Brown Canadian Bacon and add to potatoes. In a skillet, put vinegar, water, egg substitute, salt and pepper. Cook until mixture thickens. Add sweetener, potatoes, Canadian bacon, onion, green pepper and celery. Heat through.
Yield: 8 servings

Approximate Per Serving:
**Calories: 105
Fat. 2.2 g
Cholesterol: 14 mg
Carbohydrates: 11 g
Protein: 7 g
Sodium: 495 mg**

Diabetic Exchanges: 1/2 bread; 1 meat; 1 vegetable

Choose your vinegar with as much care as you choose a husband; quality vinegar should have a bouquet and a flavor all its own.

Italian Broccoli-Cauliflower Salad

(Recipe contains approximately 23% fat)

1 bunch broccoli, cut in
  bite-sized pieces
1 head cauliflower, cut in
  bite-sized pieces
1/2 lb. fresh mushrooms,
  cleaned & sliced
1 can water chestnuts,
  drained & sliced

12 lg. pitted ripe olives,
  quartered
1 sm. size btl. reduced-
  calorie Italian dressing
1 pkg. Hidden Valley dry
  salad dressing mix
10 cherry tomatoes

Blend all ingredients, except tomatoes, and pour Italian dressing and dry dressing over mixture. Blend well and refrigerate overnight. A couple of hours before serving, add halved cherry tomatoes. Mix well and refrigerate.
Yield: 12 servings

Approximate Per Serving:
Calories: 58
Fat: 1.4 g
Cholesterol: 0.0 mg
Carbohydrates: 9 g
Protein: 2 g
Sodium: 202 mg

Diabetic Exchanges: 2 vegetable; 1/4 fat

Learn to measure garlic and any other seasoning in a salad with care and discrimination. Too much seasoning ruins the fresh taste of a salad.

Lettuce and Pea Salad

(Recipe contains approximately 9% fat)

1 head lettuce, chopped
   fine
1/2 c. chopped celery
1/2 c. chopped green
   pepper
1/2 c. chopped onion
1 pkg. frozen peas
1 c. reduced-calorie
   mayonnaise

1 c. "yogurt cheese"
   (see index)
2 T. sugar, or equivalent
   sweetener
8 slices no-fat American
   cheese, diced
1/4 c. bacon bits prepared
   with soy oil

In a 9x13-inch baking dish, layer lettuce, celery, green pepper, onion and peas. Blend mayonnaise, "yogurt cheese", and sugar. Carefully spread over top of salad. Top with diced cheese slices and sprinkle with bacon bits.
Yield: 10 servings

Approximate Per Serving:
Calories: 124
Fat: 1.3 g
Cholesterol: 5 mg
Carbohydrates: 19 g
Protein: 9 g
Sodium: 620 mg

Diabetic Exchanges: 1 vegetable; 1 milk; 1/2 fat

Dress salads a split second before serving time. Never allow a green leaf to wilt into submission by too long of an intimach with a dressing.

Mexican Coleslaw

(Recipe contains approximately 11% fat)

2 (16 oz.) cans red kidney
   beans, drained & rinsed
1/4 c. ripe olives, diced
1 can whole kernel corn,
   drained
1/2 c. thinly sliced celery
1/2 green pepper, chopped
1/2 c. green onion, sliced
   (include tops)
3 med. tomatoes, seeded
   & chopped

4 c. shredded cabbage
1/4 c. reduced-calorie
   mayonnaise
1/2 c. lowfat plain yogurt
2 pkt. Equal sweetener,
   or sweetener of choice
   to equal 2 tsp. sugar
1/2 pkg. dry taco mix

Put kidney beans, olives, corn, celery, green pepper, onions, tomatoes and cabbage in large mixing bowl. Blend remaining ingredients and pour over vegetables. Refrigerate until ready to use.

Yield: 12 servings

Approximate Per Serving:
Calories: 144
Fat: 1.8 g
Cholesterol: 0.0 mg
Carbohydrates: 28 g
Protein: 7 g
Sodium: 87 mg

Diabetic Exchanges: 1 bread; 2 vegetable; 1/4 milk

*Remember that the alpha and omega
of all salad dressings is simplicity.*

Mushroom Salad

(Recipe contains approximately 13% fat)

12 lg. fresh mushrooms,
    cleaned & sliced
3 green onions, sliced thin
1/2 c. celery, sliced thin
2 T. white vinegar

1/2 tsp. salt (opt.)
Dash of white pepper
1 tsp. Dijon mustard
1/3 c. no-oil Italian
    salad dressing

Put mushrooms, onions and celery in a bowl and toss. Blend vinegar, salt, pepper, mustard and salad dressing. Pour over vegetables and allow to marinate several hours, stirring several times.
Yield: 4 servings

Approximate Per Serving:
Calories: 43
Fat: 0.6 g
Cholesterol: 0.0 mg
Carbohydrates: 6 g
Protein: 2 g
Sodium: 592 mg

Diabetic Exchanges: 1 vegetable

When making a salad remember the old Spanish proverb, "Always use four people when preparing a salad. A miser for oil, a spendthrift for vinegar, a counselor for salt and madman to toss it up."

Potato Salad

(Recipe contains approximately 13% fat)

3 c. potatoes, cooked, peeled & diced (when in a hurry I peel my potatoes, dice them & boil them in a small amount of water until tender. Simply drain & use for potato salad)
1/2 c. finely-chopped celery
1/4 c. finely-chopped green pepper
1/4 c. finely-chopped onion
1 T. dill pickle relish
Egg substitute to equal 2 eggs, scrambled then chopped
1/2 tsp. seasoned salt
Potato Salad Dressing

Blend all ingredients together and chill until ready to serve.

POTATO SALAD DRESSING:

1 T. cornstarch
1 tsp. dry mustard
1/2 c. water
Egg substitute to equal 2 eggs
1/4 tsp. salt (opt.)
Dash of white pepper
1/2 c. white vinegar
6 pkt. Equal sweetener, or artificial sweetener of choice to equal 1/4 c. sugar
1 tsp. tub margarine (do not use diet)

Put cornstarch and mustard in saucepan. Gradually add water, whisking until mixture is smooth. Add egg substitute, salt and pepper. Cook over medium heat, stirring constantly until mixture thickens. Remove from heat and add vinegar and sweetener. Stir in margarine, 1/4 teaspoon at a time, stirring between each addition.

Yield: 8 servings

Approximate Per Serving:
Calories: 91
Fat: 1.3 g
Cholesterol: 0.0 mg
Carbohydrates: 10 G
Protein: 4 g
Sodium: 193 mg

Diabetic Exchanges: 2 vegetable; 1/2 meat

When buying cabbage choose heads that are heavy for size.

Quick White Bean Salad

(Recipe contains approximately 9% fat)

2 (16 oz.) cans Great
  Northern beans, drained
1/2 c. Bermuda onions,
  chopped
1 (2 oz.) jar pimento,
  drained & diced
8 cherry tomatoes,
  quartered & seeded

1 stalk celery, sliced thin
1 1/2 T. vinegar
1 1/2 T. lemon juice
Olive oil cooking spray
1/2 tsp. garlic salt (opt.)
1/4 tsp. ground pepper
2 T. chopped parsley

In a mixing bowl, put beans, onions, pimento, tomatoes and celery. Toss to blend. Mix vinegar and lemon juice and drizzle over salad to coat evenly when tossed. Spray salad with cooking spray, tossing as it is sprayed. Add remaining ingredients. Stir and chill until time to serve.

Yield: 8 servings

Approximate Per Serving:
Calories: 144
Fat: 1.5 g
Cholesterol: 0.0 mg
Carbohydrates: 23 g
Protein: 8 g
Sodium: 14 mg

Diabetic Exchanges: 1 bread; 1 vegetable; 1/2 meat;
1/4 fat

*Help a new bottle of catsup pour by putting a
drinking straw into the bottle. Remove and pour.*

Sugar-Free Overnight Lettuce Salad

(Recipe contains approximately 11% fat)

1 head lettuce, chopped
1 head cauliflower (use
   only flowerets), chopped
2 c. no-fat, no-cholesterol
   mayonnaise
1 med. sweet onion,
   chopped
1 lg. green pepper, chopped

1 (8 oz.) btl. bacon bits,
   prepared with soy oil
8 slices no-fat American
   cheese, diced
6 pkt. Equal sweetener, or
   sweetener of choice to
   equal 1/4 c. sugar
1 tsp. vinegar

In a large mixing bowl, layer lettuce, cauliflower, mayonnaise, onion and green pepper in order given. After cauliflower layer, spread mayonnaise and continue to layer vegetables. Sprinkle with bacon bits, topped with diced cheese. Sprinkle sweetener over top and sprinkle with vinegar. Allow to stand in refrigerator overnight, covered. Just before serving, toss.
Yield: 12 servings

Approximate Per Serving:
Calories: 110
Fat: 1.3 g
Cholesterol: 3 mg
Carbohydrates: 18 g
Protein: 8 g
Sodium: 1,009 mg

Diabetic Exchanges: 1 milk; 1 vegetable

*When a recipe calls for 1 cup sour cream,
use 7/8 cup plain nonfat yogurt.*

Vegetable Toss

(Recipe contains approximately 31% fat)

2 c. broccoli flowerets
2 c. cauliflowerets
1 c. diced celery
1 c. cherry tomatoes, halved
1 bunch green onions, sliced thick
10 ripe olives, pitted & sliced
1/4 c. carrots, diced
1/4 c. radishes, sliced
1 (3.5 oz.) jar bacon bits, prepared in soy oil
1 c. "Free" Italian dressing

In a large mixing bowl, put all of vegetables and bacon bits. Toss gently. Pour dressing over vegetables and toss. Chill at least 6 hours before serving.
Yield: 8 servings

Approximate Per Serving:
Calories: 90
Fat: 3.1 g
Cholesterol: 0.0 mg
Carbohydrates: 13 g
Protein: 7 g
Sodium: 605 mg

Diabetic Exchanges: 1/2 bread; 1 vegetable; 1/2 meat; 1/4 fat

One tablespoon plain unflavored gelatin dissolved in two cups fruit juice will replace one 3-ounce package flavored gelatin.

Fruit Salads

Easy Apple Salad
(Recipe contains approximately 2% fat)

1 Granny Smith apple,
   cored & diced
1 Delicious apple, cored
   & diced
1 T. lemon juice
1 can fruit cocktail, drained
   (reserve juice)

1 c. diced celery
1/4 c. reduced-calorie
   mayonnaise
2 T. juice from fruit
   cocktail
1 T. sugar, or equivalent
   artificial sweetener

In a large mixing bowl, put diced apples and add lemon juice, tossing apples to coat. Add fruit cocktail and celery. Blend and set aside. Blend mayonnaise, fruit cocktail juice and sugar. Pour over apple mixture. Blend. Chill.
Yield: 8 servings

Approximate Per Serving:
Calories: 60
Fat: 0.1 g
Cholesterol: 0.0 mg
Carbohydrates: 15 g
Protein: Tr. g
Sodium: 103 mg

Diabetic Exchanges: 1 1/2 fruit

One cup evaporated milk will yield three cups whipped.

Easy, Tasty Fruit Salad

(Recipe contains approximately 10% fat)

1 (11 oz.) can mandarin oranges, drained

1 (20 oz.) can pineapple chunks, canned in own juice

3 bananas, peeled, sliced & tossed in a little lemon juice

2 Delicious apples, unpeeled, diced & tossed in lemon juice

1 box sugar-free instant vanilla pudding

1 c. skim milk

1/3 c. orange juice concentrate, thawed

3/4 c. lowfat vanilla or banana yogurt

In a large mixing bowl, put drained mandarin oranges and pineapple chunks. Add banana slices and diced apples. Blend and set aside. In a small mixing bowl put pudding and add milk, orange juice concentrate and yogurt. Beat with whisk until smooth. Add to fruit and blend. Chill.
Yield: 10 servings

Approximate Per Serving:
Calories: 141
Fat: 1.5 g
Cholesterol: 2 mg
Carbohydrates: 35 g
Protein: 2 g
Sodium: 118 mg

Diabetic Exchanges: 1 milk; 2 fruit

One teaspoon lemon juice can be substituted with 1/2 teaspoon vinegar.

Fruit En Wine

(Recipe contains approximately 3% fat)

1 c. fresh peach slices
1 c. fresh strawberries, halved
1 c. red seedless grapes, halved
1 lg. banana, sliced
1 c. bing cherries, seeded & halved

1/2 c. white wine (can use unsweetened grape juice)
1/2 c. unsweetened orange juice
1 T. lemon juice
2 T. honey
1/2 tsp. cinnamon, ground

Put prepared fruit in a bowl and toss to blend. Blend wine, orange juice, lemon juice, honey and cinnamon. Pour over fruit and toss to blend. Chill at least 1 hour before serving.

Yield: 8 servings

Approximate Per Serving:
**Calories: 102
Fat: 0.3 g
Cholesterol: 0.0 mg
Carbohydrates: 20 g
Protein: 1 g
Sodium: 2 mg**

Diabetic Exchanges: 2 1/2 fruit

Cranberries grind better when frozen. Simply wash the berries; pat dry and freeze in a plastic bag.

Fruit Salad with Fruit Dressing

(Recipe contains approximately 4% fat)

2 (20 oz.) cans pineapple
chunks (reserve juice)
2 (11 oz.) cans mandarin
oranges

4 med. red Delicious
apples, chopped
4 bananas, peeled &
sliced

DRESSING:
1 1/2 c. pineapple juice
3 T. cornstarch
2 T. lemon juice

2/3 c. orange juice
2 pkt. Equal or equivalent
sweetener of choice

Drain pineapple and oranges and reserve juice. Put juice in saucepan. Add cornstarch and whisk to blend. Add lemon and orange juice and cook, stirring constantly, until mixture thickens. Boil for 1 minute. Pour hot dressing over fruit. Cool, then refrigerate for at least 1 hour before serving. **Yield: 12 servings**

Approximate Per Serving:
Calories: 126
Fat: 0.6 g
Cholesterol: 0.0 mg
Carbohydrates: 32 g
Protein: 1 g
Sodium: 3 mg

Diabetic Exchanges: 3 fruit

Marshmallows will not dry out if stored in the freezer.

Holiday Cranberry Fluff—Sugar-Free

(Recipe contains approximately 11% fat)

2 c. raw cranberries, ground
3 c. mini marshmallows
18 pkt. Equal sweetener, or
   sweetener of choice to
   equal 3/4 c. sugar
2 c. diced unpeeled apples,
   tossed in a little lemon
   juice

1 c. seedless green grapes
1 pkg. Estee sugar-free
   whipped topping (pre-
   pared), or whipped topping of choice (see
   index)

Combine ground cranberries and marshmallows. Add sweetener. Cover with plastic wrap and refrigerate overnight. In the morning add apples, grapes and salt, if desired. Stir to blend. Fold in Estee whipped topping. Chill.

Yield: 10 servings

Approximate Per Serving:
Calories: 147
Fat: 1.8 g
Cholesterol: 0.0 mg
Carbohydrates: 13 g
Protein: Tr. g
Sodium: 58 mg

Diabetic Exchanges: 1 1/4 fruit

*Submerging a lemon in hot water for 15 minutes
before squeezing will yield almost twice the juice.*

Sugar-Free Cranberry Sauce

(Recipe contains approximately 3% fat)

4 c. raw cranberries,
washed & sorted
2 c. unsweetened orange
juice

24 pkt. Equal sweetener,
or sweetener of choice
to equal 1 cup sugar (if
not sweet enough add
more sweetener)

Put cranberries and orange juice in a saucepan and bring to boil. Cover with lid and boil about 5 minutes or until cranberries pop. Remove from heat. Cool slightly, then add sweetener. Stir to blend.
Yield: about 4 cups sauce

Approximate Per 1/4 Cup Serving:
Calories: 31
Fat: 0.1 g
Cholesterol: 0.0 mg
Carbohydrates: 6 g
Protein: Tr. g
Sodium: 4 mg

Diabetic Exchanges: 1/2 fruit

Cover peeled potatoes with cold water to which a few drops of vinegar has been added. Keep refrigerated and they will last 3-4 days.

Gelatin Salads

Apple Salad
(Recipe contains approximately 26% fat)

1 (3 oz.) pkg. sugar-free
   lemon gelatin
1 c. boiling water
3/4 c. cool water

1/2 c. "light" sour cream
2 Granny Smith apples,
   cored but not peeled

Put gelatin in mixing bowl and stir in boiling water, stirring until gelatin has dissolved. Add cool water. Refrigerate until mixture is the texture of egg whites. Stir in sour cream, blending until mixture is of even texture. Fold in apples. Pour into serving dish (or dishes) and chill until firm.
Yield: 8 servings

Approximate Per Serving:
Calories: 42
Fat: 1.2 g
Cholesterol: 0.0 mg
Carbohydrates: 6 g
Protein: 2 g
Sodium: 24 mg

Diabetic Exchanges: 1/2 fruit; 1/4 milk

Use a vegetable peeler to cut orange or lemon rind peels.
They come off without the white membrane.

Bowl Full of Holiday Gelatin

(Recipe contains approximately 10% fat)

1 (3 oz.) pkg. lime gelatin,
 sugar-free
1 (3 oz.) pkg. lemon gelatin,
 sugar-free
1 c. mini marshmallows
3/4 c. "yogurt cheese"
 (see index)
1 c. boiling water
1 sm. can crushed pine-
 apple, undrained

1 pkg. Estee sugar-free
 whipped topping (pre-
 pared, or sugar-free
 whipped topping of
 choice (see index)
1 (3 oz.) pkg. raspberry
 gelatin (can use straw-
 berry or cherry), sugar-free
1 (10 oz.) pkg. frozen raspberries, unsweetened

Prepare lime gelatin per package directions and pour into a 9x13-inch pan. Refrigerate until set. In a mixing bowl put lemon gelatin, marshmallows, "yogurt cheese" and 1 cup boiling water. Whisk until gelatin is dissolved and mixture is smooth. Fold in pineapple and whipped topping, stirring gently until blended. Spread over green gelatin and chill until set. Prepare raspberry gelatin with 1 cup boiling water. Add frozen raspberries and stir until mixture begins to thicken and raspberries are thawed. Pour over whipped topping layer and chill until set.

Yield: 16 servings

Approximate Per Serving:
Calories: 62
Fat: 0.7 g
Cholesterol: 1 mg
Carbohydrates: 8 g
Protein: 2 g
Sodium: 8 mg

Diabetic Exchanges: 1/2 fruit; 1/4 milk

Cranberry Mousse

(Recipe contains approximately 12% fat)

1 c. cranberry juice
  cocktail
1 (3 oz.) pkg. sugar-free
  raspberry gelatin
1 (16 oz.) can cran-raspberry
  sauce

1 pkg. Estee sugar-free
  whipped topping (pre-
  pared) or whipped top-
  ping of choice (see
  index)

Put cranberry juice in saucepan and heat just to boiling. Remove from heat and stir in gelatin, stirring until dissolved. In a mixing bowl, beat cran-raspberry sauce with an electric mixer on "high" for 1 minute. Gently fold cranberry juice mixture into sauce and chill 2 1/2 hours or until thickened, but not set. Fold in whipped topping until smooth and well blended. Spoon into serving dish or individual desserts. Chill.

Yield: 8 servings

Approximate Per Serving:
Calories: 159
Fat: 2.2 g
Cholesterol: 0.0 mg
Carbohydrates: 34 g
Protein: 1 g
Sodium: 27 mg

Diabetic Exchanges: 2 1/2 fruit; 1/2 milk

A soup ladle works great for filling small molds or pastry shells with gelatin, custard or other liquids.

Cranberry Salad

(Recipe contains approximately 3% fat)

1 (3 oz.) pkg. lemon-flavored gelatin, sugar-free	1 1/2 c. boiling water
	1 orange
	1/2 c. raw cranberries
2 T. sugar or equivalent sweetener	1/2 c. finely-chopped celery
	1 lg. apple, chopped

Dissolve gelatin in boiling water and add sugar (sweetener). Put in refrigerator until mixture is the consistency of egg whites. Grind peeled orange and cranberries. Add celery and apple; fold into chilled gelatin mixture. Pour into mold or individual serving dishes.

Yield: 8 servings

Approximate Per Serving:
Calories: 28
Fat: 0.1 g
Cholesterol: 0.0 mg
Carbohydrates: 5 g
Protein: 1 g
Sodium: 9 mg

Diabetic Exchanges: 1/2 fruit

To keep salads from getting soggy, place an inverted saucer in the bottom of the salad bowl.

Creamy Cranberry Salad

(Recipe contains approximately 24% fat)

2 (3 oz.) pkg. sugar-free
   raspberry gelatin
1 c. boiling water
1 c. cool water
1 c. cranberries, washed,
   stemmed & sorted

1/4 c. water
1 pkg. Estee sugar-free
   whipped topping, or
   sugar-free whipped
   topping of choice

Dissolve gelatin in boiling water and add cool water. Cook cranberries in 1/4 cup water until they pop, about 5 minutes. Add to gelatin mixture. Put in refrigerator until mixture begins to thicken. Fold in prepared Estee topping and chill until firm in a 9x9-inch square pan..
Yield: 9 servings

Approximate Per Serving:
Calories: 26
Fat: 0.7 g
Cholesterol: 0.0 mg
Carbohydrates: 5 g
Protein: 5 g
Sodium: 7 mg

Diabetic Exchanges: 1/4 fruit; 1/4 milk

Affix a cup hook under a cabinet or windowsill near the kitchen sink to hang rings and watches for safekeeping while doing dishes.

Delicious Mandarin Orange Salad

(Recipe contains approximately 18% fat)

1 c. boiling water
1 pkg. sugar-free orange-
 flavored gelatin
1 c. cool water
1 (11 oz) can mandarin
 oranges, drained

1 pkg. Estee sugar-free
 whipped topping, or
 sugar-free lowfat
 topping of choice

Dissolve gelatin in boiling water. Add cool water and put in refrigerator until mixture becomes the texture of egg whites. Stir in mandarin oranges and prepared whipped topping. Put into serving dish and refrigerate until firm.

Yield: 4 servings

Approximate Per Serving:
Calories: 83
Fat: 1.7 g
Cholesterol: 0.0 mg
Carbohydrates: 22 g
Protein: 10 g
Sodium: 13 mg

Diabetic Exchanges: 2 fruit

To clean your blender, put soap or detergent and a small amount of hot water into the bowl; blend for a minute, drain, rinse and dry.

Eggnog Cranberry Salad

(Recipe contains approximately 15% fat)

1 (3 oz.) pkg. vanilla pudding mix (not instant), sugar-free
1 (3 oz.) pkg. lemon-flavored gelatin, sugar-free
2 T. lemon juice
1 (3 oz.) pkg. raspberry gelatin, sugar-free
1 (16 oz.) can whole cranberry sauce
1/2 c. chopped celery
1 pkg. Estee sugar-free whipped topping (prepared, or whipped topping of choice (see index)
1/2 tsp. ground nutmeg

In a saucepan, put pudding mix, lemon gelatin and 2 cups water. Cook over medium heat until mixture begins to boil. Remove from heat and stir in lemon juice. Cool, then refrigerate until mixture thickens and begins to set. Dissolve raspberry gelatin in 1 cup boiling water, stirring constantly. Beat in cranberry sauce, then stir in celery. Chill until partially set, then fold in whipped topping and nutmeg. Chill mixture until partially set. Pour 1/2 pudding mixture into an 8x8-inch pan. Top with cranberry layer and add remaining pudding mixture. Chill overnight.
Yield: 12 servings

Approximate Per Serving:
Calories: 91
Fat: 1.5 g
Cholesterol: 0.0 mg
Carbohydrates: 20 g
Protein: 2 g
Sodium: 41 mg

Diabetic Exchanges: 2 fruit; 1/4 meat

When cutting marshmallows or dates, dip scissors into water and cut wet - they won't stick.

Festive Strawberry Salad

(Recipe contains approximately 9% fat)

1 (3 oz.) box strawberry-
flavored gelatin, sugar-
free
1 1/4 c. water

1 (10 oz.) box frozen strawberries, unsweetened,
thawed & drained (reserve
juice)
1 pt. nonfat frozen yogurt,
sugar-free

Put gelatin in mixing bowl and add water, reserved strawberry juice and frozen yogurt. Stir until smooth. Cool. When mixture begins to set, add strawberries. Pour into serving dish or individual dishes and chill.
Yield: 6 servings

Approximate Per Serving:
Calories: 101
Fat: 1.0 g
Cholesterol: 5
Carbohydrates: 19 g
Protein: 4 g
Sodium: 46 mg

Diabetic Exchanges: 2 fruit; 1/2 meat

*Keep a toothbrush around the kitchen sink - use
when cleaning beaters, graters, etc.*

Holiday Fruit Salad

(Recipe contains approximately 2% fat)

2 (3 oz.) pkg. sugar-free
   lemon-flavored gelatin
2 c. hot water
1 1/2 c. cold water
1 (8 oz.) can crushed pineapple, canned in own
   juice

2 c. homestyle sugar-
   free cranberry sauce
   (see index)
2 c. apples, peeled &
   diced
1 c. celery, diced

Dissolve gelatin in hot water. Add cold water, then pineapple. Chill. When mixture starts to thicken, add cranberry sauce, apples and celery. Pour into a 12 x 7 1/2-inch pan. Chill until firm. Cut into squares.
Yield: 8 servings

Approximate Per Serving:
Calories: 46
Fat: 0.1 g
Cholesterol: 0.0 mg
Carbohydrates: 9 g
Protein: 2 g
Sodium: 13 mg

Diabetic Exchanges: 1 fruit

Fresh lemon juice will remove onion odor from hands.

Jelled Peach Mold

(Recipe contains approximately 2% fat)

1 lg. can peaches, canned
in own juice, drained
(reserve juice)
1 box sugar-free lemon-
flavored gelatin

6 pkt. Equal sweetener, or
sweetener of choice to
equal 1/4 cup sugar
1/2 tsp. nutmeg

Drain peaches and process in blender until puréed. Set aside. Put peach juice in saucepan, adding enough water to make 1 cup liquid. Bring to boil. Remove from stove and add gelatin. Stir until gelatin dissolves. Add nutmeg, sweetener and puréed peaches. Blend. Pour into molds (one mold or individual molds). Chill until set.

Yield: 6 servings

Approximate Per Serving:
Calories: 56
Fat: 0.1 g
Cholesterol: 0.0 mg
Carbohydrates: 12 g
Protein: 2 g
Sodium: 10 mg

Diabetic Exchanges: 1 fruit

*Place thin-skinned fruits into a bowl, cover with
boiling water and allow to set for one minute.
Peel will come right off. May need paring knife for some.*

Peach of a Salad

(Recipe contains approximately 1% fat)

2 (3 oz.) pkg. sugar-free
   orange-flavored gelatin
3 1/2 c. water (divided)
1 env. unflavored gelatin
1 c. evaporated skim milk
24 pkt. Equal or sweetener
   of choice to equal 1 c. sugar

1 tsp. vanilla extract
1 (8 oz.) pkg. no-fat cream
   cheese, softened
2 c. sliced peaches,
   canned in own juice

Prepare 1 package of gelatin in 2 cups water as indicated on package. Pour into a 9x13x2-inch pan and chill until set. Soften envelope unflavored gelatin in 1/2 cup cool water. Heat evaporated skim milk and add softened gelatin. Heat until gelatin melts. Cool slightly, then add sweetener and vanilla. Put cream cheese into mixing bowl and gradually pour in warm milk mixture, whisking until mixture is smooth. Completely cool, then pour over set gelatin layer. Dissolve remaining package of orange gelatin in 1 cup boiling water. Add sliced peaches along with liquid. Pour over second layer and chill until set. Cut into squares and serve on lettuce leaf.

Yield: 12 servings

Approximate Per Serving:
Calories: 71
Fat: 0.1 g
Cholesterol: 4 mg
Carbohydrates: 10 g
Protein: 7 g
Sodium: 305 mg

Diabetic Exchanges: 1/4 milk; 1 fruit

To substitute for marshmallow creme,
melt 16 large marshmallows.

Quick Raspberry Salad

(Recipe contains approximately 8% fat)

1 (3 oz.) pkg. raspberry
   gelatin, sugar-free
1 c. boiling water
1 (10 oz.) pkg. frozen raspberries, unsweetened

1 c. unsweetened applesauce
1 c. prepared Estee sugar-
   free whipped topping,
   tinted green
6 maraschino cherries

Dissolve gelatin in boiling water. Add frozen raspberries and stir until thawed. Stir in applesauce. Pour into small stemmed dessert sherbets. Chill. Top with a dollop of tinted whipped topping and a cherry.
Yield: 6 servings

Approximate Per Serving:
Calories: 92
Fat: 0.8 g
Cholesterol: 0.0 mg
Carbohydrates: 23 g
Protein: 2 g
Sodium: 11 mg

Diabetic Exchanges: 2 fruit; 1/4 milk

Red and Green Holiday Salad

(Recipe contains approximately 23% fat)

2 (3 oz.) pkg. strawberry
   gelatin
2 c. boiling water
1 lg. pkg. frozen strawberries

2 bananas, sliced
1 sm. can crushed pineapple
2 c. "lite" whipped topping,
   tinted green

Dissolve gelatin in boiling water and add frozen strawberries. Stir until strawberries thaw and mixture begins to thicken. Add sliced bananas and undrained pineapple. Pour mixture into a 9x13-inch baking dish and chill until set. Top with whipped topping that has been tinted green. Garnish with maraschino cherry halves, if desired.
Yield: 16 servings

Approximate Per Serving:
Calories: 47
Fat: 1.2 g
Cholesterol: 0.0 mg
Carbohydrates: 7 g
Protein: 1 g
Sodium: 5 mg

Diabetic Exchanges: 1 fruit

Pasta & Rice Salads

Cheese, Pea and Pasta Salad

(Recipe contains approximately 18% fat)

1 (10 1/2 oz.) pkg. frozen
tiny green peas
Egg substitute to equal
2 eggs, scrambled &
chopped
1/4 c. chopped sweet
pickles
1/2 c. celery, chopped
4 green onions, sliced;
use part of green
1/2 c. mozzarella cheese,
lowfat, grated

1/3 c. "yogurt cheese"
(see index) (can use
plain lowfat yogurt)
3 T. no-fat, no cholesterol
mayonnaise
1/2 tsp. salt
1/4 tsp. pepper
3 T. minced fresh parsley
1 c. tiny shell macaroni
that has been cooked

Pour boiling water over peas and allow to stand for 1 minute. Drain well.
Combine peas with chopped scrambled egg substitute, pickles, celery,
green onions and cheese. Toss gently. Blend yogurt, mayonnaise, salt,
pepper and parsley. Stir into shell macaroni, then add pea mixture, blending
gently. Chill for at least 1 hour.
Yield: 6 servings

Approximate Per Serving:
Calories: 123
Fat: 2.5 g
Cholesterol: 5 mg
Carbohydrates: 14 g
Protein: 7 g
Sodium: 426 mg

Diabetic Exchanges: 1 bread; 1 meat

Crab and Pasta Salad

(Recipe contains approximately 8% fat)

1 can crabmeat, flaked
   & sorted
1 c. cooked small shell
   macaroni
1 can water chestnuts,
   drained & chopped
1/2 c. diced celery

1/4 c. green pepper
2 T. pimento, chopped
1/4 c. no-fat, no choles-
   terol mayonnaise
1/2 c. reduced-calorie
   buttermilk dressing

In a mixing bowl, put crabmeat, macaroni, chestnuts, celery, green pepper and pimento. Blend mayonnaise and buttermilk dressing and pour over pasta mixture. Blend well and refrigerate.
Yield: 6 servings

Approximate Per Serving:
Calories: 75
Fat: 0.7 g
Cholesterol: 23 mg
Carbohydrates: 12 g
Protein: 6 g
Sodium: 410 mg

Diabetic Exchanges: 1/2 meat; 3/4 bread

When recipe calls for sour cream, substitute by blending 1 cup low fat cottage cheese, 1 Tbl. milk, 1 Tbl. lemon juice. Store in refrigerator until needed.

Fiesta Salad

(Recipe contains approximately 8% fat)

4 c. shell macaroni, cooked
  per pkg. directions
1 (2 oz.) jar chopped
  pimento
1 can whole kernel corn,
  drained
1/2 c. diced green pepper
1/2 c. diced red pepper
1 T. parsley, minced

1/3 c. sweet pickle relish
1/2 c. no-fat, no-choles-
  terol mayonnaise
1 c. "yogurt cheese"
  (see index)
1 1/2 tsp. seasoned salt
1 tsp. sugar
1 T. vinegar
1/4 tsp. pepper

In a large mixing bowl, put macaroni, pimento, corn, green and red pepper, parsley and pickle relish. Blend mayonnaise, yogurt cheese, seasoned salt, sugar, vinegar and pepper. Pour over pasta mix and blend well. Refrigerate at least overnight.

Yield: 10 servings

Approximate Per Serving:
**Calories: 143
Fat: 1.2 g
Cholesterol: 1 mg
Carbohydrates: 34 g
Protein: 5 g
Sodium: 348 mg**

Diabetic Exchanges: 1 bread; 1/2 milk; 1 vegetable; 1/4 fat

Four ounces of cheese equals one cup shredded.

Layered Spaghetti Salad

(Recipe contains approximately 19% fat)

1 (16 oz.) pkg. thin
    spaghetti, break in 2"
    pieces & cook per pkg.
    directions
12 salad tomatoes, halved
8 radishes, sliced
2 carrots, diced
10 ripe olives, chopped
1 green pepper, chopped
1/4 c. Parmesan cheese
1 (16 oz.) btl. "Free" Italian
    dressing or "no oil"
    Italian dressing

Drain and cool spaghetti and then put half into 9x13-inch glass baking dish that has been lightly sprayed with cooking spray. Top with half of vegetables and sprinkle with 2 tablespoons of Parmesan cheese. Repeat layers. Pour Italian dressing evenly over salad. Cover with plastic wrap and allow to marinate overnight.

Yield: 12 servings

Approximate Per Serving:
Calories: 187
Fat: 3.9 g
Cholesterol: 1 mg
Carbohydrates: 34 g
Protein: 6 g
Sodium: 412 mg

Diabetic Exchanges: 2 bread; 1 vegetable; 1 fat

To make your own mustard, process in blender: 1/3 cup flour, 1/2 cup sugar, 1 tablespoon salt, 3/4 cup dry mustard, 1 1/2 cups white or wine vinegar, 1 green onion and dash of sugar. Blend until smooth.

Mac and Fruit Combo Salad

(Recipe contains approximately 12% fat)

1 c. cooked shell macaroni
2 c. mini marshmallows
1 can crushed pineapple,
   drained (reserve juice),
   unsweetened
1 can mandarin oranges,
   drained
1 c. pineapple juice (reserved from pineapple), use
   enough water to make a
   cup

1 T. flour
Pinch of salt
Egg substitute to equal
   2 eggs
18 pkt. Equal sweetener, or
   sweetener of choice to
   equal 3/4 cup sugar
1 pkg. Estee sugar-free
   whipped topping,
   prepared

In a large mixing bowl, put macaroni, marshmallows, pineapple and mandarin oranges. Stir to blend. Set aside. In a medium saucepan put pineapple juice, flour, salt and egg substitute. Cook until thickened, stirring constantly. Remove from stove, cool slightly and add sweetener. Cool, then fold in whipped topping and fold dressing into macaroni mixture. Chill.
Yield: 8 servings

Approximate Per Serving:
Calories: 129
Fat: 1.7 g
Cholesterol: 0.0 mg
Carbohydrates: 21 g
Protein: 1 g
Sodium: 20 mg

Diabetic Exchanges: 1 1/2 fruit, 1/2 bread, 1/2 fat

Toss salads well so you can use less dressing which is healthier.

Rice Salad Entrée

(Recipe contains approximately 6% fat)

3 c. cooked brown rice
2 green onions, sliced thin
1 c. carrots, grated
1 1/2 c. frozen peas
1/4 c. pimento, diced
1 (12-slice) pkg. nonfat
American cheese, diced
1 c. cooked chicken
breast, diced

1 T. dry Italian salad
dressing mix
3/4 c. no-fat, no choles-
terol mayonnaise
1/2 tsp. vinegar
1/2 tsp. seasoned salt
(opt.)
1/8 tsp. pepper

Put cooked rice in large mixing bowl and add onions, carrots, peas, pimento, diced cheese and chicken breast. Blend remaining ingredients and pour over rice mixture, tossing to blend. Chill. Serve on lettuce leaf.
Yield: 10 servings

Approximate Per Serving:
**Calories: 163
Fat: 1.0 g
Cholesterol: 15 mg
Carbohydrates: 15 g
Protein: 25 g
Sodium: 652 mg**

Diabetic Exchanges: 1/4 bread; 2 vegetable; 2 meat

Prepare ingredients such as greens, chopped onions, celery, carrots and radishes ahead of time. Store in separate airtight containers for quick use in a tossed salad.

Siesta Pasta Salad

(Recipe contains approximately 21% fat)

8 oz. vegetable spiral
   noodles
1 red onion, sliced thin &
   separated into rings
2 tomatoes, seeded & diced
1 green pepper, chopped

1 c. black beans, rinsed
   if canned
1 c. frozen corn, cooked
   & drained
1/2 avocado, diced
1 1/2 c. salsa
Fresh cilantro

Cook pasta according to package directions. Drain and cool. In a large mixing bowl, pour pasta, onion rings, tomato, green pepper, beans, corn and avocado. Toss with 3/4 cup salsa. Add chopped cilantro and serve with remaining salsa.

Yield: 12 servings

Approximate Per Serving:
Calories: 152
Fat: 3.5 g
Cholesterol: 0.0 mg
Carbohydrates: 25 g
Protein: 6 g
Sodium: 19 mg

Diabetic Exchanges: 1 1/2 bread; 1 vegetable; 1 fat

*The darker, outer leaves of lettuce are
higher in calcium, iron and Vitamin A.*

Tuna and Macaroni Salad

(Recipe contains approximately 15% fat)

4 c. salad macaroni, cooked
1 (10 oz.) pkg. frozen peas
1 (6 1/2 oz.) can water-
    packed tuna, drained
1 c. celery, finely diced
2 T. onion, chopped
1/4 c. sweet pickle, finely
    chopped

2 T. lemon juice
2 T. vinegar
1 T. canola oil
1 tsp. garlic salt or powder
1 c. "yogurt cheese" (see
    index) (can use plain
    lowfat yogurt)

Combine macaroni, peas, tuna, celery, onion and pickle. Blend lemon juice, vinegar, oil and garlic salt with yogurt. Pour dressing over macaroni mixture and toss lightly to blend. Allow to stand in refrigerator 2 hours before serving. Stir before serving.

Yield: 10 servings

Approximate Per Serving:
Calories: 151
Fat: 2.5 g
Cholesterol: 12 mg
Carbohydrates: 22 g
Protein: 11 g
Sodium: 100 mg

Diabetic Exchanges: 3/4 bread; 1 vegetable; 1/2 protein; 1/2 milk

Save sweet pickle juice. Store it in the refrigerator and use small amounts to thin dressings for salads.

Salad Dressings

Cottage Cheese Dilly Dressing

(Recipe contains approximately 18% fat)

1/2 c. lowfat cottage cheese
1/2 c. skim milk
1/4 c. lemon juice
1/2 tsp. seasoned salt (opt.)
1/2 tsp. paprika

1 tsp. dried dill
Egg substitute to equal 1 egg, scrambled & chopped up
1/2 lg. green pepper, finely chopped

Put cottage cheese, skim milk and lemon juice in blender. Allow to stand 3 minutes, then process until smooth. Add remaining ingredients and process briefly. Put into airtight container and chill.
Yield: about 1 1/2 cups

Approximate Per Serving:
Calories: 10
Fat: 0.2 g
Cholesterol: 4 mg
Carbohydrates: 1 g
Protein: 1 g
Sodium: 67 mg

Diabetic Exchanges: Free food—no countable exchanges for 1 tablespoon

Cleaning Copper - Just make paste of vinegar and salt.
Put on, let stand a few minutes and rinse off.

Herbed Yogurt Dressing

(Recipe contains approximately 25% fat)

1 c. plain lowfat yogurt	1 tsp. dry mustard
2 T. vinegar	1/4 tsp. Worcestershire sauce
1 green onion, finely	1/2 tsp. seasoned salt
chopped	1/4 tsp. garlic powder
1 tsp. celery seeds	1/2 tsp. Italian seasoning

Put all ingredients into mixing bowl and beat until smooth. Put into airtight container with lid and refrigerate.

Yield: about 1 cup

Approximate Per Serving:
Calories: 11
Fat: 0.3 g
Cholesterol: 0.0 mg
Carbohydrates: 1 g
Protein: 1 g
Sodium: 81 mg

Diabetic Exchanges for 1 tablespoon: free food

French Dressing

(Recipe contains approximately 0% fat)

1 c. tomato sauce	1/2 tsp. seasoned salt
2 T. vinegar	(opt.)
2 T. lemon juice	1/4 tsp. garlic powder
2 T. finely-chopped onion	1/8 tsp. black pepper
2 T. finely-chopped	
green pepper	

Combine all ingredients in a jar. Shake well to blend. Refrigerate. Shake well each time before using.

Yield: about 1 1/2 cups

Approximate Per Serving:
Calories: 4
Fat: 0.0 g
Cholesterol: 0.0 mg
Carbohydrates: 0.0 g
Protein: 1 g
Sodium: 106 mg

Diabetic Exchange Per 2 Tablespoons: Free food

French Dressing with Capers

(Recipe contains approximately 4% fat)

1 (8 oz.) btl. "Free" French
  dressing
Egg substitute to equal 1
  egg, scrambled, then
  chopped fine

1 T. capers, drained
1 green onion, diced
  very fine

Blend all ingredients and put into glass container with tight-fitting lid and store in refrigerator.
Yield: 1 cup

Approximate Per Tablespoon:
**Calories: 21
Fat: 0.1 g
Cholesterol: 0.0 mg
Carbohydrates: 4 g
Protein: Tr. g
Sodium: 156 mg**

Diabetic Exchanges: 1/4 bread

Suped Up Low-Cal French Dressing

(Recipe contains approximately 17% fat)

1 (8 oz.) btl. "Free" French
  dressing
Egg substitute to equal
  2 eggs, scrambled, then
  chopped up fine

10 sm. stuffed green
  olives, chopped
1 T. minced onion

Blend in all ingredients and put into airtight glass jar.
Yield: 1 1/4 cups

Approximate Per Tablespoon:
**Calories: 21
Fat: 0.4 g
Cholesterol: 0.0 mg
Carbohydrates: 3 g
Protein: 1 g
Sodium: 169 mg**

Diabetic Exchanges: 1/4 bread

Zingy French Dressing

(Recipe contains approximately 9% fat)

1 btl. "Free" French dressing
Egg substitute to equal
   1 egg, scrambled, then
   chopped fine
1 T. minced parsley or 1/2
   tsp. dried parsley

1 T. minced celery
1 green onion, chopped fine
1 tsp. Dijon mustard
1/2 tsp. Worcestershire
   sauce

Blend all ingredients and put into glass container with tight-fitting lid. Store in refrigerator. Use within a few days. This is great on potato salad.
Yield: about 1 1/4 cups

Approximate Per Serving:
Calories: 20
Fat: 0.2 g
Cholesterol: 0.0 mg
Carbohydrates: 3 g
Protein: 1 g
Sodium: 138 mg

Diabetic Exchanges: 1/4 milk

Lowfat Home-Style Mayonnaise

(Recipe contains approximately 13% fat)

2 T. flour
4 T. water
Egg substitute to equal
   2 eggs
1 c. vinegar

1/2 tsp. salt
1/2 c. water
24 pkt. Equal sweetener or
   sweetener of choice to
   equal 1 c. sugar

Blend flour with 4 tablespoons water until smooth. Add egg substitute, vinegar, salt and 1/2 cup water. Cook over medium heat until mixture thickens. Cool slightly, then add sweetener, blending well.
Yield: about 2 cups

Approximate Per Serving:
Calories: 7
Fat: 0.1 g
Cholesterol: 0.0 mg
Carbohydrates: 1 g
Protein: Tr. g
Sodium: 40 mg

Diabetic Exchanges: Free in limited amounts

Curried Mayonnaise

(Recipe contains only a trace of fat)

1 med. onion, minced	1 T. curry powder
1/2 c. minced green pepper	1 c. water
1/3 c. minced celery	1 c. no-fat, no choles-
2 frozen chicken stock	terol mayonnaise
cubes	Salt & pepper, to taste

In a saucepan, put onion, green pepper, celery and frozen stock cubes. Sauté until vegetables are tender. Stir in curry powder, blending well. Add water; bring to boil. Simmer 15 minutes. Pour mixture through fine sieve, pressing down on vegetables to retrieve all liquid. Discard vegetables and allow liquid to cool. In a mixing bowl, blend 1/3 cup of curry mixture with 1 cup mayonnaise. Add salt and pepper if desired. Store remaining curry mixture in airtight container until ready to use.

Yield: 1 1/2 cups

Approximate Per Tablespoon:
Calories: 12
Fat: Tr. g
Cholesterol: 0.0 mg
Carbohydrates: 3 g
Protein: Tr. g
Sodium: 139 mg

Diabetic Exchanges: Free food in limited amounts

Dill Mayonnaise

(Recipe contains approximately 0% fat)

1 c. reduced-calorie mayonnaise,	1/4 tsp. Worcestershire sauce
no fat and cholesterol	Dash of Tabasco sauce
3 tsp. lemon juice	1/8 tsp. pepper
3 tsp. dried dill weed	Dash of seasoned salt (opt.)

Mix all ingredients together and chill. This will keep for several weeks in the refrigerator.

Yield: about 1 cup

Approximate Per Tablespoon:
Calories: 13
Fat: 0.0 g
Cholesterol: 0.0 mg
Carbohydrates: 3 g
Protein: 0.0 g
Sodium: 206 mg

Diabetic Exchanges Per Tablespoon: Free food

Green Mayonnaise

(Recipe contains only a trace of fat)

2 c. no-fat, no-cholesterol
   mayonnaise
2 T. minced parsley
1 T. snipped chives

1 T. minced fresh tarragon
   or 1/2 tsp. dried tarragon
1 tsp. snipped dill
1/4 tsp. dried chervil

Put mayonnaise into bowl and fold in remaining ingredients, stirring with whisk until well blended.
Yield: about 2 1/2 cups

Approximate Per Tablespoon:
Calories: 10
Fat: Tr. g
Cholesterol: 0.0 mg
Carbohydrates: 2 g
Protein: 0.0 g
Sodium: 152 mg

Diabetic Exchanges: Free food in limited amounts

Horseradish Mayonnaise

(Recipe contains only a trace of fat)

2 c. no-fat, no-cholesterol
   mayonnaise

Juice from 1/2 lemon
1/4 c. horseradish

Put mayonnaise into mixing bowl and add lemon juice and horseradish. Blend until even in color and texture. Store in airtight jar.
Yield: 2 1/4 cups

Approximate Per Tablespoon:
Calories: 12
Fat: Tr. g
Cholesterol: 0.0 mg
Carbohydrates: 3 g
Protein: Tr. g
Sodium: 171 mg

Diabetic Exchanges: Free food in limited amounts

Mustard Mayonnaise
(This is great for potato salad)
(Recipe contains approximately 2% fat)

3/4 c. no-fat, no-cholesterol
   mayonnaise
Juice of 1/2 lemon

1 1/2 T. Dijon-style mustard
1/3 c. evaporated milk

Put mayonnaise into a mixing bowl and add lemon juice and mustard. Blend with wire whisk until even in texture and color. Fold in milk. Put into airtight jar and store in the refrigerator.
Yield: 1 cup

Approximate Per Tablespoon:
**Calories: 54
Fat: 0.1 g
Cholesterol: 0.0 mg
Carbohydrates: 3 g
Protein: Tr. g
Sodium: 165 mg**

Diabetic Exchanges: 1/4 milk

Watercress Mayonnaise
(Recipe contains no fat)

1 1/2 c. no-fat, no cholesterol mayonnaise
3/4 c. chopped watercress
   leaves
1 T. snipped dill

1 tsp. lemon juice
1 tsp. grated onion
1/4 tsp. salt
1/8 tsp. white pepper

Put mayonnaise into a blender and add remaining ingredients. Process until mixture is even in color. Store in airtight jar.
Yield: 1 1/2 cups

Approximate Per Tablespoon:
**Calories: 13
Fat: 0.0 g
Cholesterol: 0.0 mg
Carbohydrates: 3 g
Protein: 0.0 g
Sodium: 212 mg**

Diabetic Exchanges: Free food in limited amounts

Mayonnaise Tartar Sauce

(Recipe contains approximately 5% fat)

1 1/2 c. no-fat, no-choles-
    terol mayonnaise
3 green onions, minced
Egg substitute to equal
    1 egg, scrambled, then
    chopped up fine
1 T. capers, minced
1 T. minced parsley
1 T. minced onion

1/2 tsp. dried chervil
1 tsp. dried tarragon
1 tsp. Dijon-style mustard
1 tsp. lemon juice
1/2 pkt. Equal, or sweet-
    ener to equal 1 tsp. of
    sugar
1/4 tsp. salt (opt.)
1/8 tsp. white pepper

Put mayonnaise into mixing bowl. Add remaining ingredients and fold until mixture is of even color and texture. Store in airtight glass jar.
Yield: 1 1/2 cups

Approximate Per Tablespoon:
Calories: 17
Fat: 0.1 g
Cholesterol: 0.0 mg
Carbohydrates: 3 g
Protein: Tr. g
Sodium: 217 mg

Diabetic Exchanges: Free food in limited amounts

Lowfat Tartar Sauce

(Recipe contains approximately 10% fat)

1 c. no-fat, no-cholesterol
    mayonnaise
3 T. vinegar
4 med. chopped olives
1 T. capers

1 T. chopped dill pickles
1/8 tsp. pepper
1/4 tsp. seasoned salt
    (opt.)
1 tsp. Dijon mustard

Put all ingredients into mixing bowl and blend well. Store in airtight container. This will keep well for several weeks.
Yield: 1 1/2 cups

Approximately Per 2 Tablespoons:
Calories: 9
Fat: 0.1 g
Cholesterol: 0.0 mg
Carbohydrates: 2 g
Protein: 0.0 g
Sodium: 165 mg

Diabetic Exchanges: 1 tablespoon is free food

Notes & Recipes

Sugar -Free
and
Low-Sugar
Desserts

Desserts

Keeping Foods Sugar-Free and Low in Sugar
(This Chapter is Dedicated to the Many Diabetics Throughout the Country)

In this chapter you will find only sugar-free and low sugar foods that are also low in fat.

Since I have spent so much time testing and developing the foods in this chapter it is very special to me.

I am particularly proud of my Basic Cake Recipe. I spent many months and a great deal of time developing this cake. Many, many cakes hit the garbage can shortly out of the oven.

My quest was to find a way to bake a cake by incorporating the sweetener into the cake after it had been baked.

I had seen this done in a jellyroll type cake put out by Equal.

However, I found it difficult to develop a basic cake that would work for a variety of recipes. I am very proud of the one I have developed.

The reason for doing this is that Equal is the only sweetener I have found that does not leave an over-hang in the mouth.

The problem is that you can't bake with Equal. It turns bitter, loses its sweetness and is very offensive to the taste buds when exposed to high temperature.

In this chapter I have used all Equal as a sweetener. In each recipe you are given the choice of using Equal or using a sweetener of your own choice. The amount of sugar being replaced is also given. If you prefer to use sugar, simply use the amount given to replace the sweetener.

The candies in the chapter are also sugar-free. They are not exactly the candies that are sugar based. However, they are good and usually very welcome when sugar has been scratched from your score card.

Sugar is a simple carbohydrate and is not considered the best food in the world you can eat. This is due mainly to the fact that sugar contains almost no nutrients. It is often referred to as the "empty food".

Try some of the sugar-free and low sugar food in this chapter unless there is a reason for not using artificial sweeteners.

Although aspartame has been approved by the Food and Drug Administration the department does warn that it should not be consumed by the very young and by pregnant women.

Sugar-Free & Low Sugar Foods

Pies & Pie Crusts

Apple Pie Filling
(Recipe contains approximately 4% fat)

6 c. Granny Smith apples, peeled, cored & sliced	1/4 tsp. cardamom (opt.)
	1/4 tsp. salt (opt.)
2 c. unsweetened apple juice	2 T. cornstarch
1 tsp. cinnamon	24 pkt. Equal sweetener, or sweetener of choice to
1/4 tsp. nutmeg	equal 1 c. sugar

Put apple slices, 1 cup apple juice, cinnamon, nutmeg, cardamom and salt in saucepan; cook until apples are tender, stirring frequently. Add cornstarch to remaining cup of apple juice, blending with wire whisk until smooth. Add mixture to apple slices and cook until mixture thickens and becomes transparent, stirring constantly. Remove from stove and cool to room temperature. Add sweetener; blend. Pour into baked pie crust; serve in pudding dishes or in anything calling for apple pie filling
Yield: 8 servings

Approximate Per Serving (Crust Not Included):
Calories: 97
Fat: 0.4 g
Cholesterol: 0.0 mg
Carbohydrates: 19 g
Protein: Tr. g
Sodium: 68 mg

Diabetic Exchanges: 2 fruit

Apricot Pie Filling

(Recipe contains approximately 2% fat)

2 (16 oz.) cans apricot
   halves, water-packed or
   canned in natural juices
2 T. cornstarch
1/4 tsp. almond extract

1/4 tsp. cinnamon
24 pkt. Equal artificial
   sweetener, or sweetener
   of choice to equal 1 c.
   sugar

Drain apricots very well. It is best to pour apricot halves into strainer and allow to drip over pan for 10 minutes. Reserve 1 cup juice. In 1 cup juice, add cornstarch and beat with wire whisk until well blended. Cook over medium heat, stirring constantly until mixture thickens and becomes transparent. Add apricots and simmer 5 minutes. Remove from heat and add almond and cinnamon. Allow to cool to lukewarm and add sweetener. Pour into 9-inch baked pie crust or use in any recipe calling for apricot pie filling.

Yield: 8 servings

Approximate Per Serving (does not include pie crust):
Calories: 76
Fat: 0.2 g
Cholesterol: 0.0 mg
Carbohydrates: 16 g
Protein: 1 g
Sodium: 5 mg

Diabetic Exchanges: 1 1/2 fruit

*To keep pastry board or bowl from sliding around
on counter top, place a wet dishcloth under it.*

Cherry Pie Filling

(Recipe contains approximately 1% fat)

2 (16 oz.) cans sweetened
   tart cherries
1 T. cornstarch
1/2 tsp. almond extract

24 pkg. Equal artificial
   sweetener, or sweetener
   of choice to equal 1 cup

Drain cherries, very well. It is best to pour cherries in strainer and allow juice to drain out for about 10 minutes. Reserve 1 cup of juice. Combine 1 cup juice and cornstarch, beating with wire whisk until well blended. Cook over medium heat, stirring constantly, until mixture thickens and becomes transparent. Simmer for additional minute. Remove from heat and add almond and drained cherries. Allow to cool to lukewarm and add sweetener. Pour into 9-inch baked pie crust. Or use in any recipe calling for cherry pie filling.

Yield: 8 servings

Approximate Per Serving (does not include pie crust):
Calories: 111
Fat: 0.1 g
Cholesterol: 0.0 mg
Carbohydrates: 12 g
Protein: 2 g
Sodium: 17 mg

Diabetic Exchanges: 1 1/4 fruit

*Never shake a measuring utensil level; level off
with a spatula or the straight edge of a knife.*

Cheese Pie A'la Fruit

(Recipe contains approximately 17% fat)

1 (8 oz.) pkg. no-fat cream
  cheese, softened
9 pkt. Equal sweetener, or
  sweetener of choice to
  equal 1/3 cup sugar
1 pkg. Estee whipped topping
  (prepared), or sugar-free
  whipped topping of choice
  (see index)

1 recipe cherry pie filling
  (see index)
1 graham cracker crust
  (see index)

Beat cheese and sweetener until creamy. Beat in whipped topping. Spoon into prepared graham cracker crust. Top with pie filling and chill at least 3 hours.
Yield: 8 servings

Approximate Per Serving:
Calories: 243
Fat: 4.6 g
Cholesterol: 5 mg
Carbohydrates: 28 g
Protein: 8 g
Sodium: 545 mg

Diabetic Exchanges: 1 bread; 1 fruit: 1 milk; 1 fat

When making custard-type pies, bake at a high temperature for about 10 minutes to prevent a soggy crust. Finish baking at a lower temperature.

Chocolate Pie Filling

(Recipe contains approximately 22% fat)

1/4 c. cornstarch	2 tsp. tub margarine
1/2 tsp. salt (opt.)	18 pkt. Equal sweetener or
1/4 c. cocoa	sweetener of choice to
2 c. skim milk	equal 3/4 cup sugar
2 tsp. vanilla extract	

Combine cornstarch, salt and cocoa in a saucepan. Slowly add skim milk, stirring until smooth. Cook over medium heat to a boil; boil 2 minutes. Stir constantly while pudding cooks. Remove from heat and add vanilla and margarine. Cover saucepan with a saucer and cool 10 minutes. Add sweetener. Pour into dessert dishes or a baked pie shell; or use in any recipe calling for chocolate pie filling.

Yield: 8 servings

Approximate Per Serving:
Calories: 62
Fat: 1.5 g
Cholesterol: 8 mg
Carbohydrates: 8 g
Protein: 3 g
Sodium: 176 mg
Diabetic Exchanges: 3/4 milk; 1/2 fat

Put a layer of marshmallows in the bottom of a pumpkin pie before adding the filling. The marshmallows rise to the top during baking and make a nice topping.

Date-Cream Pie—Sugar-Free

(Recipe contains approximately 21% fat)

1/4 c. cornstarch
1 tsp. salt (opt.)
2 c. "light" sour cream
Egg substitute to equal
   2 eggs
2 c. dates, quartered
1 tsp. lemon juice

12 pkt. Equal sweetener, or
   artificial sweetener of
   choice to equal 1/2 c.
   sugar
1 (9") baked lowfat pie
   crust
1 pkg. Estee sugar-free
   whipped topping, or
   sugar free whipped topping of choice

In a saucepan, put cornstarch and salt. Stir in sour cream, whisking until mixture is smooth. Cook in double boiler, stirring constantly until mixture is smooth. This can also be cooked in microwave. When mixture has thickened, add a little hot mixture to egg substitute, then pour egg substitute into hot mixture. Add dates and stir well. Cool. Add lemon juice and sweetener; pour into baked pie crust. Prepare whipped topping and spread over pie within an hour of serving.

Yield: 8 servings

Approximate Per Serving:
Calories: 317
Fat: 7.3 g
Cholesterol: 0.0 mg
Carbohydrates: 39 g
Protein: 11 g
Sodium: 427 mg

Diabetic Exchanges: 1 milk; 1 bread; 1 fruit; 2 fat

Rinse a pan in cold water before
scalding milk to prevent sticking.

Easy Sugar-Free Pumpkin Pie

(Recipe contains approximately 19% fat)

1 (9") baked pie crust,
  lowfat (see index)
1 pkg. butterscotch sugar-
  free instant pie filling
1 3/4 c. skim milk
1 c. canned pumpkin
6 pkt. Equal sweetener, or
  sweetener of choice to
  equal 1/4 c. sugar

1/2 tsp. cinnamon
1/4 tsp. cardamom (opt.)
1/4 tsp. nutmeg
1/4 tsp. ginger
1 pkg. Estee sugar-free
  whipped topping

Prepare pudding with skim milk. Stir in pumpkin, Equal, cinnamon, cardamom, nutmeg and ginger. Pour into baked pie crust and chill several hours. Prepare whipped topping and spread over pie.
Yield: 8 servings

Approximate Per Serving:
Calories: 135
Fat: 2.9 g
Cholesterol: 1 mg
Carbohydrates: 21 g
Protein: 8 g
Sodium: 137 mg

Diabetic Exchanges: 1 bread; 1/2 milk; 1 fat

*Before measuring shortening, dip spoon in hot water -
the fat will slip out more easily.*

Eggnog Pie, Sugar-Free

(Recipe contains approximately 27% fat)

1 tsp. unflavored gelatin	1 tsp. vanilla
1 T. cold water	12 pkt. Equal sweetener, or
1 c. skim milk	sweetener of choice to
2 T. cornstarch	equal 1/2 c. sugar
1/4 tsp. salt	2 c. whipping topping, not
Egg substitute to equal	to exceed 0.5 grams of
2 eggs	fat per tablespoon
1 T. tub margarine	1 baked oil pie shell
2 T. rum or 1 tsp. rum	(see index)
flavoring	Dash of nutmeg

Put cold water in small bowl and sprinkle gelatin over it. Allow to soak for 5 minutes. Scald the milk and remove from stove. Blend cornstarch, salt and egg substitute. Add small amount of scalded milk to egg mixture, then pour mixture into milk. Add rum and put mixture on stove and bring to boiling point; simmer, but do not boil until mixture thickens. Remove from stove and add margarine and softened gelatin. Add vanilla and cool. Add sweetener. When completely cool, add Cool Whip. Pour into pie shell and sprinkle top with nutmeg. Chill before serving.

Yield: 8 servings

Approximate Per Serving:
Calories: 61
Fat: 1.8 g
Cholesterol: 1 mg
Carbohydrates: 4 g
Protein: 3 g
Sodium: 103 mg

Diabetic Exchanges: 1/4 milk; 1/2 fat

Ten graham crackers make one cup fine crumbs.

Frozen Yogurt Lemon Pie—Sugar-Free

(Recipe contains approximately 22% fat)

1 (16 oz.) can fruit cocktail, water-packed or canned in own juice, drain & reserve juice
1 (3 oz.) pkg. sugar-free lemon-flavored gelatin
1/2 c. water
2 c. sugar-free, lowfat frozen yogurt
1 pkg. Estee sugar-free whipping topping, or sugar-free whipped topping of choice
36 vanilla wafers

In a small saucepan, put reserved juice, water and sugar-free gelatin. Bring to a boil. Remove from stove and stir until gelatin has dissolved. Soften yogurt slightly, then fold into gelatin mixture, stirring until gelatin thickens and frozen yogurt melts. Fold in fruit cocktail. Line a 9-inch pie plate with cookies, both sides and bottom. Pour fruit mixture over cookies and refrigerate for at least 6 hours. Before serving, top with sugar-free whipped topping.

Yield: 8 servings

Approximate Per Serving:
Calories: 167
Fat: 2.9 g
Cholesterol: 2 mg
Carbohydrates: 31 g
Protein: 8 g
Sodium: 178 mg

Diabetic Exchanges: 1/2 bread; 1 milk; 1 fruit; 1/4 fat

When out of vanilla, use a little grated lemon or orange rind for flavoring or try a pinch of cinnamon or nutmeg.

Glazed Sugar-Free Strawberry Pie

(Recipe contains approximately 17% fat)

1 c. water
2 T. cornstarch
1 pkg. sugar-free straw-
 berry gelatin
3 to 4 drops red food coloring

24 pkt. Equal, or sweetener
 of choice to equal 1 c. sugar
1 pt. fresh strawberries,
 stemmed, cleaned & halved
1 lowfat pie crust (see index)

Put water and cornstarch in saucepan and whisk until smooth. Put on stove over medium heat and cook until mixture thickens. Remove from stove and stir in gelatin and food coloring. Cool slightly, then stir in sweetener. Line baked pie crust with fresh strawberries and pour glaze over berries. Chill before serving.

Yield: 8 servings

Approximate Per Serving:
Calories: 109
Fat: 2.1 g
Cholesterol: 0.0
Carbohydrates: 17 g
Protein: 3 g
Sodium: 139 mg

Diabetic Exchanges: 3/4 bread; 3/4 fruit; 1/2 fat

Grasshopper

(Recipe contains approximately 17% fat)

1 (9") baked, lowfat pie
 crust (see index)
2 pkg. sugar-free instant
 pudding (can use cooked,
 if desired)
4 c. skim milk

1/2 tsp. mint flavoring
2 to 3 drops green food
 coloring
1 pkg. Estee sugar-free
 whipped topping

Prepare pudding using skim milk and add mint flavoring. Add food coloring. Pour into baked 9-inch pie crust. Prepare whipped topping. Add 1 drop of food coloring so topping will be lighter than pie. Spread over pie.

Yield: 8 servings

Approximate Per Serving:
Calories: 156
Fat: 2.9 g
Cholesterol: 2 mg
Carbohydrates: 22 g
Protein: 9 g
Sodium: 214 mg

Diabetic Exchanges: 1 bread; 1/4 milk; 1 fat

Holiday Raspberry Frozen Yogurt Pie

(Recipe contains approximately 26% fat)

1 c. graham cracker crumbs
2 T. sugar, or equivalent
   artificial sweetener
2 T. tub margarine, melted
1 T. orange juice
1 (6 oz.) pkg. raspberry-
   flavored gelatin, sugar-
   free

1 c. hot water
1 (10 oz.) pkg. frozen raspberries, sugar-free
2 c. nonfat vanilla frozen
   yogurt (can use ice
   milk), sugar-free

Blend graham cracker crumbs, sugar, melted margarine and orange juice. Press into pie plate. Bake 10 minutes in 350° preheated oven. Mix gelatin and hot water until gelatin is dissolved. Add frozen raspberries and stir until dissolved. Add frozen yogurt and stir until smooth. Pour into cooled crust and refrigerate.
Yield: 8 servings

Approximate Per Serving:
Calories: 165
Fat: 4.8 g
Cholesterol: 3 mg
Carbohydrates: 33 g
Protein: 5 g
Sodium: 82 mg

Diabetic Exchanges: 1/2 bread; 1/2 milk; 2 fruit; 1/2 fat

When out of corn syrup, use one cup of sugar plus 1/4 cup water.

Mandarin Orange Pie

(Recipe contains approximately 22% fat)

1 (9") graham cracker pie
    crust (see index)
2 (3 oz.) pkg. sugar-free
    orange-flavored gelatin
2 c. boiling water, less 2 T.
2 c. sugar-free, lowfat
    yogurt, slightly softened
2 T. orange juice
    concentrate

1 (11 oz.) can mandarin
    oranges, drained
1 pkg. Estee sugar-free
    whipped topping, or
    sugar-free whipped
    topping of choice
    (see index)

Put gelatin in mixing bowl and add boiling water. Stir until gelatin has dissolved. Add frozen yogurt and orange juice concentrate, stirring until melted. Fold in drained mandarin oranges. Pour into graham cracker pie crust. Chill. Serve with 2 tablespoons whipped topping

Yield: 8 servings

Approximate Per Serving:
Calories: 195
Fat: 4.8 g
Cholesterol: 1 mg
Carbohydrates: 27
Protein: 9 g
Sodium: 139 mg

Diabetic Exchanges: 1 bread; 1 fruit; 1 meat; 1/2 fat

*Add a bit of sugar (without stirring) to
milk to prevent it from scorching.*

Peach Pie Filling

(Recipe contains approximately 1% fat)

2 (16 oz.) cans sliced
    peaches, water-packed
    or in natural juice
2 T. cornstarch
1/2 tsp. almond extract

1/4 tsp. cinnamon
24 pkt. Equal artificial
    sweetener or sweetener
    of choice to equal 1 c.
    sugar

Drain peaches very well. It is best to pour peach slices into strainer and allow to drip over pan for 10 minutes. Reserve 1 cup juice. In 1 cup juice, add cornstarch and beat with wire whisk until well blended. Cook over medium heat, stirring constantly, until mixture thickens and becomes transparent. Add peaches and simmer 5 minutes. Remove from heat and add almond and cinnamon. Allow to cool to lukewarm and add sweetener. Pour into 9-inch baked pie crust. Cool to room temperature or serve chilled. Or use in any recipe calling for peach pie filling.

Yield: 8 servings

Approximate Per Serving:
Calories: 71
Fat: 0.1 g
Cholesterol: 0.0 mg
Carbohydrates: 15 g
Protein: 1 g
Sodium: 5 mg

Diabetic Exchanges: 1 1/2 fruit

Twenty-two vanilla wafers equals one cup crumbs.

Pumpkin Pie on a Cloud

(Recipe contains approximately 18% fat)

1 pkg. Estee sugar-free
   whipped topping (pre-
   pared), or sugar-free
   whipped topping of
   choice to equal 2 c.
1 lowfat pie crust, baked
   (see index)
1 env. unflavored gelatin
1/4 c. cold water
1 1/4 c. pumpkin
1 1/4 c. evaporated skim
   milk

Egg substitute to equal
   1 egg
1/2 tsp. salt (opt.)
1/2 tsp. cinnamon
1/2 tsp. nutmeg
1/4 tsp. ginger
1/2 tsp. cardamom (opt.)
1/2 tsp. vanilla
24 pkt. Equal sweetener, or
   artificial sweetener of
   choice to equal 1 c.
   sugar
2 egg whites

Put prepared topping in pie shell and refrigerate. Sprinkle unflavored gelatin over water and set aside to soften. In a double boiler, put pumpkin, milk, egg substitute, salt, cinnamon, nutmeg, ginger and cardamom. Cook in double boiler until slightly thickened, stirring constantly. Add gelatin and vanilla; stir until gelatin dissolves. Remove from heat; chill until slightly thickened. Add 12 packets Equal sweetener. Beat egg whites until soft peaks form. Add 12 packets Equal. Fold into pumpkin mixture, stirring until of even color. Pour into pie plate, leaving a 1-inch rim of whipped topping showing. Chill until ready to serve.

Yield: 8 servings

Approximate Per Serving:
Calories: 164
Fat: 3.2 g
Cholesterol: 1 mg
Carbohydrates: 24 g
Protein: 11 g
Sodium: 241 mg

Diabetic Exchanges: 1 bread; 1 milk; 1/2 fat

Vanilla Cream Pie Filling—Sugar-Free

(Recipe contains approximately 12% fat)

1/2 c. cornstarch
1 tsp. salt (opt.)
4 c. skim milk
1 tsp. vanilla extract
1 tsp. almond extract

2 tsp. tub margarine
24 pkt. Equal sweetener, or
   sweetener of choice to
   equal 1 c. of sugar

In a saucepan put cornstarch and salt. Gradually add skim milk, stirring until smooth. Put on stove and over medium heat bring to boil. Boil 2 minutes. Remove from stove and stir in extracts and margarine. Cover and allow to stand 10 minutes. Stir in sweetener. Pour into 8 dessert dishes or baked pie shell.

Yield: 8 servings

Approximate Per Serving:
Calories: 80
Fat: 1.1 g
Cholesterol: 2 mg
Carbohydrates: 10 g
Protein: 4 g
Sodium: 341 mg

Diabetic Exchanges For Pudding: 1 milk

*Machine stitch circles on your pastry cloth
to indicate crust sizes you most often use.*

Baking Powder Pastry Dough

(Recipe contains approximately 30% fat)

2 c. flour, whole wheat
    blend, unbleached or
    enriched all-purpose
    flour
1 T. sugar
1 tsp. double-acting baking
    powder

1 tsp. salt
1/4 c. tub margarine, cold
Egg substitute to equal
    2 eggs

Put flour, sugar, baking powder and salt into a large mixing bowl. Cut in margarine until mixture resembles meal. Slowly add egg substitute, tossing with a fork. Form into a ball and knead lightly. Form dough into a ball; dust lightly with flour and chill for at least 1 hour before rolling out.

Yield: 2 pie crusts

Approximate Per Crust:
Calories: 742
Fat: 24.9 g
Cholesterol: 0.0 mg
Carbohydrates: 101 g
Protein: 19 g
Sodium: 1,471 mg

Diabetic Exchanges: 7 bread; 3 protein; 3 fat

Yield: 16 servings

Approximate Per Serving:
Calories: 46
Fat: 1.5 g
Cholesterol: 0.0 mg
Carbohydrates: 6 g
Protein: 1 g
Sodium: 91 mg

Diabetic Exchanges: 1/2 bread, 1/4 fat

Graham Cracker Pie Crust

(Recipe contains approximately 41% fat)

1 1/2 c. graham cracker
   crumbs
2 T. tub margarine

1/2 tsp. cinnamon, if
   desired
Cooking spray

Combine crumbs and melted tub margarine (and cinnamon, if using) and blend until margarine is evenly distributed into crumbs. Press firmly into a 9-inch pie plate. The bottom of a glass sprayed with cooking spray makes pressing the crumbs in place easier. Once the crumbs are pressed firmly into pie plate, spray crust very lightly with cooking spray. Bake in 350° preheated oven for 8 minutes and cool. Or chill 1 hour before filling without baking. Both methods work well.

Yield: 1 crust or 8 servings

Approximate Per Serving:
Calories: 81
Fat: 3.7 g
Cholesterol: 0.0 mg
Carbohydrates: 8 g
Protein: 1 g
Sodium: 98 mg

Diabetic Exchanges: 1/2 bread; 1 fat

Note: This crust should be filled with a lowfat filling to offset the high fat in the crust.

Glue rubber fruit-jar rings under each corner of your pastry board so it won't slide around when you roll out pie crust.

Lowfat Pie Crust

(Recipe contains approximately 27% fat)

2 c. enriched all-purpose
  flour
1/4 tsp. salt
1/4 c. vegetable spread
  (no more than 7 grams
  fat per tablespoon)

2 to 4 T. water, as needed
(do not use more than
needed, this is what
makes pie crusts very
tough—this & over-
handling)

Put flour and salt in mixing bowl and cut in vegetable spread. Tossing with a fork, add water, a tiny bit at a time. Form into ball and refrigerate dough for 15 minutes. Roll out (very thinly) between floured wax paper.
Yield: 2 crust

Approximate Per Crust:
Calories: 1,260
Fat: 37.6 g
Cholesterol: 0.0 mg
Carbohydrates: 190 g
Protein: 26 g
Sodium: 710 mg

Approximate Per Serving (8 servings per crust):
Calories: 79
Fat: 2.4 g
Cholesterol: 0.0 mg
Carbohydrates: 12 g
Protein: 2 g
Sodium: 44 mg

Diabetic Exchanges For 1 Serving: 3/4 bread; 1/4 fat

*Sprinkle your pastry board with 3-4 tablespoons
of quick rolled oats before rolling out dough to give
crust a "nutty" flavor and add a little extra nutrition.*

Mashed Potato Pie Crust

(Recipe contains approximately 12% fat)

2 lg. red potatoes, peeled & boiled	1/8 tsp. white pepper 1/2 c. onions, minced
1 T. skim milk	Cooking spray
1/4 tsp. salt (opt.)	

Mash boiled potatoes, adding milk, salt, pepper and minced onion. Beat until fluffy. Spray a 9-inch pie plate with vegetable oil and pour potatoes into pie plate. With a spatula or the back of a spoon, form a crust, leaving a nice well in center for filling. Bake in 375° preheated oven for 20 minutes. Spray with vegetable spray and bake another 15 minutes. Fill with desired filling and rebake, if necessary.

Yield: 1 (9-inch) crust

Approximate Per Crust:
Calories: 268
Fat: 3.6 g
Cholesterol: 0.0 mg
Carbohydrates: 59 g
Protein: 8 g
Sodium: 559 mg

Approximate Per Serving (serves 6):
Calories: 45
Fat: 0.6 g
Cholesterol: 0.0 mg
Carbohydrates: 10 g
Protein: 1 g
Sodium: 93 mg

Diabetic Exchanges: 2/3 bread

Use your onion chopper to make graham cracker crumbs. The crumbs won't crumble and will be finer than when rolled with a rolling pin.

Oatmeal Crust

(Recipe contains approximately 38% fat)

1 c. raw quick-cooking
  oats
1/3 c. enriched all-purpose
  flour
2 T. brown sugar, firmly
  packed

2 T. tub margarine, melted
3 T. water
Cooking spray

In a bowl, combine oats and flour, blending until even in texture. Stir in brown sugar. With a fork, toss in margarine and water. Press mixture into 9-inch pie plate, on bottom and sides. Bake in 375° preheated oven for 8 to 10 minutes. Cool before filling.
Yield: 8 servings

Approximate Per Crust:
Calories: 760
Fat: 32.0 g
Cholesterol: 0.0 mg
Carbohydrates: 112 g
Protein: 24 g
Sodium: 404 mg

Approximate Per Serving:
Calories: 95
Fat: 4.0 g
Cholesterol: 0.0 mg
Carbohydrates: 14 g
Protein: 3 g
Sodium: 51 mg

Diabetic Exchanges: 1 bread; 3/4 fat

A blow dryer works well to thoroughly dry washed canisters.
Prevents rust and keeps food dry and fresh.

Sugar-Free Cakes, Frostings, Sauces & Glazes

Cakes

Angel Layer Cake—Low Sugar

(Recipe contains approximately 2% fat)

6 egg whites, room temp.
1/2 tsp. cream of tartar
Dash of salt
1/3 c. sugar
1/4 tsp. vanilla extract

1/4 tsp. almond extract
(can use vanilla for
almond)
1/2 c. sifted flour, (sift
4 times, then measure)

Beat egg whites in a large mixing bowl until frothy. Add cream of tartar and salt; beat until soft peaks form. Gradually add sugar, no more than 1 tablespoon at a time, beating until stiff. Add vanilla and almond; beat another 30 seconds. With a metal spoon, gently fold in flour, in 3 additions. Pour batter into an ungreased 9-inch cake pan. Bake in a 325° preheated oven for 30 minutes. Cool in pan on wire rack for 40 minutes. Remove from pan and finish cooling on wire rack.
Yield: 12 servings

Approximate Per Serving:
Calories: 49
Fat: 0.1 g
Cholesterol: 0.0 mg
Carbohydrates: 10 g
Protein: 4 g
Sodium: 45 mg

Diabetic Exchanges: 1/2 meat; 1/2 bread

Angel Pudding Cake

(Recipe contains approximately 11% fat)

1 angel layer cake (see index)   1 3/4 c. skim milk
1 pkg. instant sugar-free
  pudding, any flavor

Bake angel layer cake and cool. With serrated knife, cut cake in half horizontally. Put half of cake on serving plate and frost with prepared pudding. Set second layer on top of first and frost cake with remaining prepared pudding.
Yield: 12 servings

Approximate Per Serving:
Calories: 79
Fat: 0.1 g
Cholesterol: 1 mg
Carbohydrates: 18 g
Protein: 9 g
Sodium: 87 mg

Diabetic Exchanges: 1/2 bread; 1/2 milk

For plump, juicy raisins in cakes and breads, soak raisins in hot water before adding to batter. Be sure to squeeze out well.

Applesauce Cake—Sugar-Free

(Recipe contains approximately 17% fat)

1/2 c. tub margarine, do not
  use diet margarine
Egg substitute to equal
  2 eggs or 4 egg whites
1 c. unsweetened
  applesauce
1 tsp. vanilla
2 c. enriched all-purpose
  flour
2 tsp. baking powder

1/2 tsp. baking soda
1/4 tsp. salt
1 tsp. ground cinnamon
1/4 tsp. ground cloves
1/4 tsp. ground allspice
1/4 c. raisins
1/4 c. boiling water
24 pkt. Equal sweetener, or
  sweetener of choice to
  equal 1 c. sugar

In a mixing bowl, put margarine, egg substitute, applesauce and vanilla. Beat with electric beater at low speed for 3 minutes. Blend flour, baking powder, baking soda, salt, cinnamon, cloves and allspice. Stir into egg substitute mixture with a wooden spoon until flour is moistened. Fold in raisins. Pour into 9x9-inch square pan that has been sprayed with vegetable oil. Bake in 350° oven for 45 to 50 minutes or until done. Remove from oven. Poke holes into cake with fork. Blend boiling water and Equal; drizzle slowly over cake, evenly. Cool. Frost.

APPLE CREAM FROSTING:

1 (8 oz.) pkg. low-calorie
  cream cheese, softened
1/2 c. plain, lowfat yogurt
2 T. apple juice concentrate,
  thawed

14 pkt. Equal sweetener, or
  sweetener of choice to
  equal 10 T. sugar

Blend all ingredients, mixing well. Spread on cake.
Yield: 12 servings

Approximate Per Serving:
Calories: 227
Fat: 4.4 g
Cholesterol: 4 mg
Carbohydrates: 37 g
Protein: 8 g
Sodium: 492 mg

Diabetic Exchanges: 1 bread; 1 fruit; 1 milk; 1 fat

Banana Cake—Low Sugar

(Recipe contains approximately 22% fat)

1/3 c. sugar
2 T. unsweetened
   applesauce
2 T. canola oil
Egg substitute to equal
   1 egg
1 1/2 c. enriched all-
   purpose flour
1 tsp. baking powder

1/4 tsp. nutmeg
Dash of salt
1 c. very ripe mashed
   banana
1 T. orange juice
   concentrate, thawed
1/2 tsp. vanilla extract
1/2 tsp. almond extract
Cooking spray

In a mixing bowl, put sugar, applesauce, oil and egg substitute. Beat at medium speed until mixture is smooth. Set aside. In a second bowl, combine flour, baking powder, nutmeg and salt. Set this mixture aside. Blend mashed banana, orange juice concentrate, vanilla and almond until well blended. Beginning and ending with flour, add flour mixture and banana mixture to oil mixture. Beat until just blended. DO NOT OVER-BEAT. Pour into an 8x8-inch square pan, lightly sprayed with cooking spray. Bake in 350° preheated oven for 25 minutes or until done. Cool in pan. Frost with Vanilla Cream Frosting (see index).
Yield: 9 servings

Approximate Per Serving:
Calories: 158
Fat: 3.9 g
Cholesterol: 0.0 mg
Carbohydrates: 29 g
Protein: 3 g
Sodium: 50 mg

Diabetic Exchanges: 1 bread; 1 fruit; 1 fat

Keep raisins and other fruits evenly distributed throughout cakes by dusting with flour before adding to batter.

Banana Chocolate Cake

(Recipe contains approximately 20% fat)

1 1/2 c. enriched all-purpose flour	2 T. unsweetened applesauce
2 T. unsweetened cocoa	Egg substitute to equal 1 egg
1 1/2 tsp. baking powder	
1/4 tsp. cinnamon	1 c. very ripe mashed bananas
2 T. tub margarine, softened	2/3 c. skim milk
1/4 c. sugar	1/2 tsp. vanilla

Blend flour, cocoa, baking powder and cinnamon; set aside. In a mixing bowl, cream margarine and sugar until light and fluffy. Add applesauce. Add egg substitute and mashed banana; blend well. Beginning and ending with flour, add flour mixture alternately with milk. Add vanilla and blend. Spoon batter into 9x9-inch baking pan that has been sprayed with cooking spray and bake in 350° preheated oven for 25 to 30 minutes, or until done. Cool in pan on wire rack. Frost with Chocolate Cream Frosting (see index).
Yield: 12 servings

Approximate Per Serving:
Calories: 114
Fat: 2.5 g
Cholesterol: Tr. mg
Carbohydrates: 21 g
Protein: 2 g
Sodium: 47 mg

Diabetic Exchanges: 1 bread; 1/2 fruit; 1/2 fat

To loosen cake layers or cookies left in pan too long, return to oven (350 degrees) for 2 minutes, them remove immediately.

Basic Low-Sugar Cake

(Recipe contains approximately 20% fat)

1/4 c. tub margarine
    (do not use diet)
1/4 c. sugar
1/4 c. unsweetened
    applesauce
1 tsp. vanilla extract
1 tsp. almond extract
    (can use vanilla, if
    preferred)

2 c. flour, whole wheat
    blend, unbleached or
    enriched all-purpose
1/2 tsp. salt
1 T. baking powder
1/3 c. dry milk granules
    (nonfat)
1 c. apple juice con-
    centrate, thawed
6 egg whites

In a large mixing bowl, beat margarine until fluffy. Add sugar and beat until well blended and smooth. Add applesauce, vanilla and almond; blend. In a second bowl, put flour, salt, baking powder and dry milk. Blend. Beginning with flour mixture, add to sugar mixture alternately with apple juice concentrate, ending with flour mixture. Beat egg whites until stiff and with a metal spoon very gently fold into batter. Divide batter between two 8-inch cake pans that have been lightly sprayed with cooking spray or pour into prepared 9x13-inch baking dish. Bake in 350° preheated oven for 30 to 35 minutes or until cake is done and springs back when pressed on with fingers. Leave in cake pans 10 minutes before removing from pan. Frost or serve as desired.

Yield: 10 servings

Approximate Per Serving:
Calories: 221
Fat: 5.0 g
Cholesterol: Tr. mg
Carbohydrates: 38 g
Protein: 5 g
Sodium: 254 mg

Diabetic Exchanges: 1 bread; 1 milk; 1 fruit; 1 fat

Basic Sugar-Free Cake

(Recipe contains approximately 22% fat)

1/4 c. tub margarine
(do not use diet)
1/4 c. unsweetened
applesauce
1 tsp. vanilla extract
1 tsp. almond extract (can
use 2 tsp. vanilla, if
preferred)
2 c. flour, whole wheat
blend, unbleached or
enriched all-purpose

1/2 tsp. salt (opt.)
1 T. baking powder
1/3 c. dry milk granules
1 c. unsweetened apple
juice concentrate,
thawed
6 egg whites
18 pkt. Equal sweetener, or
sweetener of choice to
equal 3/4 cup sugar
1/4 c. boiling water

In a mixing bowl, blend margarine, applesauce, vanilla and almond. Blend until smooth. In a separate bowl, blend flour, salt, baking powder and milk granules. Add dry ingredients to first mixture alternately with apple juice concentrate. Beat only until smooth—DO NOT OVERBEAT. Beat egg whites until stiff and gently fold into batter. Pour into two 9-inch cake pans or a 9x13-inch pan that have sprayed with cooking spray. Bake in 350° preheated oven for 30 to 35 minutes or until cake springs back when touched. Blend sweetener and boiling water. Poke holes into cake (or cakes) with fork at 1/2-inch intervals and slowly drizzle sweet liquid over it. Leave in pan 10 minutes, then remove from pan.
Yield: 10 servings

Approximate Per Serving:
Calories: 209
Fat: 5.0 g
Cholesterol: Tr. mg
Carbohydrates: 33 g
Protein: 5 g
Sodium: 237 mg

Diabetic Exchanges: 1 bread; 1 fruit; 1/2 milk; 1 fat

Basic Sugar-Free Chocolate Cake

(Recipe contains approximately 24% fat)

1 basic sugar-free cake, prepared & baked per directions, see index

To dry ingredients of basic cake add:

1/2 c. cocoa   **1/4 tsp. cinnamon**

Yield: 10 servings

Approximate Per Serving:
Calories: 220
Fat: 5.8 g
Cholesterol: Tr. mg
Carbohydrates: 36 g
Protein: 6 g
Sodium: 237 mg

Diabetic Exchanges: 1 bread; 1 1/2 fruit; 1/2 milk; 1 fat

Boston Cream Pie

(Recipe contains approximately 15% fat)

1 banana cake, low sugar (see index)

1 sm. pkg. vanilla sugar-free instant pudding

1 sm pkg. chocolate sugar-free instant pudding

3 3/4 c. skim milk

Bake banana cake per recipe directions. Can use 8-inch square or 8-inch round cake pan. Cool, then remove cake from pan and slice in half horizontally. Put 1/2 of cake on serving plate. Prepare vanilla pudding with 2 cups skim milk and spread over first layer. Pudding will probably have to set about 5 minutes before this can be done. Prepare chocolate pudding with 1 3/4 cups milk. Refrigerate for 5 minutes, then frost cake with chocolate pudding. Chill in refrigerator.

Yield: 9 servings

Approximate Per Serving:
Calories: 268
Fat: 4.6 g
Cholesterol: 2 mg
Carbohydrates: 56 g
Protein: 20 g
Sodium: 308 mg

Diabetic Exchanges: 2 bread; 2 milk; 1 fat

Cherry Topped Cake

(Recipe contains approximately 15% fat)

1 Basic Sugar-Free Cake,
  see index
1 (16 oz.) can unsweetened
  tart cherries
2 tsp. cornstarch

1/4 tsp. almond extract
12 pkt. Equal sweetener,
  or sweetener of choice
  to equal 1/2 c. sugar

Bake Basic Sugar-Free Cake in a 9x13-inch or 10-inch round cake pan. Leave a 9x13-inch cake in pan after baking. Remove 10-inch round cake to serving dish. Drain cherries and put juice in 1-cup measure. Add water, if needed, to make 1/2 cup liquid. Put juice and cornstarch in saucepan. Cook over medium heat, stirring constantly, until liquid thickens and becomes transparent. Simmer 1 additional minute. Remove from stove and add almond extract. Cool to lukewarm and add sweetener and cherries. Chill 20 minutes, then pour over top of cake.

Yield: 16 servings

Approximate Per Serving:
Calories: 165
Fat: 2.8 g
Cholesterol: Tr. mg
Carbohydrates: 24 g
Protein: 4 g
Sodium: 139 mg

Diabetic Exchanges: 1 bread; 1/2 milk; 1 fruit; 1/2 fat

Note: Peach or apple pie fillings work well on this also, see index for recipes.

Make the paper lining for the bottom of the cake pan a little smaller than the bottom of the pan. The lining will be easier to remove.

Cherry Topped Individual Cheese Cakes

(Recipe contains approximately 12% fat)

1 (8 oz.) pkg. no-fat cream style cheese
3 T. apple juice concentrate, thawed
12 pkt. Equal sweetener, or sweetener of choice to equal 1/2 c. sugar

1 pkg. Estee sugar-free whipped topping (prepared), or sugar-free whipped topping of choice
12 vanilla wafers
1/2 recipe Cherry Pie Filling, see index

Put softened cream cheese in mixing bowl and add apple juice concentrate and Equal. Beat at medium speed until light and fluffy. Fold in prepared whipped topping. Line 12 (2 1/2-inch) muffin tins with paper baking cups. Place 1 vanilla wafer in each cup. Fill with cheese mixture. Smooth off top and chill for 1 hour. Prepare Cherry Pie Filling and put on top of cheese mixture. Chill at least 1 hour before serving. If preferred, fresh fruit can be used on top of cheese mixture.
Yield: 12 servings

Approximate Per Serving:
Calories: 107
Fat: 1.4 g
Cholesterol: 3 mg
Carbohydrates: 16 g
Protein: 4 g
Sodium: 308 mg

Diabetic Exchanges: 1/4 milk; 1/2 bread; 1/2 fruit; 1/4 fat

To frost cupcakes, dip tops in soft icing and twirl slightly.

Chilled Pineapple Cake

(Recipe contains approximately 31% fat)

2 T. tub margarine
12 pkt. Equal sweetener, or
   sweetener of choice to
   equal 1/2 c. sugar
Egg substitute to equal
   2 eggs
1 c. Grape-Nuts cereal

1 (20 oz.) can crushed
   pineapple, water-packed
   or canned in natural
   juices (include juice)
48 vanilla wafers, crushed
   into crumbs

In a mixing bowl, cream margarine, sweetener and egg substitute, beating with an electric beater until smooth. With a wooden spoon, stir in pineapple and Grape-Nuts. Set aside. Crush vanilla wafers. In a 7x11-inch shallow dish, put 1/3 of crumbs and top with half of pineapple mixture. Top with another 1/3 of crumbs. Add remaining pineapple mixture, then remaining crumbs. Cover and chill for at least 8 hours. Cut into squares.
Yield: **12 servings**

Approximate Per Serving:
Calories: 163
Fat: 5.7 g
Cholesterol: 0.0 mg
Carbohydrates: 23 g
Protein: 5 g
Sodium: 336 mg

Diabetic Exchanges: 1 bread; 1 fruit; 1 fat

To make an angel food cake much taller than your cake pan, pin a strip of aluminum foil around top of pan; pour in batter and bake as usual.

Christmas Cake

(Recipe contains approximately 22% fat)

1 Basic Sugar-Free Cake,
  see index
1/2 c. boiling water
1/2 pkg. raspberry-flavored
  sugar-free gelatin

1/2 pkg. lime-flavored
  sugar-free gelatin
1 pkg. Estee sugar-free
  whipped topping

Prepare two 8-inch cake layers according to recipe directions. Turn one out onto serving plate after baking and poke holes in top with fork at 1/2-inch intervals. Blend 1/4 cup boiling water and red gelatin; slowly drizzle over cake. Top layer with whipped topping and set second layer on top of first layer. Poke second layer with holes; blend green gelatin and boiling water and drizzle over top layer. Frost cake with whipped topping. If desired, garnish with red and green maraschino cherries.

Yield: 10 servings

Approximate Per Serving:
Calories: 225
Fat: 5.6 g
Cholesterol: Tr. mg
Carbohydrates: 37 g
Protein: 10 g
Sodium: 244 mg

Diabetic Exchanges: 1 bread; 1 fruit; 1 milk; 1 fat

For an even cake, fill cake pans two-thirds full and spread batter well into corners and sides, leaving a slight hollow in the center.

Chocolate-Chocolate Trifle

(Recipe contains approximately 17% fat)

1 Basic Sugar-Free Chocolate Cake, see index	4 c. skim milk
2 pkg. instant sugar-free chocolate pudding	2 pkg. Estee whipped topping, or sugar-free topping of choice

Bake cake per package directions. Cool. Tear cake into small pieces and put 1/3 of cake in clear glass bowl (can also use punch bowl). Top with 1/3 of pudding, then 1/3 whipped topping. Repeat layers twice. Chill at least 8 hours before serving.
Yield: 16 servings

Approximate Per Serving:
Calories: 192
Fat: 3.6 g
Cholesterol: 1 mg
Carbohydrates: 35 g
Protein: 13 g
Sodium: 274 mg

Diabetic Exchanges: 1 bread; 1 milk; 1/2 fruit; 1/2 fat

Instead of using one square of unsweetened chocolate, substitute 3 tablespoons cocoa plus 3 tablespons tub margarine.

Easy Fresh Peach Cheesecake

(Recipe contains approximately 27% fat)

1 1/4 c. fine graham cracker crumbs
6 pkt. Equal, or sweetener of choice to equal 1/4 c. sugar
3 T. tub margarine, melted
1 (8 oz.) pkg. "light" cream cheese, room temp.

2 c. skim milk
1 (3 1/2 oz.) pkg. sugar-free instant lemon pudding*
3 peaches, sliced
1 T. lemon-flavored sugar-free gelatin, more if desired

Blend graham cracker crumbs, sweetener and margarine. Mix well and press firmly into 9-inch pie plate. Chill for at least 1 hour. Beat cream cheese and milk until smooth. Add instant pudding and beat until the consistency of pudding. Pour into chilled crust. Chill until firm. When about ready to serve, peel and slice peaches and arrange peach slices on top of cheesecake. Sprinkle with lemon-flavored gelatin and chill another 30 minutes.
Yield: 8 servings

Approximate Per Serving:
Calories: 193
Fat: 5.7 g
Cholesterol: 6 mg
Carbohydrates: 22 g
Protein: 9 g
Sodium: 527 mg

Diabetic Exchanges: 1 bread; 1/2 milk; 1/2 meat; 1 fat

*If you can't get instant lemon pudding, use instant vanilla pudding and add a package of sugar-free lemonade.

A cake is done if it shrinks slightly from the sides of the pan or if it springs back when touched lightly with the finger.

Fruit Trifle

(Recipe contains approximately 17% fat)

1 Basic Sugar-Free Cake
2 (3 1/2 oz.) pkg. instant
   sugar-free vanilla pudding
4 c. skim milk
1 qt. fresh strawberries,
   sliced
12 pkt. Equal, or sweetener
   of choice to equal 1/2 cup
   sugar, stirred into sliced
   strawberries

1 kiwi, peeled, sliced;
   slices halved
1 pkg. Estee whipped top-
   ping, or sugar-free topping of choice

Bake cake per package directions. Cool. Tear cake in small pieces and put 1/3 of cake in clear glass bowl (can also use punch bowl). Top with 1/3 of pudding. Layer 1/3 strawberries over pudding and top with 1/3 whipped topping. Put a row of kiwi around edge of bowl, then repeat layers twice. Top with 2 to 3 whole berries. Chill at least 8 hours before serving.
Yield: 16 servings

Approximate Per Serving:
Calories: 204
Fat: 3.8 g
Cholesterol: 1 mg
Carbohydrates: 39 g
Protein: 13 g
Sodium: 275 mg

Diabetic Exchanges: 1 bread; 1 milk; 1 fruit; 1/4 fat

*Unless instructed differently, a cake should
not be frosted until completely cool.*

Individual Low-Sugar Cheesecakes

(Recipe contains approximately 28% fat)

3/4 c. lowfat cream-style
    cottage cheese, drained
8 oz. ricotta cheese
1/3 c. sugar
Egg substitute to equal
    2 eggs

1 tsp. vanilla extract
Fresh peach slices
12 vanilla wafers
12 maraschino cherries

Put cottage cheese in a blender and process until smooth. Pour into medium mixing bowl. With an electric mixer, blend puréed cottage cheese and ricotta cheese until smooth. Add sugar gradually. Beat in egg substitute and vanilla extract. Line 12 (2 1/2-inch) muffin pans with paper baking cups. Place a vanilla wafer in each cup. Spoon mixture into muffin cups, making sure top surface is even. Bake in 350° preheated oven for 20 minutes or until set. DO NOT OVERBAKE. Centers should still be creamy when removed from oven. Remove from muffin pan and cool on rack. Chill. Just before serving remove paper liners and top with fresh peach slices and a maraschino cherry.

Yield: 12 servings

Approximate Per Serving:
Calories: 90
Fat: 2.8 g
Cholesterol: 18 mg
Carbohydrates: 11 g
Protein: 6 g
Sodium: 115 mg

Diabetic Exchanges: 1/2 bread; 1 protein

*When creaming margarine and sugar always wash
the bowl in hot water first to hasten creaming.*

Lemon Cake—Sugar-Free

(Recipe contains approximately 22% fat)

1 Basic Sugar-Free Cake,
   see index
1 pkg. sugar-free lemon-
   flavored gelatin

1/2 c. boiling water
1 pkg. Estee sugar-free
   whipped topping

Prepare cake as directed and bake in 9x13-inch baking pan for 30 to 35 minutes or until done. Do not use 4 tablespoons of boiling water mixed with 18 packets Equal. Instead, mix lemon-flavored gelatin with 1/2 cup boiling water. Polk holes in cake with fork at 1/2-inch intervals and slowly drizzle lemon mixture over cake. Cool completely, then top with packet of prepared Estee sugar-free whipped topping.

Yield: 18 servings

Approximate Per Serving:
**Calories: 125
Fat: 3.1 g
Cholesterol: Tr. g
Carbohydrates: 21 g
Protein: 5 g
Sodium: 134 mg**

Diabetic Exchanges: 1/2 bread; 1/2 fruit; 1/2 milk; 3/4 fat

*Use thread instead of a knife when a cake is to be cut
while still hot. This also works well on sheet cakes.*

Pineapple Cheesecake

(Recipe contains approximately 25% fat)

1 c. graham cracker crumbs
2 T. tub margarine, melted
1 pkg. unflavored gelatin
1/2 c. apple juice concentrate, thawed
1/2 c. boiling water
1 (16 oz.) ctn. lowfat cream-style cottage cheese, drained
12 pkt. Equal sweetener, or sweetener of choice to equal 1/2 c. sugar

1 T. lemon juice
1 tsp. vanilla
1 (8 oz.) can crushed pineapple, canned in own juice
1 T. water
2 tsp. cornstarch
6 pkt. Equal sweetener, or sweetener of choice to equal 1/4 c. sugar

In a mixing bowl, put graham cracker crumbs and tub margarine. Blend until of even consistency. Press into bottom of 8-inch springform pan that has been sprayed with cooking spray. Chill for 1 hour.

Sprinkle unflavored gelatin over thawed apple juice concentrate. Allow to stand 2 minutes to soften. Add boiling water and stir until gelatin dissolves. In a blender, process cottage cheese, artificial sweetener, lemon juice and vanilla. Process until smooth. Add gelatin mixture and process until well blended. Pour into springform pan that has been sprayed with cooking spray. Chill until solidly set.

In a saucepan, put crushed pineapple, water and cornstarch. Cook over medium heat, stirring constantly, until mixture comes to a boil. Remove from heat and cool. Stir in artificial sweetener and spread over cheesecake. Chill at least an hour before serving.

Yield: 10 servings

Approximate Per Serving:
Calories: 110
Fat: 3.1 g
Cholesterol: 17 mg
Carbohydrates: 16 g
Protein: 4 g
Sodium: 106 mg

Diabetic Exchanges: 1 bread; 1/4 meat; 1/2 fat

Pineapple Filled Cake

(Recipe contains approximately 18% fat)

1 Basic Sugar-Free Cake,
  see index
1 sm. can crushed pine-
  apple, drained (water
  packed or canned in
  natural juice)

1 pkg. instant sugar-free
  vanilla pudding
1 3/4 c. skim milk

Bake Basic Sugar-Free Cake in two 8-inch cake pans that have been sprayed with cooking spray. Remove from oven, poke with holes and drizzle with water-Equal as directed. Allow to stand 10 minutes, then remove from pans. Prepare instant sugar-free vanilla pudding with skim milk and add crushed pineapple. Put 1 layer of cake on serving dish and top with half of pudding mixture. Set second layer over pudding and top with remaining pudding mixture. Chill several hours before serving.
Yield: 12 servings

Approximate Per Serving:
Calories: 211
Fat: 4.2 g
Cholesterol: 1 mg
Carbohydrates: 38 g
Protein: 4 g
Sodium: 276 mg

Diabetic Exchanges: 2 bread; 1 fruit; 3/4 fat

When doing any sort of baking, you will get better results if cookie sheets, muffin tins or cake pans are preheated.

Pineapple Upside-Down Cake

(Recipe contains approximately 19% fat)

1 Basic Sugar-Free Cake,
   see index
1 lg. can pineapple slices,
   drained (use water-
   packed pineapple, or
   pineapple canned in
   natural juice)

6 pkt. Equal sweetener, or
   sweetener of choice to
   equal 2 T. sugar

Cut pineapple slices in half and arrange in a 10-inch cake pan that has been sprayed with cooking spray. Prepare Basic Sugar-Free Cake and pour over pineapple halves. Bake in 350° preheated oven for 25 to 30 minutes or until done. Remove from oven and drizzle with boiling water and Equal per cake recipe directions. Allow to cool slightly, then remove from pan onto serving dish. Sprinkle pineapple halves with 6 packets Equal.
Yield: 12 servings

Approximate Per Serving:
Calories: 194
Fat: 4.2 g
Cholesterol: Tr. mg
Carbohydrates: 31 g
Protein: 4 g
Sodium: 198 mg

Diabetic Exchanges: 1 bread; 1 fruit; 1/2 milk; 1 fat

*Clean clothespins provide cool handles to steady
a cake when removing from a hot oven.*

Sugar-Free Banana Cake

(Recipe contains approximately 21% fat)

1 Basic Sugar-Free Cake, prepared & baked per package directions

Substitute 1 c. very ripe mashed bananas for applesauce
Decrease apple juice concentrate by 1/4 cup

Yield: 10 servings

Approximate Per Serving:
Calories: 217
Fat: 5.1 g
Cholesterol: Tr. mg
Carbohydrates: 35 g
Protein: 5 g
Sodium: 237 mg

Diabetic Exchanges: 1 bread; 1 fruit; 1/2 milk; 1 fat

Strawberry Cake Deluxe

(Recipe contains approximately 22% fat)

1 Basic Sugar-Free Cake (see index)
1 1/2 c. boiling water
2 pkg. sugar-free strawberry-flavored gelatin

1 (10 oz.) pkg. unsweetened, frozen strawberries
1 pkg. Estee sugar-free whipped topping, or Sugar-Free Whipped Topping (see index)

Bake Basic Sugar-Free Cake in 9x13-inch pan for 25 to 35 minutes. Omit boiling water and Equal drizzle. Instead blend 1/2 cup boiling water with 1 package sugar-free strawberry-flavored gelatin. Mix until gelatin is dissolved. Poke holes in cake with fork at 1/2-inch intervals. Slowly pour strawberry mixture over cake evenly. Dissolve second package of strawberry gelatin in 1 cup boiling water and add frozen strawberries, stirring until strawberries are thawed. Set in refrigerator for 10 minutes. Prepare 1 package of whipped topping and spread over cake. Top with strawberry mixture. Chill.
Yield: 18 servings

Approximate Per Serving:
Calories: 129
Fat: 3.1 g
Cholesterol: Tr. mg
Carbohydrates: 21 g
Protein: 5 g
Sodium: 134 mg

Diabetic Exchanges: 1 bread; 1 fruit; 1/2 fat

Sugar-Free Cake with Mother's Nutmeg Dip

(Recipe contains approximately 28% fat)

1 Basic Sugar-Free Cake	1/2 tsp. nutmeg
2 T. tub margarine	6 pkt. Equal sweetener, or
2 T. flour	sweetener of choice to
Dash of salt	equal 1/4 cup sugar
1 1/2 c. water	

Bake cake in 10-inch round pan. Allow to cool after drizzling with water and Equal. Turn out onto serving plate and set aside. In a small saucepan, blend margarine and flour. Cook over medium heat for about 3 minutes to cook flour. Add salt and very slowly whisk in water until mixture is smooth. Cook over medium heat until mixture thickens. Remove from heat and add nutmeg and sweetener. Pour over cake. Can be served warm, or chilled and served cold.

Yield: 12 servings

Approximate Per Serving:
Calories: 198
Fat: 6.1 g
Cholesterol: Tr. mg
Carbohydrates: 29 g
Protein: 4 g
Sodium: 275 mg

Diabetic Exchanges: 1 bread; 1 fruit; 1/2 milk; 1 fat

Use a thread instead of a knife when cutting a hot cake.

Frostings

Chocolate Cream Frosting

(Recipe contains approximately 16% fat)

1 (8 oz.) pkg. fat-free cream
   cheese (less than 1 gram
   fat per ounce)
12 pkg. Equal sweetener, or
   sweetener of choice to
   equal 1/2 c. sugar

2 T. cocoa
1/8 tsp. cinnamon
1 pkg. Estee sugar-free
   whipped topping,
   prepared

In a mixing bowl, beat cream cheese until fluffy, about 5 minutes. Add sweetener, cocoa and cinnamon and blend well. Add whipped topping and blend quickly. Refrigerate for 5 minutes, then frost cake. Frosts a 9x13-inch cake or one 8 or 9-inch layer cake.
Yield: 16 servings

Approximate Per Serving:
Calories: 28
Fat: 0.5 g
Cholesterol: 3 mg
Carbohydrates: 4 g
Protein: 5 g
Sodium: 215 mg

Diabetic Exchanges: 1/3 milk

When creaming margarine and sugar, rinse the bowl with boiling water first and it will cream faster.

Lemon Cream Frosting

(Recipe contains approximately 13% fat)

1 (8 oz.) pkg. fat-free cream cheese (less than 1 gram fat per ounce)
12 pkt. Equal sweetener, or sweetener of choice to equal 1/2 cup sugar
1 T. lemon juice
1/4 tsp. grated lemon zest
1/2 tsp. lemon extract
1 pkg. Estee sugar-free whipped topping (prepared), or whipping topping substitute of choice (see index)

In a mixing bowl, beat cream cheese until fluffy, about 5 minutes. Beat in sweetener, lemon juice, lemon zest and lemon extract. Quickly beat in whipped topping. Refrigerate 5 minutes before frosting cake. Frosts one 9x13-inch cake or an 8 or 9-inch layer cake.
Yield: 16 servings

Approximate Per Serving:
Calories: 27
Fat: 0.4 g
Cholesterol: 3 g
Carbohydrates: 4 g
Protein: 5 g
Sodium: 108 mg

Diabetic Exchanges: 1/2 milk

To substitute for one ounce bitter chocolate, blend four tablespoons cocoa plus 3 tablespoons tub margarine.

Vanilla Cream Frosting

(Recipe contains approximately 13% fat)

1 (8 oz.) pkg. fat-free cream
cheese (less than 1 gram
fat per ounce)

12 pkt. Equal sweetener, or
sweetener of choice to
equal 1/2 cup sugar

1 pkg. Estee sugar-free
whipped topping (pre-
pared)

In a mixing bowl, beat cream cheese until fluffy, about 5 minutes. Beat in sweetener. Add whipped topping and quickly beat in. Refrigerate 5 minutes, then frost cake. Frosts one 9x13-inch cake or one 8-inch layer cake.

Yield: 16 servings per recipe

Approximate Per Serving:
Calories: 27
Fat: 0.4 g
Cholesterol: 3 mg
Carbohydrates: 4 g
Protein: 5 g
Sodium: 215 mg

Diabetic Exchanges: 1/2 milk

*When a recipe calls for powdered sugar (1 cup) and you
are out, put 1 cup granulated sugar and 2 tablespoons
cornstarch in blender and process until very fine.*

Sauces & Glazes

Chocolate Sauce—Sugar-Free

(Recipe contains approximately 21% fat)

3 T. cocoa
4 tsp. cornstarch
1/8 tsp. salt
1 1/2 c. skim milk
1 T. tub margarine

2 tsp. vanilla
12 pkt. Equal sweetener, or
artificial sweetener of
choice to equal 1/2 c.
sugar

In a saucepan, put cocoa, cornstarch and salt. Blend. Gradually add skim milk, stirring until smooth. Add tub margarine and cook over medium heat, stirring constantly, until mixture boils. Boil 2 minutes; remove from heat and add vanilla and sweetener. Pour into container with lid; cool to room temperature, then chill. Best if served at room temperature.
Yield: 1 1/2 cups or 12 (2 tablespoons) servings

Approximate Per Serving:
Calories: 26
Fat: 0.6 g
Cholesterol: 1 mg
Carbohydrates: 3 g
Protein: 1 g
Sodium: 41 mg

Diabetic Exchanges: 1/4 milk

When recipe calls for cake flour, you can substitute
1 cup all-purpose flour minus 2 tablespoons and
add 2 tablespoons of cornstarch. Blend and sift.

Deluxe Pineapple Sauce—Sugar-Free

(Recipe contains approximately 8% fat)

Dash of salt (opt.)
3 T. cornstarch
2 c. pineapple juice, unsweetened
1 c. unsweetened orange juice

18 pkt. Equal sweetener, or artificial sweetener of choice to equal 3/4 cup sugar
1 pkg. Estee sugar-free whipped topping
1 sm. can crushed pineapple, drained

Put cornstarch in saucepan with salt. Gradually add pineapple juice, stirring until mixture is smooth. Add orange juice. Cook over medium heat until mixture thickens. Add sweetener. Cool to room temperature. Prepare whipped topping. Start beating thickened juice mixture, then slowly add prepared whipped topping, beating until blended. Add crushed pineapple. Serve over cake.

Yield: 12 servings

Approximate Per Serving:
Calories: 69
Fat: 0.6 g
Cholesterol: 0.0 mg
Carbohydrates: 14 g
Protein: 3 g
Sodium: 24 mg

Diabetic Exchanges: 1 fruit; 1/4 milk

When the recipe calls for a four-cup baking dish, use: a 9-inch pie plate, an 8 x 1 1/4-inch layer cake pan or a 7 3/8 x 3 5/8 x 2 1/4-inch loaf pan.

Orange Sauce—Sugar-Free

(Recipe contains approximately 1% fat)

2 T. cornstarch
1/8 tsp. salt
1/4 c. orange juice
  concentrate
1 3/4 c. water

6 pkg. Equal sweetener, or
  sweetener of choice to
  equal 1/4 cup sugar
1 (11 oz.) can mandarin
  oranges, drained

In a small saucepan, put cornstarch and salt. Dissolve orange juice concentrate in water and gradually add to cornstarch mixture, stirring until mixture is smooth. Cook over medium heat until mixture is thickened and transparent. Simmer an additional 2 minutes. Remove from stove and stir in sweetener. Fold in mandarin oranges. Serve over cake warm, or over sugar-free ice cream or frozen yogurt at room temperature.

Yield: 8 servings

Approximate Per Serving:
Calories: 65
Fat: 0.1 g
Cholesterol: 0.0 mg
Carbohydrates: 9 g
Protein: Tr. g
Sodium: 36 mg

Diabetic Exchanges: 1 fruit

When a recipe calls for one pound of sugar, use 2 cups sugar.

Orange Glaze

(Recipe contains approximately 18% fat)

1/4 c. cornstarch
1 c. orange juice
1 tsp. lemon juice
2 tsp. tub margarine
2 T. grated orange rind

Pinch of salt
24 pkt. of Equal, or sweet-
    ener of choice to equal
    1 cup sugar

Put cornstarch in saucepan and gradually add orange juice, stirring until mixture is smooth. Add lemon juice, margarine, grated orange rind and pinch of salt. Cook over medium heat until mixture thickens. Remove from heat and add sweetener. Serve over cake or ice cream.

Yield: 1 cup or 16 tablespoons

Approximate Per Serving:
Calories: 25
Fat: 0.5 g
Cholesterol: 0.0 mg
Carbohydrates: 2 g
Protein: Tr. g
Sodium: 21 mg

Diabetic Exchanges: 1/4 fruit

Vanilla Glaze

(Recipe contains no fat)

1/4 c. cold water
1 1/2 tsp. cornstarch
Dash of salt

12 pkt. Equal sweetener
1 tsp. vanilla

Put cold water and cornstarch in a small saucepan and blend until smooth. Add salt. Cook over medium heat until mixture thickens and becomes clear. Remove from heat and add sweetener and vanilla. Brush over cookies or a cake. If using on a cake, double the recipe.

Yield: enough for 3 dozen cookies; double recipe will do a 9x13-inch cake

Approximate Per Serving:
Calories: 100
Fat: 0.0 g
Cholesterol: 0.0 mg
Carbohydrates: 0.0 g
Protein: 0.0 g
Sodium: 266 mg

Diabetic Exchanges: Free food when used on cookies or cake

Cookies & Bars

Cookies

Apple Oatmeal Cookies

(Recipe contains approximately 19% fat)

1/3 c. raisins
3/4 c. apple juice concentrate, heated to boiling
1/2 c. tub margarine, do not use diet
1/2 c. unsweetened applesauce
Egg substitute to equal 2 eggs

1 tsp. vanilla extract
2 c. enriched all-purpose flour
1 tsp. cinnamon
1 tsp. baking powder
1/2 tsp. baking soda
2 c. rolled oats

Combine raisins and hot apple juice concentrate and set aside until mixture cools to room temperature and raisins plump. In a large mixing bowl, put margarine and applesauce and cream with electric beater to soften, and until mixture becomes fluffy. Add egg substitute, 1/4 cup at a time, beating after each addition. Add vanilla extract and beat an additional minute.

Stir together flour, cinnamon, baking powder and baking soda with wire whisk until blended. Add oats to creamed mixture, stirring with wooden spoon. Blend well. Stir in flour mixture, raisins and juice, stirring just until flour is moist. Do not overstir. Drop by heaping tablespoonful onto cookie sheet that has been sprayed with cooking oil. With bottom of glass that has been sprayed with cooking oil, flatten cookie to a circle 2 inches in diameter. Bake in 375° preheated oven for 10 to 12 minutes. With a fork, poke several holes into cookies. Brush with glaze; remove from cookie sheet and cool on rack.

GLAZE:
1/4 c. apple juice concentrate, heated

18 pkt. Equal sweetener, or sweetener of choice to equal 3/4 cup sugar

Yield: 36 large cookies (1 per serving)

Continued on follwoing page

Continued from preceding page

Approximate Per Serving:
Calories: 91
Fat: 1.9 g
Cholesterol: Tr. mg
Carbohydrates: 18 g
Protein: 2 g
Sodium: 20 mg

Diabetic Exchanges 1 bread; 1/2 fat

Carrot and Pineapple Cookies with Dates
(Low Sugar)
(Recipe contains approximately 29% fat)

2 c. enriched all-purpose
    flour
1 1/2 tsp. baking powder
1 1/2 tsp. cinnamon
1 tsp. nutmeg
1/4 c. tub margarine,
    softened
1/4 c. brown sugar, firmly
    packed
Egg substitute to equal
    1 egg

1/4 c. unsweetened
    applesauce
1/2 tsp. vanilla
1 c. shredded carrots
1 sm. can unsweetened
    crushed pineapple,
    drained (1 cup)
1/2 c. dates, finely
    chopped
Cooking spray

In a mixing bowl, put flour, baking powder, cinnamon and nutmeg. Stir with whisk until even in color; set aside. In a second mixing bowl, put margarine and beat until fluffy. Cream in brown sugar, beating at medium speed. Add egg substitute and beat until mixture is smooth. Add applesauce and vanilla; beat. With a wooden spoon, stir in flour mixture. Add carrots, pineapple and dates; blend well. At 2-inch intervals, drop by teaspoonfuls onto baking sheets that have been lightly sprayed with cooking spray. Bake in 350° preheated oven for 12 minutes or until nicely browned.
Yield: 60 cookies

Approximate Per Cookie:
Calories: 28
Fat: 0.9 g
Cholesterol: 0.0 mg
Carbohydrates: 6 g
Protein: 1 g
Sodium: 19 mg

Diabetic Exchanges (3 cookies): 1 bread; 1/2 fruit

Cream Puffs

(Recipe contains approximately 21% fat)

1 c. enriched all-purpose flour	2 T. tub margarine
1/4 tsp. salt	Egg substitute to equal 2 eggs
1 c. water	1 egg white

Combine flour and salt; set aside. Combine water and margarine in a large saucepan and bring to a boil. Turn heat to low and add flour mixture, stirring constantly until mixture leaves the sides of the pan. Remove from heat and cool 4 minutes. Add egg substitute, 1/4 cup at a time, stirring until well blended between each addition. Add egg white and stir until smooth. Spray baking sheet with cooking spray and drop dough by teaspoonfuls onto baking sheet. Bake in 400° preheated oven for 25 minutes or until crisp and nicely browned. Cool on racks. When cool, fill with lowfat sugar-free pudding.

Yield: 24 puffs

Approximate Per Puff, Filled with Lowfat, Sugar-Free Pudding:
Calories: 48
Fat: 1.1 g
Cholesterol: 0.0
Carbohydrates: 8 g
Protein: 4 g
Sodium: 86 mg

Diabetic Exchanges: 1/4 bread; 1/3 milk; 1/4 fat

*One pound of powdered sugar equals
3 1/2 cups powdered sugar.*

Date Cookies

(Recipe contains approximately 30% fat)

1 c. finely crushed graham cracker crumbs
1/2 c. enriched all-purpose flour
3 T. nonfat dry milk granules
1/2 tsp. baking soda
1/2 tsp. salt
Egg substitute to equal 3 eggs
1/4 c. apple juice concentrate, unsweetened
1/4 c. tub margarine, softened (do not use diet)
1/4 c. unsweetened applesauce
1/2 c. chopped dates
1/4 c. water
18 pkt. Equal sweetener, or sweetener of choice to equal 3/4 cup sugar

Put graham cracker crumbs, flour, dry milk, baking soda and salt in a mixing bowl. Stir with wire whisk until mixture is well blended. Add egg substitute, apple juice concentrate, margarine and applesauce. Beat at medium speed for 1 minute. With a wooden spoon, stir in dates. Drop by tablespoonfuls onto cookie sheet sprayed with cooking spray and bake in 375° preheated oven for 10 to 12 minutes or until lightly browned. Mix water and Equal and brush over cookies after removing from oven. Cool on wire rack.

Yield: 24 cookies (1 cookie per serving):

Approximate Per Serving:
Calories: 85
Fat: 2.9 g
Cholesterol: 1 mg
Carbohydrates: 11 g
Protein: 1 g
Sodium: 88 mg

Diabetic Exchanges: 1 bread; 1/2 fat

One and one-third cups packed brown sugar equals one cup of granulated sugar.

Date Drop Cookies

(Recipe contains approximately 17% fat)

2 T. tub margarine
2 T. brown sugar, or
  equivalent sweetener
1/4 c. unsweetened
  applesauce
2 T. apple juice concentrate
Egg substitute to equal
  1 egg

1 tsp. vanilla
1 c. enriched all-purpose
  flour
1/2 tsp. baking soda
1/2 tsp. ground cinnamon
1/8 tsp. nutmeg
3/4 c. oatmeal, uncooked
3/4 c. chopped dates
Cooking spray

Cream margarine and sugar until fluffy. Add applesauce, apple juice, egg substitute and vanilla. Blend until smooth. Blend flour, baking soda, cinnamon and nutmeg; add. Blend well. Stir in oatmeal and dates. Drop by teaspoonfuls onto cookie sheet that has been sprayed with cooking spray. Bake in 350° preheated oven for 12 to 14 minutes. Cool on rack.
Yield: 42 cookies

Approximate Per Cookie:
Calories: 47
Fat: 0.9 g
Cholesterol: 0.0 mg
Carbohydrates: 7 g
Protein: 1 g
Sodium: 9 mg

Diabetic Exchanges (2 cookies): 1 bread; 1/4 fat

Sometimes toothpicks are too short to test a cake for doneness.
When this happens use an uncooked piece of spaghetti.

Date N' Apple Cookies

(Recipe contains approximately 29% fat)

3 T. tub margarine,
  softened
3 T. brown sugar, firmly
  packed
2 T. honey
Egg substitute to equal
  1 egg
1 tsp. vanilla
1 c. enriched all-purpose
  flour

1/2 tsp. baking soda
1/2 tsp. cinnamon
1/4 tsp. cardamom (opt.)
1/8 tsp. nutmeg
3/4 c. raw old-fashioned
  oats
1/2 c. grated Red Delicious
  apple
1/4 c. chopped dates
Cooking spray

In a mixing bowl, beat margarine until fluffy. Slowly add brown sugar. Add honey and beat. Add egg substitute and beat. Add vanilla. In a second bowl, put flour, baking soda, cinnamon, cardamom, nutmeg and oats. Blend until even in color and texture. Stir into first mixture. Add apples and dates. Blend until evenly mixed. Spray cookie sheets with cooking spray and drop batter by teaspoonfuls about 2 inches apart onto cookie sheets. Bake in 350° preheated oven for 12 to 14 minutes or until done. Cool on rack.
Yield: 42 cookies

Approximate Per Serving:
Calories: 34
Fat: 1.1 g
Cholesterol: 0.0 mg
Carbohydrates: 5 g
Protein: 1 g
Sodium: 13 mg

Diabetic Exchanges (3 cookies): 1 bread; 1/4 fat

Split cupcakes and frost instead of frosting top when to be used for lunches. This way frosting will not stick to wrap.

Glazed Chocolate Low-Sugar Cookies

(Recipe contains approximately 32% fat)

1 3/4 c. flour
2 tsp. baking powder
1/2 tsp. salt (opt.)
1/2 tsp. cinnamon
2 T. cocoa
1/4 c. sugar

1/2 c. apple juice concentrate
1/4 c. water
1/4 c. canola oil
Egg substitute to equal
1 egg

In a small mixing bowl, put flour, baking powder, salt, cinnamon and cocoa. Stir with whisk to blend; set aside. In a medium mixing bowl, put sugar, apple juice concentrate, water, oil and egg substitute. Blend well. Stir in dry ingredients, blending just until flour is moist. Drop by teaspoonfuls onto a baking sheet that has been sprayed with vegetable oil. Bake 10 to 12 minutes or until done.

GLAZE:
1/4 c. water
1 1/2 tsp. cornstarch
Dash of salt

1 tsp. vanilla
12 pkt. Equal sweetener, or
sweetener of choice to
equal 1/2 cup sugar

Put water and cornstarch in pan and whisk until smooth. Add salt. Cook over medium heat until thick and clear. Remove from heat and add vanilla and sweetener. When cookies come out of oven, and while still hot, brush each cookie with glaze.
Yield: 34 cookies

Approximate Per Serving:
Calories: 50
Fat: 1.8 g
Cholesterol: 0.0 mg
Carbohydrates: 7 g
Protein: 1 g
Sodium: 42 mg

Diabetic Exchanges: 1/2 bread; 1/2 fat

Krispie Date Balls—Sugar-Free

(Recipe contains approximately 26% fat)

1/2 c. tub margarine (do not use diet)	1 pkg. chopped dates
Egg substitute to equal 1 egg	24 pkt. of Equal sweetener, or sweetener of choice to equal 1 cup sugar
1 tsp. vanilla	3 c. Rice Krispies cereal

Put margarine, egg substitute, vanilla and dates in a saucepan and boil for 10 minutes. Remove from stove and add sweetener. Stir in cereal. Chill for about 1 hour. Form into balls.
Yield: 50 balls

Approximate Per Ball:
Calories: 26
Fat: 0.7 g
Cholesterol: 0.0 mg
Carbohydrates: 3 g
Protein: Tr. g
Sodium: 45 mg

Diabetic Exchanges (3 cookies): 1 bread

A pair of pinking shears makes an ideal cookie cutter or pastry trimmer to trim the edges of pies, to cut fancy sandwiches and to cut odd-shaped cookies. Keep a pair of pinking shears just for kitchen use.

Low-Sugar Oatmeal Cookies

(Recipe contains approximately 17% fat)

1 T. tub margarine
1/4 c. firmly-packed brown
    sugar, or sugar substitute
1/3 c. applesauce
Egg substitute to equal
    1 egg
1 tsp. vanilla extract

1/2 c. enriched all-purpose
    flour
1/2 c. quick-cooking oats,
    uncooked
1/4 tsp. baking powder
1/4 tsp. baking soda
3/4 c. Rice Krispies cereal

Cream margarine and add sugar, beating until light and fluffy. Add applesauce and beat until smooth and well blended. Add egg substitute and vanilla; blend. Combine flour, oats, baking powder and baking soda. Gradually add to creamed mixture. Stir in cereal. Drop dough from teaspoon onto ungreased cookie sheets. Bake in 350° preheated oven for 8 to 10 minutes. Cool on wire racks.

Yield: 32 cookies

Approximate Per Serving:
Calories: 27
Fat: 0.5 g
Cholesterol: 0.0 mg
Carbohydrates: 5 g
Protein: 1 g
Sodium: 18 mg

Diabetic Exchanges (3 cookies): 1 bread

For oatmeal that's piping hot, stir in 1/3 cup instant dry milk per serving and a little extra water as the cereal cooks.

No-Bake Apple-Peanut Butter Balls

(Recipe contains approximately 30% fat)

1/2 c. skim milk	3 T. instant nonfat dry milk
1/3 c. apple juice concen-	granules
trate	1 tsp. vanilla
1/4 c. creamy peanut butter	3 c. oat bran flakes cereal
from refrigerator section	1 c. Rice Krispies cereal
of store, pour off any oil	
from top of jar before	
dipping out peanut butter	

Combine milk, apple juice concentrate, peanut butter and milk granules in a saucepan. Cook over medium heat, stirring constantly until mixture is hot. Remove from stove and add vanilla. In a large mixing bowl put cereal. Mix, then pour peanut butter mixture over cereal, stirring until cereal is evenly coated. Spray hands lightly with cooking spray and shape into 1 1/2-inch balls. Place on cookie sheet and put in refrigerator until chilled through.
Yield: 16 balls

Approximate Per Ball:
Calories: 74
Fat: 2.5 g
Cholesterol: Tr. mg
Carbohydrates: 14 g
Protein: 3 g
Sodium: 136 mg

Diabetic Exchanges: 1 bread

For a quick cake decoration, press an animal-shaped cookie cutter into the center of an iced cake. Tint shape with contrasting food colors.

Pineapple Oatmeal Cookies

(Recipe contains approximately 22% fat)

1 1/2 c. sifted enriched
   all-purpose flour
2 tsp. baking powder
1/2 tsp. salt
1/2 tsp. cinnamon
2 c. rolled oats
1 c. unsweetened crushed
   pineapple, drained very,
   very well

1/4 c. tub margarine
1/4 c. sugar
1/4 c. brown sugar
Egg substitute to equal
   2 eggs
1/2 c. skim milk

Sift together flour, baking powder, salt and cinnamon. Stir in rolled oats and crushed pineapple; set aside. In a large mixing bowl, cream margarine and sugars until fluffy. Add egg substitute, 1/4 cup at a time. With a wooden spoon, stir in flour mixture and milk alternately. Drop by teaspoonfuls onto a cookie sheet that has been sprayed with cooking spray. Bake in 375° preheated oven for 12 to 15 minutes or until golden brown. Remove from sheet and cool on wax paper.

Yield: 36 cookies

Approximate Per Serving:
Calories: 71
Fat: 1.7 g
Cholesterol: Tr. mg
Carbohydrates: 12 g
Protein: 2 g
Sodium: 69 mg

Diabetic Exchanges: 3/4 bread; 1/4 milk

Before creaming hard margarine, put beaters
in hot water for a few minutes.

Sugarless Fruit Cookies

(Recipe contains approximately 24% fat)

1 c. flour, whole wheat
   blend, unbleached or
   enriched all-purpose
1 c. oatmeal
1 tsp. baking soda
1 tsp. baking powder
1/2 tsp. cinnamon
1/4 tsp. ground cardamom
1/4 tsp. nutmeg
1/3 c. tub margarine

1/4 c. orange juice con-
   centrate, thawed
1/4 c. apple juice con-
   centrate, thawed
Egg substitute to equal
   2 eggs
1 c. raisins
1/2 c. apples, peeled,
   cored & diced
1/2 c. chopped dates

In a large mixing bowl, combine flour, oatmeal, baking soda, baking powder, cinnamon, cardamom and nutmeg. Cut in margarine. Add orange juice concentrate, apple juice concentrate and egg substitute. Stir in raisins, apples and dates. Refrigerate dough 4 hours. Drop by teaspoonfuls onto cookie sheet that has been sprayed with cooking spray. Bake in 350° preheated oven for 10 to 12 minutes. Watch closely as these burn quickly when done. Store in refrigerator.

Yield: 4 dozen

Approximate Per Cookie:
Calories: 50
Fat: 1.6 g
Cholesterol: 0.0 mg
Carbohydrates: 7 g
Protein: 1 g
Sodium: 18 mg

Diabetic Exchanges (2 cookies): 1 bread; 1/2 fruit; 1/4 fat

An ice bucket makes a good cookie jar.

Sugar-Free Cocoa Drops

(Recipe contains approximately 21% fat)

1 c. raisins	2 c. flour
1/2 c. apple juice concen- trate	2 c. oatmeal
	1 T. baking soda
1/4 c. tub margarine	4 T. cocoa
1 c. applesauce	1 tsp. cinnamon
1 tsp. vanilla	1/2 tsp. salt
Egg substitute to equal 1 egg	

Put raisins, apple juice concentrate, margarine and applesauce in saucepan and bring to boil. Remove from heat and cover. Allow to stand 10 minutes. Remove lid and allow mixture to cool. When cool, add vanilla add egg substitute. In a large mixing bowl, put remaining ingredients. Add raisin mixture, stirring until well blended. Drop on baking sheets that have been sprayed with cooking spray. Bake in 350° preheated oven for 12 to 15 minutes. Cool on rack.

Yield: 6 dozen cookies

Approximate Per Cookie:
Calories: 39
Fat: 0.9 g
Cholesterol: 0.0 mg
Carbohydrates: 7 g
Protein: 1 g
Sodium: 24 mg

Diabetic Exchanges: 1/2 bread

Clean the tip of a cake-decorating tube
by using a pipe cleaners as a brush.

Sugar-Free Date Filled Cookie

(Recipe contains approximately 29% fat)

1/2 c. canola oil	2 tsp. baking powder
1/3 c. tub margarine	3 c. flour, unbleached,
Egg substitute to equal	whole wheat blend or
2 eggs	enriched all-purpose
1 tsp. vanilla extract	10 pkt. Equal sweetener,
1 tsp. almond extract	or sweetener of choice

With an electric beater, cream together oil and margarine until smooth. Add egg substitute, vanilla extract and almond extract. Beat until smooth. Blend together baking powder and flour and stir into liquid mixture with wooden spoon. Chill for at least 1 hour. Roll out on lightly floured surface to 1/8-inch thickness. Cut with 2-inch cookie cutter to make 72 rounds.

FILLING:

2 c. chopped dates	1/4 c. orange juice
1/2 c. water	concentrate

Put above ingredients in saucepan and cook for 10 to 15 minutes or until thick. Put a scant teaspoonful on 24 cookies and top with a second cookie round. Press fork around edge of 2 cookie rounds to seal together. Place on baking sheet and bake in 400° oven for 8 to 10 minutes or until lightly browned. Watch carefully so as not to overbrown. Remove from oven and sprinkle with Equal.
Yield: 24 cookies

Approximate Per Cookie:
Calories: 185
Fat: 5.9 g
Cholesterol: 0.0 mg
Carbohydrates: 21 g
Protein: 3 g
Sodium: 50 mg

Diabetic Exchanges: 1 bread; 1 fruit; 1 fat

Sugar-Free Raisin Drops

(Recipe contains approximately 22% fat)

3/4 c. water	Egg substitute to equal
3/4 c. apple juice	2 eggs
concentrate	2 c. flour
1/4 c. oil	1 tsp. baking soda
1/4 c. applesauce	1/8 tsp. salt
2 c. raisins	1 tsp. baking powder
1 tsp. vanilla	1 tsp. cinnamon

In a saucepan, put water, apple juice concentrate, oil, applesauce and raisins. Bring to boil. Remove from stove; add vanilla and cover. Set aside for 10 minutes. Remove lid and cool. When cool, add egg substitute. In a large mixing bowl, put flour, soda, salt, baking powder and cinnamon. Stir with whisk to blend. Add raisin mixture, stirring with wooden spoon until well blended. Drop onto baking sheets that have been sprayed with cooking spray. Bake in 400° preheated oven for 8 minutes.
Yield: 60 large cookies

Approximate Per Cookie:
Calories: 46
Fat: 1.1 g
Cholesterol: 0.0 mg
Carbohydrates: 9 g
Protein: 1 g
Sodium: 15 mg

Diabetic Exchanges: 1/2 bread; 1/4 fat

Crisp Cookies: For thin unbroken cookies, remove cookies from oven after 6 minutes of baking. Slide spatula under each cookie, then return to oven to finish baking.

Sugar-Free Raisin Filled Fold-Overs

(Recipe contains approximately 28% fat)

1/4 c. canola oil
1/4 c. unsweetened
   applesauce
1/3 c. tub margarine
Egg substitute to equal
   2 eggs
1 tsp. vanilla extract
1 tsp. almond extract

2 tsp. baking powder
1 tsp. cinnamon
3 c. flour, unbleached,
   whole wheat blend or
   enriched all-purpose
10 pkt. Equal sweetener,
   or sweetener of choice

With an electric mixer, blend oil, applesauce and margarine. Add egg substitute, beating until smooth. Blend in vanilla and almond extracts. Blend together baking powder, cinnamon and flour; stir into liquid mixture with wooden spoon. Chill for at least 1 hour. Roll out on floured surface to 1/8-inch thick and cut with 2-inch cutter. Place scant teaspoon of filling on each round. Fold over and seal by pressing edge firmly with tines of fork. Place on baking sheet and bake at 400° for 8 to 10 minutes or until lightly browned. Remove from oven and sprinkle with sweetener. Cool on rack.

RAISIN FILLING:
3 c. raisins

1/2 c. orange juice
   concentrate

Put ingredients in saucepan and cook until mixture becomes thick.
Yield: 48 cookies

Approximate Per Serving:
Calories: 87
Fat: 2.7 g
Cholesterol: 0.0 mg
Carbohydrates: 14 g
Protein: 1 g
Sodium: 22 mg

Diabetic Exchanges: 1 bread; 1/2 fruit; 1 fat

Bars

Apple-Brownies

(Recipe contains approximately 31% fat)

1 1/4 c. enriched all-
purpose flour
1/2 c. sugar
1/4 c. unsweetened cocoa
1 1/2 tsp. baking powder
1/2 tsp. cinnamon
1/4 tsp. salt
1/4 tub margarine, melted
(not diet margarine)

1/4 c. unsweetened
applesauce
Egg substitute to equal
2 eggs
2 tsp. vanilla
1 c. peeled & grated apples
Cooking spray

In a mixing bowl, put flour, sugar, cocoa, baking powder, cinnamon and salt. Blend with wire whisk until well blended and even in color. Add margarine, applesauce, egg substitute and vanilla. Beat at medium speed until well blended. Add grated apples, stirring them in with wooden spoon. Pour batter into 9x9-inch square baking pan that has been lightly sprayed with cooking oil. Bake in 325° preheated oven for 25 to 30 minutes or until done. Cool in pan on rack. Cut in 16 squares.
Yield: 16 servings

Approximate Per Serving:
Calories: 104
Fat: 3.6 g
Cholesterol: 0.0 mg
Carbohydrates: 17 g
Protein: 2 g
Sodium: 53 mg

Diabetic Exchanges: 1 bread; 1/4 fruit; 1/2 fat

Bran and Applesauce Bars

(Recipe contains approximately 27% fat)

1 c. enriched all-purpose
   flour
2/3 c. Bran Buds, 100%
   Bran or All-Bran
1/2 c. rolled oats
1/2 tsp. salt (opt.)
1/2 tsp. baking soda
1 tsp. baking powder
1 tsp. cinnamon
1/4 tsp. nutmeg
1/2 tub margarine (do
   not use diet)

Egg substitute to equal
   2 eggs
1 tsp. vanilla
1/2 c. chopped dates
1 c. unsweetened apple-
   sauce, room temp.
1/2 c. apple juice concentrate, heated to boiling
18 pkt. Equal sweetener, or
   artificial sweetener of
   choice to equal 3/4 cup
   sugar

In a mixing bowl, put flour, bran, oats, salt, baking soda, baking powder, cinnamon and nutmeg. With a wire whisk, mix dry ingredients until well blended. Blend margarine, egg substitute, vanilla, dates and applesauce; stir into dry ingredients with a wooden spoon, stirring just until flour is moistened. Pour into a 9x13-inch pan that has been sprayed with cooking spray and spread evenly over pan. Bake in 375° preheated oven for 25 to 30 minutes or until brown. When done, bars should pull away slightly from pan. Remove from oven and poke holes into bars with fork at 1/2-inch intervals. Mix heated apple juice concentrate and sweetener. Slowly drizzle over bars. Cut into 15 squares.
Yield: 15 servings

Approximate Per Serving:
Calories: 122
Fat: 3.6 g
Cholesterol: 0.0 mg
Carbohydrates: 15 g
Protein: 3 g
Sodium: 147 mg

Diabetic Exchanges: 1 bread; 1 fat

Eclair Linda May—Sugar-Free

(Recipe contains approximately 22% fat)

1 c. enriched all-purpose
    flour
1/4 tsp. salt
1 c. water
2 T. tub margarine
Egg substitute to equal
    2 eggs
1 egg white
1 pkg. sugar-free chocolate
    instant pie filling

1 (3 oz.) pkg. no-fat cream
    cheese, softened
6 pkt. Equal sweetener, or
    sweetener of choice
1 T. cocoa
1/2 pkg. Estee sugar-free
    whipped topping,
    prepared

Combine flour and salt. Set aside. In a saucepan, put water and margarine and bring to a boil. Turn heat to low and add flour mixture, stirring constantly until mixture leaves the sides of the pan. Remove from heat and cool 4 minutes. Add egg substitute, 1/4 cup at a time, stirring until each addition is well blended. Add egg white and stir until smooth. Spray baking sheet with cooking spray. Put mixture in pasty bag and with large piping tube, pipe ribbons of 3 inches. If desired, put large spoonful on baking sheet and shape into 3-inch ribbon with back of spoon. Bake in 400° preheated oven for 20 to 25 minutes or until crisp and nicely browned. Cool on racks. When cool, make split in side of eclair and fill with prepared chocolate pudding. Blend cream cheese and sweetener, beating with electric blender until fluffy. Beat in cocoa, then fold in whipped topping. Frost filled eclairs.
Yield: 12 eclairs

Approximate Per Eclair:
Calories: 118
Fat: 2.9 g
Cholesterol: 2 mg
Carbohydrates: 20 g
Protein: 10 g
Sodium: 217 mg

Diabetic Exchanges: 1 milk, 1/2 bread, 1/2 fat

Sugar-Free Brownies

(Recipe contains approximately 34% fat)

1/4 c. tub margarine, melted
3/4 c. applesauce, unsweetened
Egg substitute to equal 4 eggs
2 tsp. vanilla
1 1/2 c. enriched all-purpose flour

8 T. cocoa
1/4 tsp. cinnamon
3 T. boiling water
18 pkt. Equal sweetener, or sweetener of choice to equal 3/4 cup sugar

Put melted margarine in saucepan and stir in unsweetened applesauce. Add egg substitute 1/4 cup at a time, stirring between each addition. Add vanilla. Blend flour, cocoa and cinnamon. Stir into applesauce mixture, just until moistened. Pour into 7x11-inch baking pan that has been sprayed with cooking spray. Bake in 350° oven for 20 to 25 minutes. Remove from oven and poke holes into brownies with a fork. Mix sweetener and boiling water. Drizzle over brownies, allowing liquid to go into holes. Cool and cut.
Yield: 25 servings

Approximate Per Serving:
Calories: 45
Fat: 1.7 g
Cholesterol: 0.0 mg
Carbohydrates: 6 g
Protein: 1 g
Sodium: 26 mg

Diabetic Exchanges: 1/4 bread; 1/4 fruit; 1/4 fat

For a crispy cookie coating, sprinkle a mixture of flour and sugar on pastry board before rolling out dough.

Raisin Bars

(Recipe contains approximately 22% fat)

1/2 c. raisins
1 c. apple juice
1/4 c. soft margarine, soft-
    ened (do not use diet
    margarine)
1/2 c. unsweetened
    applesauce
5 egg whites
2 1/4 c. enriched all-
    purpose flour

1 tsp. baking soda
1/2 tsp. salt (opt.)
1 tsp. cinnamon
1/4 c. apple juice concen-
    trate, heated to boiling
18 pkt. Equal sweetener, or
    sweetener of choice to
    equal 3/4 c. sugar

Put raisins and apple juice in saucepan and bring to boil. Set aside until cooled to room temperature. Beat margarine and applesauce with electric mixer until light and fluffy. Add egg whites, one at a time, beating between each addition. Sift together flour, soda, salt and cinnamon. Add to creamed mixture along with raisins and liquid. Stir with wooden spoon until flour is moistened. Spread evenly over surface of a 9x13-inch baking pan that has been sprayed with cooking spray. Bake in a 350° preheated oven for 25 to 30 minutes or until browned. Blend apple juice concentrate and sweetener and brush over bars. Cut into 20 squares.
Yield: 10 servings

Approximate Per Serving:
Calories: 104
Fat: 2.5 g
Cholesterol: 0.0 mg
Carbohydrates: 18 g
Protein: 2 g
Sodium: 94 mg

Diabetic Exchanges: 1 bread; 1/4 fruit; 1/2 fat

*For a nice summer dessert, put a scoop of
sugar free frozen yogurt in each melon half.*

Ice Cream Bars

(Recipe contains approximately 20% fat)

3 c. Rice Chex
18 pkt. Equal sweetener, or
   sweetener of choice to
   equal 3/4 cup sugar

3 T. tub margarine, melted
8 c. lowfat sugar-free
   frozen yogurt, softened

Crush Rice Chex; put into bowl and add sweetener and melted margarine. Blend well. Press half of mixture into a 9x13-inch baking dish. Top with all of frozen yogurt, spreading evenly. Top with remaining Rice Chex mixture. Cover and freeze until solid. Cut into squares and serve cold.
Yield: 16 servings

Approximate Per Serving:
Calories 120
Fat: 2.7 g
Cholesterol: 3 mg
Carbohydrates: 15 g
Protein: 3 g
Sodium: 95 mg

Diabetic Exchanges: 1 bread; 1 fat

Cool cookies in a single layer to prevent them from sticking together.

Sugar-Free Ice Cream Bars

(Recipe contains approximately 15% fat)

3 c. lowfat, sugar-free
frozen chocolate yogurt
1 pkg. Estee whipped top-
ped, prepared per pkg.
directions
2 pkg. chocolate sugar-free
instant pudding mix

1/2 c. refrigerator-style
peanut butter, oil
poured off
1 1/2 c. Grape-Nuts

Soften frozen yogurt to mixing consistency; add whipped topping, pudding and peanut butter. Blend well. Stir in Grape-Nuts. Pour into a 9x9-inch pan that has been lightly sprayed with cooking spray. Spread out evenly. Freeze. Cut into bars. Wrap separately and put back into freezer. **Yield: 12 (2 1/4 x 6 1/4-inch) bars**

Approximate Per Serving:
Calories: 226
Fat: 3.8 g
Cholesterol: 3 mg
Carbohydrates: 38 g
Protein: 18 g
Sodium: 308 mg

Diabetic Exchanges: 2 milk; 1 bread

*Ten large marshmallows equals
one cup miniature marshmallows.*

Refrigerator Desserts

Apricot Refrigerator Dessert

(Recipe contains approximately 8% fat)

1 pkg. sugar-free orange-
flavored gelatin
1 c. apricot juice (can use
part water)
1 (3 oz.) pkg. "light" cream
cheese
1 lg. can apricots, drained
(reserve juice)

1 pkg. Estee sugar-free
whipped topping, or
home-style (see index)
1 can mandarin orange,
drained

Heat juice and dissolve gelatin. Cool. Blend softened cream cheese with sliced apricots. Prepare whipped topping and fold into cheese mixture. Stir in gelatin mixture and add mandarin oranges, mixing well. Pour into a 9x9-inch baking dish and refrigerate until firm.
Yield: 9 servings

Approximate Per Serving:
Calories: 89
Fat: 0.8 g
Cholesterol: 2 mg
Carbohydrates 20 g
Protein: 2 g
Sodium: 151 mg

Diabetic Exchanges: 2 fruit

When a recipe calls for a six-cup baking dish, use:
an 8 or 9 x 11 1/2-inch layer-cake pan; a
10-inch pie plate or an 8 1/2 x 3 5/8-inch loaf pan.

Basic Crepe Recipe

(Recipe contains approximately 25% fat)

1 c. enriched all-purpose
flour
Egg substitute to equal
3 eggs
2 T. "light" tub margarine
1 1/2 c. skim milk

1/2 tsp. salt (opt.)
6 pkt. Equal sweetener, or
sweetener of choice to
equal 1/4 cup sugar
1/2 tsp. vanilla

Put flour in mixing bowl and add half of egg substitute. Beat with electric beater at low speed until blended. Add remaining egg substitute and beat 5 minutes. Add margarine, skim milk, salt, sweetener and vanilla. Refrigerate batter for at least 2 hours. Batter should now be the consistency of thin cream. If too thick, add a tiny bit of milk.

Spray a 6-inch skillet with cooking spray and heat skillet. Pour 1/4 cup batter into skillet and quickly tilt pan in all directions to distribute batter over entire bottom of pan. Cook crepe until lightly browned, about 1 minute. Turn and brown second side a few seconds.

Yield: 12 servings

Approximate Per Serving:
Calories: 83
Fat: 2.3 g
Cholesterol: 1 mg
Carbohydrates: 10 g
Protein: 4 g
Sodium: 152 mg

Diabetic Exchanges: 1/4 bread; 1/2 milk; 1 fat

Ten miniature marshmallows equals one large marshmallow.

Cherry Cream Crepe Stacks

(Recipe contains approximately 8% fat)

6 crepes, see index for
  Basic Crepe
1 pkg. instant sugar-free
  vanilla pudding

2 c. skim milk
1/2 recipe Cherry Pie
  Filling (see index)

On a serving plate, put crepe and frost lightly with vanilla pudding. Repeat with layers until there is a stack of 6 crepes. On last crepe, spread cherry pie filling. Chill.

Yield: 6 servings

Approximate Per Serving:
Calories: 218
Fat: 2.0 g
Cholesterol: 1 mg
Carbohydrates: 31 g
Protein: 5 g
Sodium: 248 mg

Diabetic Exchanges: 1 bread; 1/2 milk; 1 fruit; 1 fat

Strawberry Crepe Fold-Overs—Sugar-Free

(Recipe contains approximately 26% fat)

1 recipe of Basic Crepes
  (see index)
1 c. boiling water
1 pkg. sugar-free straw-
  berry-flavored gelatin

1 (10 oz.) pkg. unsweetened strawberries (frozen)
1 pkg. Estee sugar-free
  whipped topping (can use
  home-style whipped
  topping, see index)

Prepare crepes and set aside. Dissolve gelatin in boiling water and add strawberries. Stir until berries thaw. Put into refrigerator for about 30 minutes or until mixture is the consistency of egg white. Prepare whipped topping. Put 1/2 of mixture down center of crepe and fold toward middle from both sides. Chill.

Yield: 12 filled crepes

Approximate Per Crepe:
Calories: 101
Fat: 2.9 g
Cholesterol: 1 mg
Carbohydrates: 13 g
Protein: 7 g
Sodium: 155 mg

Diabetic Exchanges: 1/2 bread; 3/4 fruit; 1/2 meat

Blueberry-Pineapple Dessert

(Recipe contains approximately 12% fat)

1 can blueberries, drained
   (reserve juice)
1 lg. can crushed pineapple,
   drained (reserve juice)
2 c. boiling water

2 pkg. strawberry-flavored
   sugar-free gelatin
1 pkg. Estee sugar-free
   topping, or sugar-free
   topping of choice to
   equal 2 cups

Drain blueberries and pineapple. Add water to juice, if necessary, to make 2 cups. Put juice in medium mixing bowl. Add boiling water to gelatin and stir until gelatin is dissolved. Add gelatin mixture to juice in bowl. Chill until mixture becomes like egg whites. Remove 3/4 cup of mixture and set aside in the refrigerator. Stir blueberries and pineapple into the remaining mixture. Put into 9x9-inch baking dish and return to refrigerator. Prepare whipped topping and fold reserved gelatin mixture into whipped topping. Spread over top of gelatin.

Yield: 9 servings

Approximate Per Serving:
Calories: 69
Fat: 0.9 g
Cholesterol: 0.0 mg
Carbohydrates: 17 g
Protein: 5 g
Sodium: 6 mg

Diabetic Exchanges: 1 fruit; 1/2 meat

When a recipe calls for an 8-cup baking dish, use:
an 8 x 8 x 2-inch square pan; an 11 x 7 x 1 1/2-inch
baking pan or a 9 x 5 x 3-inch loaf pan.

Cherry Crumb Dessert—Sugar-Free

(Recipe contains approximately 18% fat)

1 c. oatmeal
12 pkt. Equal sweetener, or
   sweetener of choice to
   equal 1/2 cup sugar
2 T. tub margarine, melted
1 pkg. sugar-free cherry-
   flavored gelatin

1 c. boiling water
1/2 recipe Cherry Pie Filling
   (see index)
2 c. lowfat, sugar-free
   frozen yogurt, slightly
   softened

Put oatmeal on a baking sheet and put into 350° preheated oven for 15 minutes, stirring every 5 minutes. Remove from oven and cool. Add sweetener and margarine, tossing to coat evenly. Reserve 1/2 cup of crumb mixture and press remainder into a 9x9-inch square baking pan. Chill for at least 30 minutes. Combine gelatin and boiling water. Add frozen yogurt and cherry pie filling. Stir until smooth. Pour over crumb crust. Chill 30 minutes, then sprinkle remaining crumbs over top.

Yield: 9 servings

Approximate Per Serving:
Calories: 190
Fat: 3.9 g
Cholesterol: 2 mg
Carbohydrates: 22 g
Protein: 5 g
Sodium: 62 mg

Diabetic Exchanges: 1 bread; 1 fruit; 1/2 milk; 1 fat

When a recipe calls for 1/4 pound marshmallows, use 16.

Chocolate-Cherry Delight—Low Sugar

(Recipe contains approximately 14% fat)

2 (3 oz.) pkg. sugar-free
   instant chocolate pudding
4 c. skim milk

28 vanilla wafers, crushed
1 recipe Cherry Pie Filling
   (see index)

Prepare pudding per package directions. Prepare cherry pie filling and cool. In a 9x9-inch baking dish, put half of chocolate pudding and top with half of cookie crumbs. Cover crumbs with half of cherry pie filling. Repeat layers. Chill for several hours before serving.

Yield: 9 servings

Approximate Per Serving:
Calories: 286
Fat: 4.3 g
Cholesterol: 2 mg
Carbohydrates: 33 g
Protein: 19 g
Sodium: 319 mg

Diabetic Exchanges: 1/2 bread; 2 milk; 1/2 fruit; 1 fat

Cool and Easy Mandarin Dessert

(Recipe contains approximately 4% fat)

2 (3 oz.) pkg. sugar-free
   orange-flavored gelatin
2 c. boiling water, less 2 T.
2 c. sugar-free, lowfat
   frozen yogurt, slightly
   softened

2 T. orange juice
   concentrate
1 (11 oz.) can mandarin
   oranges, drained

Put gelatin into mixing bowl and add boiling water. Stir until gelatin has dissolved. Add frozen yogurt and orange juice concentrate, stirring until melted. Fold in drained mandarin oranges. Pour into 1-quart mold. Chill until firm. Unmold.

Yield: 8 servings

Approximate Per Serving:
Calories: 73
Fat: 0.3 g
Cholesterol: 0.0 mg
Carbohydrates: 15 g
Protein: 4 g
Sodium: 33 mg

Diabetic Exchanges: 1/2 milk; 1 fruit

Fresh Peach Dessert—Sugar-Free

(Recipe contains approximately 4% fat)

1 c. oatmeal
12 pkt. Equal sweetener, or
   sweetener of choice to
   equal 1/2 cup sugar
2 T. tub margarine,
   melted

1 pkg. orange sugar-free
   gelatin
1 c. boiling water
2 c. sliced peaches
2 c. low fat, sugar-free
   frozen yogurt, slightly
   softened

Put oatmeal on a baking sheet and put into 350° preheated oven for 15 minutes, stirring every 5 minutes. Remove from oven and cool. Add sweetener and margarine, tossing to coat evenly. Reserve 1/2 cup of crumb mixture and press remainder into a 9-inch square baking pan. Chill for at least 30 minutes. Combine gelatin and boiling water. Add frozen yogurt and peaches. Stir until smooth. Pour over crumb crust. Chill 30 minutes, then sprinkle crumbs over top.

Yield: 9 servings

Approximate Per Serving:
Calories: 183
Fat: 4.1 g
Cholesterol: 2 mg
Carbohydrates: 28 g
Protein: 5 g
Sodium: 62 mg

Diabetic Exchanges: 1 fruit; 1 bread; 1/2 milk; 1 fat

One lemon will yield 3 to 4 tablespoons juice.

Lemon-Cheese Topped Dessert

(Recipe contains approximately 13% fat)

2 pkg. sugar-free lemon-flavored gelatin
2 c. boiling water
2 c. cool water
2 lg. bananas
1 lg. can crushed pineapple, drained (reserve juice)
Egg substitute to 2 eggs
2 tsp. tub margarine (do not use diet margarine)
1 T. flour

1 c. pineapple juice, add water to make cup, if necessary
6 pkt. Equal sweetener, or artificial sweetener of choice to equal 1/4 c. sugar
1 pkg. Estee whipped topping, or sugar-free whipped topping of choice to equal 2 cups
6 slices no-fat American cheese, diced

Put gelatin into mixing bowl and add boiling water. Stir until gelatin dissolves. Add cool water. Pour into a 9x13-inch baking dish. Put in refrigerator until the consistency of egg whites. Stir in well drained pineapple and sliced bananas. Put back into refrigerator until firm. Over a double boiler cook egg substitute, margarine, flour and pineapple juice until thick. Cool. Add sweetener. Prepare whipped topping and fold into cooled cooked mixture. Spread over firm gelatin. Sprinkle cheese over top and refrigerate until ready to serve. Cut into squares.
Yield: 15 servings

Approximate Per Serving:
Calories: 74
Fat: 1.1 g
Cholesterol: 2 mg
Carbohydrates: 11 g
Protein: 6 g
Sodium: 196 mg

Diabetic Exchanges: 1/2 milk; 1/2 fruit; 1/2 fat

Lemon Cottage Cheese Dessert

(Recipe contains approximately 21% fat)

1 pkg. sugar-free lemon-
flavored gelatin
1 c. boiling water
1 c. crushed pineapple,
drained
1 c. cottage cheese,
cream-style, drained

1 pkg. Estee sugar-free
whipped topping (pre-
pared), or sugar-free
whipped topping of
choice to equal 2 cups

In a mixing bowl dissolve gelatin in boiling water. Pour into 7x12-inch pan. Refrigerate until the consistency of egg whites. Stir in pineapple and cottage cheese; add prepared whipped topping and refrigerate until firm
Yield: 12 servings

Approximate Per Serving:
Calories: 38
Fat: 0.9 g
Cholesterol: 16 mg
Carbohydrates: 5 g
Protein: 6 g
Sodium: 80 mg

Diabetic Exchanges: 1/2 meat; 1/2 fruit

Lemon Frozen Yogurt-Gelatin Parfait

(Recipe contains approximately 5% fat)

1 pkg. sugar-free lemon-
flavored gelatin
1 c. boiling water

2 c. sugar-free frozen
yogurt, softened slightly
1 sm. can crushed pine-
apple, drained

Dissolve gelatin in boiling water, stirring until dissolved. Stir in frozen yogurt, stirring until yogurt melts and mixture is of even consistency. Add pineapple. Pour into parfait glasses and refrigerate.
Yield: 6 servings

Approximate Per Serving:
Calories: 67
Fat: 0.4 g
Cholesterol: 0.0 mg
Carbohydrates: 12 g
Protein: 4 g
Sodium: 36 mg

Diabetic Exchanges: 1/2 milk; 1 fruit

Mandarin-Frozen Yogurt Dessert— Sugar-Free

(Recipe contains approximately 20% fat)

1 c. oatmeal
12 pkt. Equal sweetener, or
   sweetener of choice to
   equal 1/2 c. sugar
2 T. tub margarine, melted
1 pkg. sugar-free orange-
   flavored gelatin

1 c. boiling water
2 (11 oz.) cans mandarin
   oranges, drained
2 c. lowfat, sugar-free
   frozen yogurt, slightly
   softened

Put oatmeal on a baking sheet and put into 350° preheated oven for 15 minutes, stirring every 5 minutes. Remove from oven and cool. Add sweetener and margarine, tossing to coat evenly. Reserve 1/2 cup of crumb mixture and press remainder into 9x9-inch square baking pan. Chill for at least 30 minutes. Combine gelatin and boiling water. Add frozen yogurt and mandarin oranges. Stir until smooth. Pour over crumb crust. Chill 30 minutes, then sprinkle remaining crumbs over top.
Yield: 9 servings

Approximate Per Serving:
Calories: 179
Fat: 3.9 g
Cholesterol: 2 mg
Carbohydrates: 29 g
Protein: 4 g
Sodium: 65 mg

Diabetic Exchanges: 1 bread; 1 fruit; 1/2 milk; 1/2 fat

*Two and one-half cups brown sugar
equals one pound brown sugar.*

Pineapple Chill—Sugar-Free

(Recipe contains approximately 22% fat)

1 c. oatmeal	1 c. boiling water
12 pkt. Equal sweetener, or sweetener of choice to equal 1/2 c. sugar	1 lg. can unsweetened, crushed pineapple, drained
2 T. tub margarine, melted	2 c. lowfat, sugar-free frozen yogurt, slightly softened
1 pkg. sugar-free raspberry-flavored sugar-free gelatin	

Put oatmeal on a baking sheet and put into 350° preheated oven for 15 minutes, stirring every 5 minutes. Remove from oven and cool. Add sweetener and margarine, tossing to coat evenly. Reserve 1/2 cup of crumb mixture. Press remainder into 9x9-inch square baking pan. Chill for at least 30 minutes. Combine gelatin and boiling water. Add frozen yogurt and pineapple. Stir until smooth. Pour over crumb crust. Chill 30 minutes, then sprinkle remaining crumbs over top.

Yield: 9 servings

Approximate Per Serving:
Calories: 162
Fat: 3.9 g
Cholesterol: 2 mg
Carbohydrates: 22 g
Protein: 4 g
Sodium: 61 mg

Diabetic Exchanges: 1 bread; 1/2 fruit; 1/2 milk; 1/2 fat

One cup honey can be substituted for one cup molasses.

Pineapple Refrigerator Dessert

(Recipe contains approximately 23% fat)

9 whole graham cracker
    sheets
1 (15 oz.) can crushed pine-
    apple, water packed or
    canned in own juices
1 pkg. sugar-free lemon-
    flavored gelatin

18 pkt. Equal sweetener, or
    artificial sweetener of
    choice to equal 3/4 cup
    sugar
1 pkg. Estee sugar-free
    whipped topping, pre-
    pared according to
    package directions

Put pineapple in saucepan with juice and add gelatin. Bring to a boil, stirring until gelatin dissolves. Remove from stove and add sweetener. Cool to room temperature, then fold into whipped topping. Line a 9x13-inch pan with crackers and pour mixture over crackers.
Yield: 12 servings

Approximate Per Serving:
Calories: 72
Fat: 1.8 g
Cholesterol: 1 mg
Carbohydrates: 13 g
Protein: 4 g
Sodium 11 mg

Diabetic Exchanges: 1/2 bread; 1/2 fruit; 1/2 fat

If a recipe calls for honey and you have none, substitute
1 1/2 cups sugar plus 1/4 cup liquid (water or apple juice).

Pumpkin Chiffon Pie

(Recipe contains approximately 29% fat)

1 c. graham cracker crumbs
2 T. tub margarine
1 pkg. instant vanilla
  pudding, sugar-free
1 c. skim milk
1 tsp. pumpkin pie spice

1 (16 oz.) can pumpkin
1 pkg. Estee sugar-free
  whipped topping, or
  sugar-free whipped
  topping of choice
  (see index)

Blend graham cracker crumbs and margarine; press into pie plate. Chill at least 30 minutes. Put pudding mix, milk, pumpkin spice and pumpkin in a mixing bowl and beat on low for 1 minute. With a spoon, fold in whipped topping. Pour into pie crust and chill at least 3 hours.
Yields: 8 servings

Approximate Per Serving:
Calories: 116
Fat: 3.7 g
Cholesterol: 1 mg
Carbohydrates: 23 g
Protein: 9 g
Sodium: 170 mg

Diabetic Exchanges: 1 bread; 1/2 milk

Quick Sugar-Free Dessert

(Recipe contains approximately 11% fat)

1 pkg. sugar-free instant
  vanilla pudding
1 (20 oz.) can unsweetened
  crushed pineapple

1 pkg. Estee sugar-free whipped
  topping, or whipped sugar-
  free topping of choice
  (see index)
1 banana, sliced

Put crushed pineapple in a mixing bowl and sprinkle pudding mix over pineapple. Add whipped topping. Stir until well blended. Add bananas. Chill.
Yield: 6 servings

Approximate Per Serving:
Calories: 104
Fat: 1.3 g
Cholesterol: 0.0 mg
Carbohydrates: 22 g
Protein: 3 g
Sodium: 64 mg

Diabetic Exchanges: 1 fruit; 1/2 milk; 1/2 fat

Raspberry Yogurt Stack

(Recipe contains approximately 19% fat)

1 1/4 c. boiling water
1 pkg. sugar-free rasp-
   berry-flavored gelatin

2 c. vanilla sugar-free,
   lowfat frozen yogurt
24 graham cracker squares

Dissolve gelatin in boiling water. Stir in slightly softened sugar-free yogurt. Stir until yogurt melts and mixture thickens. Refrigerate for about 20 minutes. Spread onto 12 graham crackers and top each with graham cracker square. Refrigerate.

Yield: 12 servings

Approximate Per Serving:
Calories: 86
Fat: 1.8 g
Cholesterol: 1 mg
Carbohydrates: 15 g
Protein: 3 g
Sodium: 29 mg

Diabetic Exchanges: 1/2 bread; 1 fruit; 1/4 fat

Store whole lemons in a tightly-sealed jar of water in the refrigerator.
They will yield much more juice than a fresh purchased lemon.

Refrigerator Pineapple-Apricot Cheesecake

(Recipe contains approximately 26% fat)

1/2 c. well-drained, crushed pineapple (reserve 1/4 c. juice)
1 1/2 c. well-drained apricot halves (reserve 1/4 c. juice)
1 tsp. salt (opt.)
2 c. cottage cheese, run through ricer or sieve
1 pkg. sugar-free lemon-flavored gelatin
6 pkt. Equal sweetener, or artificial sweetener of choice to equal 1/4 c. sugar
1 c. evaporated skim milk
1/2 c. finely-crushed graham cracker crumbs
2 T. tub margarine, melted

Place pineapple in medium mixing bowl. Run apricots through ricer or sieve, making 1 cup pulp. Add to mixing bowl and blend well with pineapple. Add salt and cottage cheese. Blend. Put gelatin in small mixing bowl. Put pineapple and apricot juice in small saucepan and bring to boil. Pour over gelatin and stir until gelatin has dissolved. Add gelatin mixture to cheese mixture, blending well. Add sweetener to milk and gently fold into cheese mixture. Pour into a lightly sprayed 9-inch springform pan. Chill overnight. Blend graham cracker crumbs and margarine; sprinkle over top.
Yield: 10 servings

Approximate Per Serving:
Calories: 109
Fat: 3.2 g
Cholesterol: 3 mg
Carbohydrates: 13 g
Protein: 7 g
Sodium: 255 mg

Diabetic Exchanges: 1 milk; 1/2 fat

When lining a baking pan with foil, fit the foil over the inverted bottom of the pan first and then fit it inside the pan.

Strawberry-Pretzel Dessert
(Shown on Cover)
(Recipe contains approximately 22% fat)

2 c. crushed pretzels
12 pkt. Equal sweetener, or sweetener of choice to equal 1/2 cup sugar
3 T. reduced-calorie margarine, fat not to exceed 7 grams per tablespoon
1 (8 oz.) pkg. no-fat cream cheese
12 pkt. Equal sweetener, or sweetener of choice to equal 1/2 cup sugar

1 pkg. Estee sugar-free whipped topping, or whipped topping of choice
1 (6 oz.) box strawberry sugar-free gelatin
2 c. boiling water
2 (10 oz.) boxes unsweetened strawberries, still frozen (if berries are whole, slice or mash & re-freeze)

Put not-too-fine crushed pretzels in mixing bowl and stir in sweetener and margarine, mixing until well blended. Press mixture into heart-shaped springform pan or 9x13-inch baking dish. Chill for 30 minutes. Combine cream cheese and 12 packets of sweetener. Prepare whipped topping and fold into cheese mixture. Pour on top of pretzel crust, smoothing out until even in pan. Allow to stand 30 minutes. Dissolve gelatin in boiling water and add frozen strawberries. Stir until strawberries thaw. Put into refrigerator until the consistency of egg whites. Pour on top of cheese layer and allow to set. Decorate with candy hearts, if desired. FOR THE DIABETIC IT WOULD BE BEST NOT TO USE THE SWEET CANDY HEARTS OR TO AVOID EATING THEM BECAUSE OF THEIR SUGAR CONTENT.

CANDY HEARTS:
1/2 of 3 oz. pkg. no-fat cream cheese
Food coloring to make hearts pink (paste is best)

3 drops of oil of peppermint
Enough powdered sugar to make stiff dough (about 2 cups)

Allow cream cheese to soften, then work powdered sugar into it; kneading to make a pie dough-like consistency. Work in peppermint oil and food coloring. Press into heart molds and turn out onto wax paper to dry. It is best to cover with soft cloth or paper towel until candy hardens a bit. Store in airtight containers. These freeze well.
Yield: 16 servings

Continued on following page

Continued from preceding page

Approximate Per Serving (candy hearts counted as decoration and not included in breakdown):
Calories: 82
Fat: 2.0 g
Cholesterol: 3 mg
Carbohydrates: 8 g
Protein: 5 g
Sodium: 304 mg

Diabetic Exchanges: 1/2 fruit; 1/2 bread; 1/2 fat

Strawberry Refrigerator Dessert
(Recipe contains approximately 17% fat)

9 whole graham cracker sheets
1 pkg. sugar-free vanilla pudding, the cooked kind
2 c. skim milk
1 pkg. strawberry-flavored sugar-free gelatin
1 c. hot water
1/3 c. cold water
1 pt. fresh strawberries, crushed (can use sugar-free frozen strawberries)
1 pkg. Estee sugar-free whipped topping, or sugar-free topping of choice

Combine vanilla pudding and milk and cook over medium heat until thick. Remove from heat; pour into bowl and cool to room temperature. Chill. Dissolve gelatin in hot water. Add cold water and strawberries. Put into refrigerator until the consistency of egg whites. With an electric beater on low speed, whip gelatin until fluffy and thick. Slowly add pudding, folding as pudding is added. Line a 9x13-inch baking dish with graham crackers and pour pudding mixture over crackers. Chill for at least 6 hours. Top with prepared whipped topping and serve.
Yield: 15 servings

Approximate Per Serving:
Calories: 78
Fat: 1.5 g
Cholesterol: 1 mg
Carbohydrates: 12
Protein: 3 g
Sodium: 18 mg

Diabetic Exchanges: 1/2 bread; 1/2 milk; 1/4 fat

Sugar-Free Heavenly Hash

(Recipe contains approximately 10% fat)

2 c. boiling water
1 (6 oz.) pkg. raspberry-
  flavored gelatin, or flavor
  of choice
1/2 c. uncooked brown rice,
  cooked per package
  directions

1 pkg. Estee sugar-free
  whipped topping, or
  sugar-free topping of
  choice to equal 2 c.
2 pkg. Equal sweetener, or
  sweetener of choice to
  equal 2 cups
1 (8 1/4 oz.) can crushed
  pineapple, drained
  (reserve juice)

Dissolve gelatin in boiling water, stirring until dissolved. Drain pineapple and add enough water, stirring until dissolved. Drain pineapple and add enough water to make 2 cups liquid. Add to gelatin. Chill until thick, but not set. Chill cooked rice in refrigerator. Into whipped topping, whip in gelatin until of an even consistency. Add sweetener, rice and drained crushed pineapple. Put into mold or serving dish and refrigerate until firm.
Yield: 12 servings

Approximate Per Serving:
Calories: 53
Fat: 0.6 g
Cholesterol: 0.0 mg
Carbohydrates: 11 g
Protein: 5 g
Sodium: 6 mg

Diabetic Exchanges: 1/2 bread; 1/2 milk

Small, handpainted tiles make attractive and inexpensive coasters for guests.

Candy

Applesauce Candy—Sugar-Free
(Recipe contains approximately 7% fat)

1 c. canned unsweetened applesauce	18 pkg. Equal sweetener, or sweetener of choice to equal 3/4 c. sugar
1 pkg. strawberry or lime flavored sugar-free gelatin	

Put applesauce in pan and bring to a boil over medium heat. Add gelatin and stir until gelatin has dissolved. Remove from heat and add sweetener. Pout into 8-inch square pan. Chill until firm. Cut into 36 squares. Allow to dry 6 to 8 hours. Keep in airtight container or in refrigerator.
Yield: 36 pieces

Approximate Per Serving:
Calories: 13
Fat: 0.1 g
Cholesterol: 0.0 mg
Carbohydrates: 4 g
Protein: 1 g
Sodium: 3 mg

Diabetic Exchanges: 1/4 fruit

Soften brown sugar by placing a slice of soft white bread in the package and closing package tightly. In a couple of hours it will be soft again.

Apricot Rum Balls
(Low Sugar)
(Recipe contains approximately 5% fat)

3/4 c. Grape-Nuts
3/4 c. finely-crushed
  graham crackers
3/4 c. finely-snipped,
  dried apricots

1/2 c. sifted powdered
  sugar
1/4 c. light Karo syrup
1 tsp. rum or rum flavoring
2 tsp. orange juice concentrate, thawed

In a mixing bowl, combine Grape-Nuts, graham cracker crumbs, apricots and powdered sugar. Stir in syrup, rum and orange juice. Form into 40 balls and roll in extra powdered sugar. Chill.
Yield: 40 balls

Approximate Per Serving:
Calories: 35
Fat: 0.2 g
Cholesterol: 0.0 mg
Carbohydrates: 6 g
Protein: Tr. g
Sodium: 16 mg

Diabetic Exchanges: 1/2 bread

Candy Fruit Balls—Low Sugar
(Recipe contains approximately 4% fat)

1/4 c. raisins
1 c. dates

10 whole figs
3 T. sugar

Grind fruit and roll into small balls. Dust with sugar. Set on baking sheet to dry. Store in airtight container.
Yield: 32 balls

Approximate Per Ball:
Calories: 42
Fat: 0.2 g
Cholesterol: 0.0 mg
Carbohydrates: 9 g
Protein: Tr. g
Sodium: 1 mg

Diabetic Exchanges: 1 fruit

Chocolate Meringue Kisses—Low Sugar

(Recipe contains approximately 8% fat)

3 egg whites, room temp.	**3 T. cocoa**
1/4 tsp. cream of tartar	**1 tsp. vanilla extract**
1/3 c. sugar	

Put egg whites and cream of tartar in a medium mixing bowl and beat at high speed until egg whites form soft peaks. Very slowly (no more than 1 tablespoon at a time) add sugar, beating after each addition. When sugar is completely dissolved into egg whites, add cocoa and vanilla and beat until mixture is stiff and glossy peaks form. With a teaspoon, drop meringue onto baking sheet that has been lined with aluminum foil and lightly sprayed with cooking spray. As meringue is dropped, bring spoon up to form a candy kiss. Bake 1 hour, or until set, in 200° preheated oven. Let cool on baking sheet before removing with spatula. Allow to dry out before storing in airtight container.

Yield: 40 kisses

Approximate Per Kiss:
Calories: 12
Fat: 0.1 g
Cholesterol: 0.0 mg
Carbohydrates: 3 g
Protein: Tr. g
Sodium: 4 mg

Diabetic Exchange: 1 kiss free

When in a hurry, soften brown sugar by putting in the microwave for a few seconds. If first few seconds does not do it, try again.

Date-Apricot Balls

(Recipe contains approximately 2% fat)

1 c. dates
1 c. apricots
1 c. raisins
2 T. orange juice concen-
trate, thawed

8 pkt. Equal sweetener, or
artificial sweetener of
choice

Run dates, apricots and raisins through grinder. Stir in juice and form into balls. Roll lightly in sweetener. Leave out on tray for an hour or so to dry out slightly. Store in airtight container in refrigerator.
Yield: 32 balls

Approximate Per Ball:
Calories: 45
Fat: 0.1 g
Cholesterol: 0.0 mg
Carbohydrates: 11 g
Protein: Tr. g
Sodium: 1 mg

Diabetic Exchanges: 1 fruit

Date Roll

(Recipe contains approximately 18% fat)

2 c. very-fine vanilla wafer
crumbs
1 c. finely-chopped dates

1/4 c. evaporated skim milk, or
amount needed to moisten
1 tsp. lemon juice

In a mixing bowl, combine vanilla wafer crumbs and dates. Blend. Add lemon juice to milk and allow to stand 2 minutes. Slowly add to crumb mixture until of a kneading consistency. You may need a spoonful more or less of milk than given in recipe. Knead until mixture is well blended. Form into roll; wrap in foil and refrigerate for at least 12 hours. Cut into 20 slices. (Can form into 2 or 3 rolls, if desired).
Yield: 20 slices

Approximate Per Slice:
Calories: 66
Fat: 1.3 g
Cholesterol: Tr. mg
Carbohydrates: 10 g
Protein: 1 g
Sodium: 71 mg

Diabetic Exchanges: 1 fruit; 1/2 fat

Drop Sugar-Free Crunchy Fudge

(Recipe contains approximately 33% fat)

6 T. tub margarine, melted	1/4 c. skim milk
6 T. unsweetened apple-	1 tsp. vanilla
sauce	2 c. flour
25 pkt. Equal sweetener,	1/4 c. cocoa
or sweetener of choice	1 tsp. baking soda
to equal 1 1/3 c. sugar	1/2 tsp. salt (opt.)
4 egg whites	3 c. Rice Krispies

In a large mixing bowl, put margarine, applesauce, Equal, egg whites, skim milk and vanilla. Beat with an electric mixer, on medium speed, for 3 minutes. In a small mixing bowl, combine flour, cocoa, baking soda and salt. Stir into first mixture with a wooden spoon. Stir in Rice Krispies. Put into refrigerator for 30 minutes to 1 hour. Drop by teaspoon onto wax paper. Allow to dry for 1 hour, then store for 24 hours in the refrigerator before consuming.

Yield: 60 servings

Approximate Per Piece:
Calories: 35
Fat: 1.3 g
Cholesterol: Tr. mg
Carbohydrates: 5 g
Protein: 1 g
Sodium: 52 mg

Diabetic Exchanges (2 cookies): 1 bread

When recipe calls for sweetened condensed milk and you are out, substitute by mixing 1 cup plus 2 tablespoons nonfat dry milk and 1/2 cup warm water. Add 3/4 cup sugar and blend until smooth.

Drop Sugar-Free Mock Fudge

(Recipe contains approximately 32% fat)

6 T. tub margarine, melted	1/4 c. skim milk
6 T. unsweetened apple- sauce	1 tsp. vanilla
	2 c. flour
25 pkt. Equal sweetener, or sweetener of choice to equal 1 1/3 c. sugar	1/4 c. cocoa
	1 tsp. baking soda
	1/2 tsp. salt (opt.)
4 egg whites	2 c. oatmeal

In a large mixing bowl, put margarine, applesauce, Equal, egg whites, skim milk and vanilla. Beat with an electric beater on medium speed for 3 minutes. In a small bowl, combine flour, cocoa, baking soda and salt. Stir into first mixture with wooden spoon. Stir in oatmeal. Put into refrigerator for 30 minutes to 1 hour. Drop by teaspoon onto wax paper. Allow to dry for 1 hour. Then store for 24 hours in the refrigerator before consuming.
Yield: 60 servings

Approximate Per Serving:
Calories: 40
Fat: 1.4 g
Cholesterol: Tr. mg
Carbohydrates: 6 g
Protein: 1 g
Sodium: 35 mg

Diabetic Exchanges (2 pieces): 1 bread

Put honey in small plastic freezer containers to
prevent sugaring. Honey thaws very quickly.

Sugar-Free Sugar Plums

(Recipe contains only a trace of fat)

1/2 c. dried apricots
1/4 c. golden raisins
1/4 c. dried apples
2 T. orange juice concen-
    trate, thawed

8 pkt. Equal sweetener,
    or artificial sweetener
    of choice

Chop finely in food processor, apricots, raisins and apples. Add orange juice concentrate while chopping. Remove from processor and form into 24 balls. Dust lightly with dry sweetener. Keep in airtight container up to 2 weeks at room temperature, or keep in refrigerator. May be frozen for several months.

Yield: 24 servings

Approximate Per Serving:
Calories: 20
Fat: Tr. g
Cholesterol: 0.0 mg
Carbohydrates: 4 g
Protein: Tr. g
Sodium: Tr. mg

Diabetic Exchanges (2 sugar plums): 1 fruit

If honey has become sugary, place
jar in a boiling pot of water.

Miscellaneous

Blueberry Ice Cream Topping

(Recipe contain approximately 5% fat)

2 c. fresh or frozen
    unsweetened blueberries
1 1/4 tsp. cornstarch
1/4 c. cold water

1 tsp. lemon juice
6 pkt. Equal sweetener, or
    sweetener of choice to
    equal 1/4 cup sugar

Place blueberries in top of double broiler. Cook over boiling water until berries are soft and juicy. Blend cornstarch and water until smooth. Stir into berry mixture and cook until clear and thickened. Remove from heat and stir in lemon juice and sweetener. Cool and keep refrigerated. Bring back to room temperature before using, for best taste.

Yield: 6 servings

Approximate Per 1/4 Cup:
Calories: 37
Fat: 0.2 g
Cholesterol: 0.0 mg
Carbohydrates: 8 g
Protein: 0.0 g
Sodium: 3 mg

Diabetic Exchanges: 1 fruit

*Use a little vinegar in rinse water when washing
hosiery and it will strengthen the stockings.*

Chocolate Topping for Ice Cream

(Recipe contains approximately 27% fat)

1/4 c. cocoa
2 T. tub margarine, melted
3 T. cornstarch
3 c. evaporated skim
   milk

1/2 tsp. salt
2 tsp. vanilla
12 pkt. Equal sweetener,
   or sweetener of choice
   to equal 1/2 cup sugar

Combine cocoa and tub margarine until smooth. Add cornstarch and stir until smooth. Stir in milk and add salt. Cook over medium heat until mixture reaches a full boil. Boil for 2 minutes. Remove from heat and add vanilla and sweetener. Cool, then keep refrigerated. For best taste bring back to room temperature before using, or heat the amount to be used in a microwave for a hot chocolate topping.

Yield: 3 cups

Approximate Per 1/4 Cup:
Calories: 84
Fat: 2.5 g
Cholesterol: 2 mg
Carbohydrates: 10 g
Protein: 5 g
Sodium: 165 mg

Diabetic Exchanges: 3/4 milk; 1/2 fat

To make your own old-fashioned cough medicine,
blend one cup honey with the juice of one lemon.

Raspberry Ice Cream Topping

(Recipe contains approximately 7% fat)

2 c. fresh or frozen rasp-
    berries, unsweetened
1 1/2 tsp. cornstarch
1/4 tsp. cold water

6 pkt. Equal sweetener,
    or sweetener of choice
    to equal 1/4 c. sugar
1/8 tsp. cinnamon

Place raspberries in top of double boiler. Cook over boiling water until berries are soft and juicy. Blend cornstarch and water until smooth. Stir into berry mixture. Cook until clear and thickened. Remove from heat and add sweetener. Stir in cinnamon. Cool and keep refrigerated. Bring back to room temperature before using, for best taste.

Yield: 1 1/2 cups

Approximate Per Tablespoon:
Calories: 27
Fat: 0.2 g
Cholesterol: 0.0 mg
Carbohydrates: 5
Protein: Tr. g
Sodium: 1 mg

Diabetic Exchanges: 1/2 fruit

Strawberry Topping for Ice Cream

(Recipe contains approximately 8% fat)

2 c. fresh or frozen straw-
    berries, unsweetened
1 1/2 tsp. cornstarch
1/4 c. cold water

6 pkt. Equal sweetener, or
    sweetener of choice to
    equal 1/4 cup sugar

Place strawberries in top of double boiler. Cook over boiling water until berries are soft and juicy. Blend cornstarch and water until smooth. Stir into berry mixture. Cook until clear and thickened. Remove from heat and add sweetener. Cool and keep refrigerated. Bring back to room temperature before using, for best taste.

Yield: 1 1/2 cups

Approximate Per Serving:
Calories: 25
Fat: 0.2 g
Cholesterol: 0.0 mg
Carbohydrates: 5 g
Protein: Tr. g
Sodium: Tr. mg

Diabetic Exchanges: 1/2 fruit

Instant Sugar-Free Cocoa Mix

(Recipe contains approximately 8% fat)

4 c. nonfat dry milk
   granules

32 pkt. Equal or equivalent
   sweetener of choice to
   equal 1 1/4 c. sugar
1/2 c. cocoa

Blend all ingredients very well. Put into airtight container and store.

To Make: Put 5 scant teaspoons of mix into cup and add a little boiling water to make a paste, then fill cup with boiling water.

Yield: 16 servings

Approximate Per Serving:
Calories: 77
Fat: 0.7 g
Cholesterol: 3 mg
Carbohydrates: 11 g
Protein: 7 g
Sodium: 93 mg

Diabetic Exchanges: 1 milk

Index

A

About Cheeses 27
Angel Biscuits 94
Angel Layer Cake 340
Angel Pudding Cake 341

Appetizers
Beef and Bean Dip 50
Christmas Eggs 51
Easy Elegant Shrimp
    Dip 52
Holiday Corn Dip 53
Manhandlers Nachos 54
Mexican Dip 55
Nacho Dip Olé 56
Oven Tortilla Chips 56
Potato Skins 263
Potted Herbed Cheese ... 57
Refried Beans 58
Stuffed Mushrooms
    Florentine 59
Surprise Meatball
    Skewers 60
Sweet and Sour
    Meatballs 61
Tostada Dip 62
Zippy Bean Dip 63

Apple Brownies, SF 385
Apple Oat Coffee
    Cake, LS 92
Apple Oatmeal
    Cookies, SF 369
Apple Pie Filling, SF 320

Apples
Apple Brownies, SF 385
Apple Date
    Cookies, SF 374

Apple Oat Coffee
    Cake, LS 92
Apple Oatmeal
    Cookies, SF 369
Apple Pie Filling, SF 320
Apple Salad, SF 290
Applesauce Cake, SF ... 342
Applesauce
    Candy, SF 410
Bran and Applesauce
    Bars, SF 386
Easy Apple Salad, SF ... 284
Easy, Tasty Fruit
    Salad 285
Low Sugar Apple
    Cinnamon Puffs, LS ... 90
Spicy Apple Shake, SF ... 72
Sweet Potato and Apple
    Scallop, LS 266

Apple Salad, SF 290
Applesauce Cake, SF 342
Apple Syrup, SF 125
Apricot Pie Filling, SF 321
Apricot Refrigerator
    Dessert, SF 392
Apricot Rum Balls, LS 411

Apricots
Apricot Pie Filling, SF 321
Apricot Refrigerator
    Dessert, SF 392
Apricot Rum Balls 411
Apricot Stuffed
    Tenderloin 218
Apricot Syrup, SF 125
Date-Apricot Balls, SF ... 413
Refrigerator Pineapple-
    Apricot Cheese-
    Cake, SF 406
Stuffed French
    Toast, SF 121
Sugar Free Sugar
    Plums, SF 416

SF - Sugar Free; LS = Low Sugar Content

Apricot Stuffed
    Tenderloin 218
Apricot Syrup 125

B

Baking Powder Biscuits 95
Baking Powder Pastry
    Dough, SF 335
Banana Cake, LS 343
Banana Chocolate
    Cake, SF 344

Bars

Apple Brownies, SF 385
Bran and Applesauce
    Bars, SF 386
Eclair Linda May, SF 387
Ice Cream Bars, SF 390
Raisin Bar, SF 389
Sugar Free
    Brownies, SF 388

Basic Crepe Recipe 393
Basic Low Sugar
    Cake, LS 345
Basic Sugar Free
    Cake, SF 346
Basic Sugar Free
    Chocolate Cake, SF 347
Bean Burgers 151
Bean and Turkey Soup 138
Beef and Bean Dip 50

Beverages

Cranberry Christmas
    Punch 67
Fresh Lemonade 67
Frozen Banana
    Daiquiris 68
Holiday Punch 68
Hot Spiced Cranberry
    Punch 69

Peppermint Refresher 69
Strawberry-Orange
    Cooler.........................70
Sweet and Spicy Tea
    Mix 70
Pumpkin Holiday
    Shake 71
Purple Passion Shake 71
Spicy Apple Shake 72
Sugar Free Pineapple
    Shake 72

Biscuits

Angel Biscuits 94
Baking Powder
    Biscuits 95
Breakfast in a Biscuit 114
Drop Raisin Biscuits 96
Lowfat Baking Powder
    Biscuits 97
Lowfat Sour Milk
    Biscuits 97

Blackberry Syrup, SF 126
Blueberry English
    Muffins, LS 85
Blueberry Ice Cream
    Topping 417
Blueberry Muffins, SF 86
Blueberry Pineapple
    Dessert, SF 395
Blueberry Preserves, SF....106
Blueberry Syrup for
    Pancakes 126

Blueberries

Blueberry English
    Muffins, LS 85
Blueberry Muffins 86
Blueberry Ice Cream
    Topping, SF..............417
Blueberry Pineapple
    Dessert, SF 395

SF - Sugar Free; LS = Low Sugar Content

Blueberry Preserves 106
Fresh Banana-Blueberry
    Bread, LS 77

Boiling Potatoes 252
Bowl Full of Holiday
    Gelatin, SF 291
Boston Cream Pie, LS 347
Bran and Applesauce
    Bar 386

Breads
About Baking Bread 73

Breakfast Muffins
and Rolls
Blueberry English
    Muffins 85
Blueberry Muffins 86
Breakfast Popovers 88
Easy Brown Sugar
    Rolls, LS 89
Low Sugar Apple Cream
    Puffs, LS 90
No Knead Cinnamon
    Rolls, LS 91
Refrigerator Bran
    Muffins, SF 87

Coffee Cakes
Apple Oat Coffee
    Cake, LS 92
Dried Fig Streusel, LS 93

Dinner Rolls
Brown and Serve Rolls ... 81
Cottage Rolls 82
Freeze Ahead Rolls 83
Oatmeal Rolls 84

Miscellaneous
Corn Bread Olé 204
Corn Waffle Bread 98

Filled Potato Dumplings .. 99
Low-fat Waffle Garlic
    Bread 100
Reservation Flat
    Bread 101
Shish Kabread 102
No End Bread Sticks 103
Whole Wheat Pizza
    Crust 104
Yeast Dumplings 105

Quick Breads
Fresh Banana-Blueberry
    Bread, LS 77
Multi-Grain Loaf 78
Pat's Beer Bread, LS 79
Zucchini Bread, SF 80

Yeast Bread
Cottage Cheese-Dilly
    Bread 74
Cracked Wheat Bread 75
Fast and Easy Onion
    Bread 76

Breakfast Fare
Angel Biscuits 94
Apple-Oat Coffee
    Cake, LS 92
Apple Syrup, SF 125
Apricot Syrup, SF 125
Baking Powder
    Biscuits 95
Blackberry Syrup, SF 126
Blueberry English
    Muffins, LS 85
Blueberry Muffins, LS 86
Breakfast in a Biscuit 114
Breakfast Popovers 88
Drop Raisin
    Biscuits, LS 96
Easy Brown Sugar
    Rolls, LS 89

SF - Sugar Free; LS = Low Sugar Content

Extra Tender
   Waffles, LS 122
Fig Streusel 93
Fresh Banana-Blueberry
   Bread, LS 77
French Toast
   Waffles, LS 123
Granola Low-Sugar 123
Granola Sugar-Free 124
Great Oatmeal
   Pancakes, SF 116
Low-Fat Baking Powder
   Biscuits, LS 97
Low-Fat Sour Milk
   Biscuits, SF 97
Low-Sugar Cinnamon
   Puffs, LS 90
Maple Cinnamon
   Syrup, LS 127
Meal on a Muffin 115
No Knead Cinnamon
   Rolls, SF 91
Oatmeal Pancakes with
   Fruit, LS 117
Oven French
   Toast, SF 120
Quick Maple Syrup 126
Refrigerator Bran
   Muffins, SF 87
Strawberry Syrup, SF 127
Stuffed French
   Toast, SF 121
Tender Low-Fat
   Pancakes 118
Whole Wheat
   Pancakes 119

Breakfast in a Biscuit 114
Breakfast Popovers 88
Broccoli and Corn
   Casserole 242
Broccoli Stuffed
   Potatoes 172
Broiled Leg of Lamb 219

Brown Bone Stock 39
Brown and Serve Rolls 81
Browned Flour 26

Brunch
   Brunch Pizza 128
   Crabmeat Quiche 129
   Crustless Quiche........... 130
   Easy Hash Brown
      Quiche 131
   Ham and Egg
      Casserole 132
   Hamburger Casserole ... 133
   Holiday No Fry
      Omelet 134
   Quick and Easy Do Ahead
      Brunch Casserole 135
   Spanish Omelet 136
   Tuna Quiche in Rice
      Crust 137

Brunch Pizza 128
Burritos in a Hurry 201
Busy Day Casserole 178

C

Cajun Seasoning 26

Cakes
   Angel Layer Cake, LS ... 340
   Angel Pudding
      Cake, LS 341
   Applesauce Cake, SF ... 342
   Banana Cake, LS 343
   Banana Chocolate
      Cake, SF 344
   Basic Low Sugar
      Cake, LS 345
   Basic Sugar-Free
      Chocolate
      Cake, SF 346
   Boston Cream Pie, LS .. 345

SF - Sugar Free; LS = Low Sugar Content

Cherry Cream Crepe
Stacks, SF 394
Cherry Topped
Cake, SF 348
Cherry Topped Individual
Cheesecakes, LS 355
Chilled Pineapple
Cake, SF 350
Christmas Cake, SF 351
Chocolate, Chocolate
Trifle, SF 352
Easy Fresh Peach
Cheesecake, SF 353
Fruit Trifle, SF 354
Individual Low Sugar
Cheesecake, LS 355
Lemon Cake, SF 356
Pineapple
Cheesecake, SF 357
Pineapple Filled
Cake, SF 358
Pineapple Upside Down
Cake, SF 359
Strawberry Cake
Deluxe, SF 360
Sugar-Free Banana
Cake, SF 360
Sugar-Free Cake with
Mother's Nutmeg
Dip, SF 361

California Casserole 245

Candy
Applesauce
Candy, SF 410
Apricot Rum Balls, LS ... 411
Candy Fruit Balls, LS 411
Date Apricot Balls, SF ... 413
Date Roll, LS 413
Drop Sugar-Free Crunchy
Fudge, SF 414
Drop Sugar-Free Mock
Fudge, SF 415

Sugar-Free Sugar
Plums, SF 416

Canteens 152
Carrot-Pineapple Cookies
with Dates, LS 370
Carrots Supreme 241

Casseroles
Brunch Casserole 135
Busy Day Casserole 178
Cheesy Manicotti 196
Chicken Enchiladas 202
Chili Relleno
Casserole 203
Easy Chicken Divan 226
Enchilada Casserole 207
Ham and Asparagus
Bake 182
Ham and Egg
Casserole 132
Hamburger
Casserole 133
Low-fat Ham, Cheese
and Macaroni 183
Macaroni Taco
Casserole 208
Mexican Lasagna 211
Mexicale Chicken and
Rice 209
Mexicale Rice
Casserole 210
Oven Baked Chicken
Hash 186
Quick and Easy Do-Ahead
Brunch Casserole 135
Spaghetti Bake 200

Cereal Party Mix 64
Charts 9-24
Cheese and Chili Pepper
Stuffed Potatoes 173
Cheese Pea and Pasta
Salad 302

SF - Sugar Free; LS = Low Sugar Content

Cheese Pie À la Fruit, SF .. 323
Cheese Soup 139
Cheese Asparagus 239
Cheesy Manicotti 196
Cheese Potatoes 253
Cherry Cream
  Stacks, SF 394
Cherry Crumb
  Dessert, SF 396
Cherry Topped Cake, SF ... 348
Cherry Topped Individual
  Cheesecakes 349

Chicken
  Chicken and Feathery
    Dumplings 150
  Chicken Breast
    Bourdeaux 221
  Chicken Breast
    Wellington 222
  Chicken Enchiladas 202
  Chicken Filled
    Potatoes 174
  Chicken Patties with
    Cranberry Sauce 179
  Chinese Chicken 190
  Cock-A-Doodle Stew 149
  Crispy Italian Chicken
    Breast 180
  Easy Chicken Divan 226
  Florentine Chicken En
    Phyllo Dough 228
  Italian Frecassed
    Chicken 198
  Mexicale Chicken and
    Rice 209
  Mexican Style Chicken
    Freciassee 213
  Oriental Chicken
    Salad 193
  Oven Baked Chicken
    Hash 186

Chicken and Feathery
  Dumplings 150
Chicken Breast
  Bordeaux 221
Chicken Breast
  Wellington 222
Chicken Enchiladas 202
Chicken Filled
  Potatoes 174
Chicken Patties with
  Cranberry Sauce 179
Chili Relleno Casserole 203
Chili Stuffed Potatoes 175
Chilled Pineapple
  Cake, SF 350
Chinese Chicken 190

Chinese Food
  Chinese Chicken 190
  Chicken Pepper
    Steak 191
  Chop Suey 192
  Oriental Chicken
    Salad 193
  Oriental Pork Fried
    Rice 194
  Shrimp Egg Foo Yung ... 195

Chinese Pepper Steak 191

Chocolate
  Basic Sugar-Free
    Chocolate
    Cake, SF 347
  Chocolate Cherry
    Delish, LS 397
  Chocolate, Chocolate
    Trifle, SF 352
  Chocolate Cream
    Frosting, SF 362
  Chocolate Meringue
    Kisses, LS 412
  Chocolate Pie
    Filling, SF 324

SF - Sugar Free; LS = Low Sugar Content

Chocolate Sauce, SF 365
Chocolate Topping for
Ice Cream, SF 418
Drop Sugar-Free Crunchy
Fudge, SF 414
Drop Sugar-Free Mock
Fudge, SF 415
Glazed Chocolate Low-
Sugar Cookies, LS ...375
Instant Sugar-Free Cocoa
Mix, SF 420
Sugar-Free Cocoa
Drops, SF 381

Chocolate Cherry
Delish 397
Chocolate, Chocolate
Trifle, SF 352
Chocolate Cream
Frosting, SF 362
Chocolate Meringue
Kisses, SF 412
Chocolate Pie Filling, SF ...324
Chocolate Sauce, SF 365
Chocolate Topping for
Ice Cream, SF 418
Chop Suey 192
Christmas Cake, SF 351
Christmas Eggs 51
Cock-A-Doodle Stew with
Oatmeal Biscuits 149
Company Green Beans 246
Cooked Vegetable
Salad 270

Cookies
Apple Oatmeal
Cookies, SF 369
Carrot and Pineapple
Cookies with
Dates, SF 370
Cream Puffs, SF 371
Date Cookies, SF 372

Date Drop
Cookies, LS 373
Date 'N' Apple
Cookies, LS 374
Glazed Chocolate Low-
Sugar Cookies, LS ...375
Krispie Date Balls, SF ...376
Low-Sugar Oatmeal
Cookies, LS 377
No-Bake Apple-Peanut
Butter Balls, SF 378
Pineapple Oatmeal
Cookies, SF.............. 379
Sugarless Fruit
Cookies, SF.............. 380
Sugar-Free Cocoa
Drops, SF 381
Sugar-Free Date-Filled
Cookies, SF.............. 382
Sugar-Free Raisin
Drops, SF 383
Sugar-Free Raisin-Filled
Fold Overs, SF 384

Cool and Easy Mandarin
Dessert, SF 397
Corn and Cabbage
Salad 272
Corn Bread Olé 204
Corn Waffle Bread 98
Cottage Cheese-Dilly
Bread 74
Cottage Cheese Dilly
Dressing 310
Cottage Rolls 82
Crab and Pasta Salad 303
Crab Enchiladas 205
Crabmeat Quiche 129
Cracked Wheat Bread 75
Cranberry Christmas
Punch, SF 67
Cranberry Mousse, SF 292
Cranberry Salad, SF 293
Cranberry Sauce, SF 289

SF - Sugar Free; LS = Low Sugar Content

Cream Cheese Substitute
for Cold Dishes 28
Cream Cheese Substitute
for Hot Dishes 29
Cream Puffs 371
Cream Substitute for Heavy
and Light Cream 29
Cream Soup Substitute 30
Cream Cranberry
Salad, SF 294
Creamy Skillet Potatoes 253
Creole Soup 140

Crepes

    Basic Crepe Recipe 393
    Cherry Cream Crepe
        Stack, SF 394
    Strawberry Crepe
        Foldovers, SF 394

Crispy Italian Chicken
Breasts 180
Croutons 42
Crown Roast of Pork with
Vegetables 220
Crustless Quiche 130
Curried Mayonnaise 314

D

Date Apricot Balls, SF 413
Date Cream Pie, SF 325
Date Cookies, SF 372
Date Drop Cookies, SF 374
Date'N' Apple
Cookies, LS 374
Date Rolls, LS 413
Delicious Ham En Milk 223
Delicious Mandarin Orange
Salad, SF 295
Delicious Scalloped
Potatoes 254
Delicious Wild Rice Soup .. 141
Delmonico Potatoes 255

Deluxe Mushroom and
Artichoke Salad 273
Deluxe Patty Melts 153
Deluxe Pineapple
Sauce, SF 366
Dill Mayonnaise 314
Dilly Potatoes 255
Drop Raisin, SF 96
Drop Sugar-Free Crunchy
Fudge, SF 414
Drop Sugar-Free Mock
Fudge, SF 415
Duck à la Orange 225

E

Easiest Ever Goulash 181
Easy Apple Salad 284
Easy Brown Sugar
Rolls, LS 89
Easy Cannelloni 197
Easy Chicken Divan 226
Easy Elegant Shrimp Dip 52
Easy Fresh Peach
Coffeecake, SF 353
Easy Hash Brown Quiche .. 131
Easy Sugar-Free Pumpkin
Pie, SF 326
Easy Scalloped Corn 243
Easy Scalloped
Tomatoes 251
Easy Taco Salad 206
Easy, Tasty Fruit
Salad, SF 285
Eclairs Linda May, SF 387
Eggnog Cranberry
Salad, SF 296
Eggnog Pie, Sugar-Free 327
Egg Substitute in the
Freezer 33
Egg Substitute on the
Shelf 34
Enchilada Casserole 207
Extra Tender Waffles 122

SF - Sugar Free; LS = Low Sugar Content

F

Fast and Easy Onion
   Bread 76
Favorite Roast in Wine
   Sauce 227
Festive Strawberry
   Salad, SF 297
Fiesta Salad 304
Fig Streusel 93
Filled Potato Dumplings 99

Fish and Seafood
   Crab and Pasta
      Salad 303
   Crab Enchiladas 205
   Crabmeat Quiche 129
   Easy Elegant Shrimp
      Dip 52
   Dr. Bob's Deluxe
      Salmon Patties 224
   Fish Fumet 40
   Grilled Fish on French
      Bread 155
   Luncheon Salmon
      Salad 184
   Mermaids 159
   Salmon Bisque 146
   Scallops Mornay 230
   Scallop Stir-Fry 231
   Seafood Jambalaya 232
   Shrimp and Scallops
      Bobby Dean 233
   Shrimp Egg Foo Yong ... 195
   Shrimp Gumbo Cajun
      Style 234
   Shrimp Stuffed
      Potatoes 176
   Tuna Quiche in Rice
      Crust 137

Fish Fumet 40
Florentine Chicken En
   Phyllo Dough 228

Freeze-Ahead Dinner
   Rolls 83
French Dressing 311
French Dressing with
   Capers 312
French Hamburger 154
French Toast Waffles 123
Fresh Banana-Blueberry
   Bread, LS 77
Fresh Peach Dessert, SF .. 398
Fresh Lemonade, SF 67

Frosting
   Chocolate Cream
      Frosting, SF 362
   Lemon Cream
      Frosting, SF 363
   Vanilla Cream
      Frosting, SF 364

Frozen Banana
   Daiquiris, SF 68
Frozen Stock Cubes 37
Frozen Yogurt Lemon
   Pie, SF 328
Fruit En Wine 286
Fruit Salad with Fruit
   Dressing, SF 287
Fruit Trifle, SF 354

G

Getting Fat Out of Ground
   Beef 5-6
Glazed Chocolate Low-
   Sugar Cookies, LS 375
Glazed Sugar-Free
   Strawberry Pie, SF 329
Graham Cracker Pie
   Crust, LS 335
Granola, Low Sugar, LS 123
Granola, Sugar Free, SF ... 124
Grasshopper Pie, SF 329

SF - Sugar Free; LS = Low Sugar Content

Great Oatmeal
   Pancakes, SF 116
Green Beans with a
   Zing 247
Green Mayonnaise 315
Grilled Fish on French
   Bread 155

H

Ham and Asparagus
   Bake 182
Ham and Egg Casserole.... 132
Hamburger Quiche 133
Herbed Yogurt Dressing 311
Holiday Corn
   Casserole 244
Holiday Corn Dip 53
Holiday Cranberry
   Fluff, SF 288
Holiday Fruit Salad, SF 298
Holiday Green Beans 348
Holiday No-Fry Omelet 134
Holiday Punch, SF 68
Holiday Raspberry Frozen
   Yogurt Pie 330
Hominy Vegetable Salad ... 274
Horseradish Mayonnaise ... 315
Hot Potato Salad 275
Hot Spicy Cranberry
   Punch, SF 69
How Much Fat and Cholesterol
   Should be Consumed 7

I

Ice Cream Bars 390

Ice Cream Toppings
   Blueberry Ice Cream
      Topping, SF 417
   Chocolate Topping for
      Ice Cream 418

Raspberry Ice Cream
   Topping, SF 419
Strawberry Ice Cream
   Topping, SF 419

Individual Cheese
   Cakes, SF 420
Instant Sugar-Free Cocoa
   Mix, SF 420
Italian Broccoli-Cauliflower
   Salad 276

Italian Foods
   Brunch Pizza 128
   Cheesy Manicotti 196
   Crispy Italian Chicken
      Breasts 180
   Easy Cannelloni 197
   Italian Broccoli-
      Cauliflower Salad 276
   Italian Fricassed
      Chicken 198
   Italian Vegetable Soup .. 142
   Lasagne-Low Fat 199
   Minestrone 144
   Pizza Cups 163
   Pizza on English
      Muffins 164
   Quick Pizza Melts 165
   Spaghetti Bake 200
   Vegetable Pasta
      Patties 171

Italian Fricassed Chicken .. 198
Italian Vegetable Soup 142
Introduction 1-3

J

Jalapeño Potatoes 256
Jelled Peach Mold, SF 299
Jell-o Pops, SF 65
Jumbo Vienna
   Sandwiches 156

SF - Sugar Free; LS = Low Sugar Content

K

Krispie Date Balls 376

L

Lasagna-Low Fat 199
Layered Spaghetti Salad ... 305
Lemon Cake, SF 356
Lemon-Cheese Topped
    Dessert, SF 399
Lemon Cottage Cheese
    Dessert, SF 400
Lemon Cream
    Frosting, SF 363
Lemon Frozen Yogurt-Gelatin
    Parfait, SF 400
Lettuce and Pea Salad 277
Lowfat Baking Powder
    Biscuits 97
Lowfat Bread Sauce 35
Lowfat Ham and Cheese
    Macaroni 183
Lowfat Home-Style
    Mayonnaise 313
Lowfat Home-Style Yogurt ... 46
Lowfat Pie Crust 337
Lowfat Sausage Patties 36
Lowfat Sour Milk Biscuits 97
Lowfat Tartar Sauce 317
Lowfat Waffle Garlic
    Bread 100
Lowfat Western Fries 257
Low Sugar Apple Cinnamon
    Puffs 90
Low Sugar Oatmeal
    Cookies, LS 377

Luncheon Entrées
    Busy Day Casserole 178
    Chicken Patties with
        Cranberry Sauce 179
    Crispy Italian Chicken
        Breasts 180

Easiest Ever Goulash ... 181
Easy Taco Salad 206
Ham and Asparagus
    Bake 182
Lowfat Ham, Cheese and
    Macaroni 183
Luncheon Salmon
    Salad 184
Mining Town Pasties 185
Old-Fashioned Goulash
    From Yesteryear 186
Oven Baked Oven
    Hash 186
Turkey Porcupines 187

Luncheon Salmon Salad 184

M

Mac and Fruit Combo 306
Macaroni Taco
    Casserole 208
Maidrites 157
Maid Rites of Yesteryear ... 158
Mandarin Orange Pie, SF .. 331
Mandarin Frozen Yogurt
    Dessert, SF 401
Manhandlers Nachos 54
Maple-Cinnamon
    Syrup, LS 127
Mashed Potato Pie
    Crust 338
Master Baking Mix 35
Mayonnaise Tartar Sauce .. 317
Meal on a Muffin 115
Mermaids 159
Mexicale Chicken and
    Rice 209
Mexicale Rice
    Casserole 210
Mexican Chili (Hot) 143
Mexican Coleslaw 278
Mexican Dip 55

SF - Sugar Free; LS = Low Sugar Content

Mexican Foods

Burritos in a Hurry 201
Cheese and Chili Pepper
   Stuffed Potatoes.......173
Chicken Enchiladas 202
Chili Relleno
   Casserole 203
Chili Stuffed
   Potatoes 175
Corn Bread Olé 204
Crab Enchiladas 205
Easy Taco Salad...........206
Enchilada Casserole 207
Jalapeño Potatoes 256
Macaroni Taco
   Casserole 208
Manhandlers Nachos 54
Mexicale Chicken and
   Rice 209
Mexicale Rice
   Casserole 210
Mexican Chili (Hot) 143
Mexican Coleslaw 278
Mexican Dip 55
Mexican Lasagna 211
Mexican Roll-Ups 212
Mexican Style Chicken
   Fricassee.................213
Mock Sangria 215
Oven Tortilla Chips 56
Refried Beans 58
Spanish Omelet 136
Sweet and Spicy
   Mexican Mix 66
Taco Bean Burgers 167
Tacos 168
Taco Salad for a
   Crowd 214
Taco Soup Olé 148
Taco Stuffed
   Potatoes 177
Tostada Dip.....................62
Zippy Bean Dip 63

Mexican Lasagna 211
Mexican Roll-Ups 212
Mexican Style Chicken
   Fricassee 213
Minestrone 144
Mining Town Pasties 185
Mixed Stock 41
Mock Pear Butter, SF 107
Mock Pork Tenderloins 160
Mock Sangria 215
Mock Sour Cream 43
Mushroom Filled Meatloaf.. 229
Mushroom Salad 279
Mushroom Wine Burgers ...161
Multi Grain Loaf 78
Mustard Mayonnaise 316

N

Nacho Dip Olé 56
No-Bake Apple Peanut
   Butter Balls, SF 378
No-End Bread Sticks 103
No-Knead Cinnamon Rolls ..91

O

Oatmeal Dinner Rolls...........84
Oatmeal Pancakes with
   Fruit 117
Oatmeal Pie Crust 339
Old Fashioned Goulash
   from Yesteryear 186
Olive Oil Substitute 36
Orange Glaze, SF 368
Orange Sauce, SF 367
Oriental Chicken Salad 193
Oriental Green Beans 249
Oriental Pork Fried Rice 194
Oven Baked Chicken
   Hash..............................186
Oven French Toast, SF 120
Oven Fried Potatoes 258
Oven Tortilla Chips 56

SF - Sugar Free; LS = Low Sugar Content

P

Parmesan Oven Fries 259
Pat's BeefrBread 79
Pat's Deviled Potatoes 259
Peach Breakfast
    Spread, SF 108
Peach of a Salad, SF 300
Peach Pie Filling, SF 332
Peas Oriental 250
Peppermint Refresher 69

Pie Crusts

Baking Powder Pastry
    Dough, SF 335
Graham Cracker Pie
    Crust, LS 336
Lowfat Pie Crust, SF 337
Mashed Potato Pie
    Crust 338
Oatmeal Pie Crust, LS .. 339

Pies and Pie Fillings

Apple Pie Filling 320
Apricot Pie Filling, SF 321
Cherry Pie Filling, SF 322
Cheese Pie À la
    Fruit, SF 323
Chocolate Pie
    Filling, SF 324
Date Cream Pie, SF 325
Easy Sugar-Free Pumpkin
    Pie, SF 326
Eggnog Pie, SF 327
Frozen Yogurt Lemon
    Pie, SF 328
Glazed Sugar-Free
    Strawberry Pie, SF ... 329
Grasshopper Pie, SF 329
Holiday Raspberry Frozen
    Yogurt Pie, SF 330
Mandarin Orange
    Pie, SF 331
Peach Pie Filling, SF 332

Pumpkin Chiffon
    Pie, LS 404
Pumpkin Pie on a
    Cloud, SF 333
Vanilla Cream Pie
    Filling, SF 334

Pineapple
    Cheesecake, SF 357
Pineapple Chill, SF 402
Pineapple Filled
    Cake, SF 358
Pineapple Hamburgers 162
Pineapple Oatmeal
    Cookies, LS 379
Pineapple Refrigerator
    Cake, SF 403
Pineapple Upside-Down
    Cake, SF 359
Pizza Cups 163
Pizza on English Muffins 164
Potato Broccoli Bake 260
Potato Dumpling 260

Potato Entrées

Broccoli Stuffed
    Potatoes 172
Cheese and Chili
    Pepper Stuffed
    Potatoes 173
Chicken Filled
    Potatoes 174
Chili Stuffed Potatoes ... 175
Shrimp Stuffed
    Potatoes 176
Taco Stuffed Potatoes .. 177

Potato Pie Crust 261
Potato Rice Balls 262

Potatoes

Boiling Potatoes 252
Broccoli Stuffed
    Potatoes 172

SF - Sugar Free; LS = Low Sugar Content

Cheese and Chili
  Pepper Stuffed
  Potatoes 173
Cheesy Potatoes 253
Chicken Filled
  Potatoes 174
Chili Stuffed
  Potatoes 175
Creamy Skillet
  Potatoes 253
Delicious Scalloped
  Potatoes 254
Delmonico Potatoes 255
Dilly Potatoes 255
Jalapeño Potatoes 256
Low-Fat Western
  Potatoes 257
Oven-Fried Potatoes 258
Parmesan Oven Fries ... 259
Pat's Deviled
  Potatoes 259
Potato-Broccoli
  Potatoes 260
Potato Dumplings 260
Potato Pie Crust 261
Potato Rice Balls 262
Potato Skins 263
Potato Soup with
  Ribbles 145
Pure and Simple
  Scalloped
  Potatoes 264
Shrimp Stuffed
  Potatoes 176
Taco Stuffed
  Potatoes 177
Zesty Mashed
  Potatoes 265

Potatoes, Sweet
Sweet Potato and Apple
  Scallop 266
Thumbprint Sweet
  Potatoes 266

Potato Salad 280
Potato Skins 263
Potato Soup with
  Ribbles 145
Potted Herbed Cheese 57
Pumpkin Chiffon Pie, LS 404
Pumpkin Holiday
  Shake, SF 71
Pumpkin Pie on a
  Cloud, SF 333
Pure and Simple Scalloped
  Potatoes 264
Purple Passion Shake, SF ... 71

Q

Quiche
  Crabmeat Quiche 129
  Crustless Quiche 130
  Easy Hashbrown
    Quiche 131
  Hamburger Quiche 133
  Tuna Quiche in Rice
    Crust 137

Quick and Easy Do Ahead
  Brunch Casserole 135
Quick Maple Syrup 126
Quick Pizza Melt 165
Quick Raspberry Salad 301
Quick Sugar-Free
  Dessert, SF 404
Quick White Bean Salad 281

R

Raisin Bars, SF 389
Raspberry Ice Cream
  Topping, SF 419
Raspberry Preserves, SF .. 109
Raspberry-Yogurt
  Stack, LS 405
Red and Green Holiday
  Salad, SF 301

SF - Sugar Free; LS = Low Sugar Content

Refried Beans 58
Refrigerator Bran
    Muffins, SF 87

Refrigerator Desserts
    Apricot Refrigerator
        Dessert, SF 392
    Basic Cream
        Recipe, SF 393
        Cherry Cream Crepe
            Stacks, SF 394
        Strawberry Crepe
            Foldovers, SF 394
    Blueberry Pineapple
        Dessert, SF 395
    Cherry Crumb
        Dessert, SF 396
    Chocolate Cherry
        Delight, LS................397
    Cool and Easy Mandarin
        Dessert, SF 397
    Fresh Peach
        Dessert, SF 398
    Lemon-Cheese Topped
        Dessert, SF 399
    Lemon Cottage Cheese
        Dessert, SF 400
    Lemon Frozen Yogurt-
        Gelatin Parfait, SF 400
    Mandarin Frozen Yogurt
        Desert, SF 401
    Pineapple Chill, SF 402
    Pineapple Chiffon
        Pie, LS 404
    Pineapple Refrigerator
        Dessert 403
    Quick Sugar-Free
        Dessert, SF 404
    Raspberry-Yogurt
        Stack, SF..................405
    Refrigerator Pineapple-
        Apricot Cheese-
            cake, SF 406

Strawberry Pretzel
    Dessert (Cover), SF..407
Strawberry Refrigerator
    Dessert, SF 408
Sugar-Free Heavenly
    Hash, SF 409

Refrigerator-Pineapple-
    Apricot Cheese-
        cake, SF 406
Reservation Flat Bread 101

Rice
    Chop Suey 192
    Delicious Wild Rice
        Soup 141
    Mexicale Rice
        Casserole 210
    Mexican Chicken and
        Rice 209
    Oriental Chicken Salad..193
    Oriental Pork Fried
        Rice 194
    Rice Salad Entrée 307
    Shrimp Egg Foo Yung ...195
    Split Pea and Rice
        Soup 147
    Steamed Rice 267
    Sugar-Free Heavenly
        Hash, SF 409
    Tuna Quiche in Rice
        Crust 137
    Turkey Porcupines 187

Rice Salad Entrée 307

Rolls

Dinner
    Brown and Serve Rolls ...81
    Cottage Rolls 82
    Freeze Ahead Dinner
        Rolls 83
    Oatmeal Rolls 84

SF - Sugar Free; LS = Low Sugar Content

Sweet

Easy Brown Sugar
    Rolls, LS 89
Low-Sugar Apple
    Cinnamon Puffs, LS ... 90
No Knead Cinnamon
    Rolls, LS 91

S

Salad Dressings

Cottage Cheese Dilly
    Dressing 310
Herbed Yogurt
    Dressing 311
French Dressing 311
French Dressing with
    Capers 312
Suped Up Low-Cal
    French Dressing 312
Zingy French Dressing .. 313
Curried Mayonnaise 314
Dill Mayonnaise 314
Green Mayonnaise 315
Horseradish
    Mayonnaise 315
Lowfat Home-Style
    Mayonnaise 313
Mustard Mayonnaise 316
Watercress
    Mayonnaise 316
Mayonnaise Tartar
    Sauce 317
Low-Fat Tartar Sauce ... 317

Salads

Fruit Salads

Cranberry Sauce, SF 289
Easy Apple Salad 284
Easy Tasty Fruit
    Salad 285
Fruit En Wine, LS 286

Fruit Salad with Fruit
    Dressing, LS 288
Holiday Cranberry,
    Fluff, SF 288
Sugar-Free Cranberry
    Sauce 289

Gelatin Salads

Apple Salad, SF 290
Bowl Full of Gelatin
    Salad, SF 291
Cranberry Mousse, SF... 292
Cranberry Salad, SF 293
Creamy Cranberry
    Salad, SF 294
Delicious Mandarin Orange
    Salad, SF 295
Eggnog Cranberry
    Salad, SF 296
Festive Strawberry
    Salad, SF 297
Holiday Fruit
    Salad, SF 298
Jelled Peach
    Mold, SF 299
Peach of a Salad, SF 300
Quick Raspberry
    Salad, SF 301
Red and Green Holiday
    Salad, SF 302

Pasta and Rice Salads

Cheese, Pea and Pasta
    Salad 302
Crab and Pasta Salad ... 303
Fiesta Salad 304
Layered Spaghetti
    Salad 305
Mac and Fruit Combo
    Salad, SF 306
Rice Salad Entrée 307
Siesta Pasta Salad 308
Tuna and Macaroni
    Salad 309

SF - Sugar Free; LS = Low Sugar Content

Vegetable Salads
Cooked Vegetable
   Salad 270
Corn and Cabbage
   Salad 272
Deluxe Mushroom and
   Artichoke Salad 273
Hominy-Vegetable
   Salad 274
Hot Potato Salad 275
Italian Broccoli-
   Cauliflower Salad 276
Lettuce and Pea Salad .. 277
Mexican Coleslaw 278
Mushroom Salad 279
Potato Salad 280
Quick White Bean
   Salad 281
Sugar-Free Overnight
   Lettuce Salad, SF 282
Vegetable Toss 283

Salmon Bisque 146

Sandwiches
Bean Burgers 151
Canteens 152
Deluxe Pattie Melts 153
French Hamburgers 154
Grilled Fish on French
   Bread 155
Jumbo Vienna
   Sandwich 156
Maidrites 157
Maidrites of
   Yesteryear 158
Mermaids 159
Mock Pork Tenderloins
   (Turkey) 160
Mushroom Wine
   Burgers 161
Pineapple
   Hamburgers 162
Pizza Cups 163

Pizza on English
   Muffins 164
Quick Pizza Melts 165
Sloppy Joe's 165
Stroganoff on French
   Bread 166
Taco Bean Burgers 167
Tacos 168
Vegetable Oven
   Burgers 170
Vegetable Pasta
   Patties 171

Sauces and Glazes
Chocolate Sauce, SF 365
Deluxe Pineapple
   Sauce, SF 366
Orange Sauce, SF 367
Orange Glaze, SF 368
Vanilla Glaze, SF 368

Sausage Patties 36
Sautéing with Stock 37
Sautéed Onion Rings 250
Scalloped Cabbage 240
Scallops Mornay 230
Scallop Stir Fry 231
Seafood Jambalaya 232
Seasoned Croutons 42
Shish-Kabread 102
Shrimp and Scallops
   Bobby Dean 233
Shrimp Egg Foo Yung 195
Shrimp Gumbo Cajun
   Style 234
Shrimp Stuffed Potatoes 176
Siesta Pasta Salad 308
Sloppy Joe's 165

Snacks
Cereal Party Mix 64
Jell-o Pops, SF 65
Sweet and Spicy Mexican
   Mix 66

SF - Sugar Free; LS = Low Sugar Content

Soups and Stews

Bean and Turkey
Soup 138
Cheese Soup 139
Creole Soup 140
Delicious Wild Rice
Soup 141
Italian Vegetable Soup .. 142
Mexican Chili (Hot) 143
Minestrone 144
Potato Soup with
Ribbles 145
Salmon Bisque 146
Split Pea and Rice
Soup 147
Taco Soup Olé 148
Cock-a-Doodle Stew
with Oatmeal
Biscuits 149
Chicken and Feathery
Dumplings 150

Sour Cream Substitute 42
Spaghetti Bake 200
Spanish Omelet 136
Spicy Apple Shake, SF 72
Split Pea and Rice
Soup 147

Special Entrées

Apricot Stuffed Pork
Tenderloin with
Vegetables 218
Broiled Leg of Lamb 219
Crown Roast of Pork
with Vegetables 220
Chicken Breast
Bordeaux 221
Chicken Breast
Wellington 222
Delicious Ham En Milk .. 223
Dr. Bob's Deluxe Salmon
Patties 224
Duck A L' Orange 225

Easy Chicken Divan 226
Favorite Round Roast in
Wine Sauce 227
Florentine Chicken En
Phyllo Dough 228
Mushroom Filled
Meatloaf 229
Scallops Mornay 230
Scallops Stir Fry 231
Seafood Jambalaya 232
Shrimp and Scallop
Bobby Dean 233
Shrimp Gumbo Cajun
Style 234
Teriyaki Salmon
Steaks 235
Turkey O'Beautiful 236

Spicy Apple Shake, SF 72
Split Pea and Rice
Soup 147

Spreads

Blueberry
Preserves, SF 106
Mock Pear
Butter, SF 107
Peach Breakfast
Spread, SF 108
Raspberry
Preserves, SF 109
Strawberry Breakfast
Spread, SF 110
Strawberry
Preserves, SF 111

Sta-Whip Whipped
Topping, SF 45
Steamed Rice 267
Stock 38
Strawberry Breakfast
Spread, SF 110
Strawberry Cake
Deluxe, SF 360

SF - Sugar Free; LS = Low Sugar Content

Strawberry Crepe
  Foldovers, SF 394
Strawberry Ice Cream
  Topping, SF 419
Strawberry-Orange
  Cooler, SF 70
Strawberrt Preserves, SF .. 111
Strawberry Pretzel
  Dessert, SF 407
Strawberry Refrigerator
  Dessert, SF 408
Strawberry Syrup, SF 127
Stroganoff on French
  Bread 166
Stuffed French Toast, SF .. 121
Stuffed Mushrooms
  Florentine 59
Substitute for Heavy or
  Light Cream 31

Substitutes
  Browned Flour 26
  Cajun Seasoning 26
  Croutons, Seasoned 42
  Cream Cheese Substitute
    for Cold Dishes 28
  Cream Cheese Substitute
    for Hot Dishes 29
  Substitute for Cream
    Soup 29-30
  Substitute for Heavy or
    Light Cream 31
  Egg Substitute in the
    Freezer 33
  Egg Substitute on the
    Shelf 34
  Master Baking Mix 35
  Mock Sour Cream 43
  Lowfat Bread Sauce 35
  Lowfat Sausage Patties .. 36
  Reduced-Fat Spread for
    Bread 31
  Seasoned Croutons 42
  Frozen Stock Cubes 37

Stock
Brown Bone Stock 39
Mixed Stock 41
Stock 38
Fish Fumet 40

Olive Oil Substitute 36
Sausage Patties 36
Thin White Sauce 43

Whipped Toppings
Sta-Whip Whipped
  Topping 45
Sugar-Free Whipped
  Topping 44
Whipped Topping
  Substitute 44
Whipped Topping
  Substitute II 45

Lowfat Yogurt 47-48
Yogurt Cheese 46
Yogurt, Making Your
  Own 46

Sugar-Free Banana
  Cake, SF 360
Sugar-Free Brownies, SF .. 288
Sugar-Free Cake with
  Mother's Nutmeg
  Dip, SF 361
Sugar-Free Cocoa
  Drops, SF 381
Sugar-Free Cranberry
  Sauce, SF 289
Sugar-Free Filled Date
  Cookies, SF 382
Sugar-Free Heavenly
  Hash, SF 409
Sugar-Free Ice Cream
  Bars, SF 391
Sugarless Fruit
  Cookies, SF 380

SF - Sugar Free; LS = Low Sugar Content

Sugar-Free Overnight Lettuce
Salad, SF 282
Sugar-Free Pineapple
Shake, SF 72
Sugar-Free Raisin
Drops, SF 383
Sugar-Free Raisin-Filled
Foldovers, SF 384
Sugar-Free Sugar
Plums, SF 416
Sugar-Free Whipped
Topping, SF 44
Suped Up French
Dressing, SF 312
Surprise Meatball
Skewers 60
Sweet Potato Apple
Scallop 266
Sweet and Sour
Meatballs 61
Sweet and Spicy Mexican
Mix 66
Sweet and Spicy Tea Mix 70
Sweet Hamburger
Relish, SF 169
Sweet Potato and Apple
Salad 266

T

Taco Bean Burger 167
Tacos 168
Taco Salad for a
Crowd 214
Taco Soup Olé 148
Taco Stuffed Potatoes 177
Taking the Fat Out of
Ground Beef 3-5
Tender Lowfat
Pancakes, SF 118
Teriyaki Salmon
Steaks 235
Thin White Sauce 43

Thumbprint Sweet
Potatoes 266
Tomatoes Provencalé 251
Tostada Dip 62
Tuna Quiche in Rice
Crust 137
Tuna and Macaroni
Salad 309
Turkey O' Beautiful 236
Turkey Porcupines 187

U

V

Vanilla Cream
Frosting, SF 364
Vanilla Cream Pie
Filling, SF 334
Vanilla Glaze, SF 368
Vegetable Oven Burgers ... 170
Vegetable Pasta
Patties 171
Vegetable Toss 283

Vegetables
Cheese Asparagus 239
Scalloped Cabbage 240
Carrots Supreme 241
Broccoli and Corn
Casserole 242
Easy Scalloped
Corn 243
Holiday Corn
Casserole 244
California Casserole 245
Company Green
Beans 246
Green Beans with a
Zing 247
Holiday Green Beans 248

SF - Sugar Free; LS = Low Sugar Content

Oriental Green Beans ...249
Peas Oriental 250
Sautéed Onion Rings 250
Easy Scalloped
    Tomatoes 251
Tomatoes Provencalé ...251
Boiling Potatoes 252
Cheesy Potatoes...........253
Creamy Skillet
    Potatoes 253
Delicious Scalloped
    Potatoes 254
Delmonico Potatoes......255
Dilly Potatoes 255
Jalapeño Potatoes 256
Low-Fat Western
    Fries 257
Oven Fried Potatoes 258
Parmesan Oven Fries ...259
Pat's Deviled
    Potatoes 259
Potato-Broccoli Bake 260
Potato Dumplings 260
Potato Pie Crust............261
Potato Rice Balls...........262
Potato Skins 263
Pure and Simple Scalloped
    Potatoes 264
Zesty Mashed
    Potatoes 265
Sweet Potato and Apple
    Scallop 266
Thumbprint Sweet
    Potatoes 266

W

Extra Tender
    Waffles, LS 122
French Toast
    Waffles 123
Watercress Mayonnaise 316
Whipped Topping
    Substitute, SF 44-45
Whole Wheat Pancakes 119
Whole Wheat Pizza
    Crust 104

Y

Yeast Dumplings...............105
Yogurt Cheese 46
Yogurt, Making Your
    Own 47-48

Z

Zesty Mashed
    Potatoes 265
Zippy Bean Dip 63
Zingy French Dressing.......313
Zucchini Bread, SF 80

SF - Sugar Free; LS = Low Sugar Content

"HEART SMART - SUGAR WISE COOKBOOK"   ORDER BLANK

NAME _____

ADDRESS_____

CITY & STATE _____   ZIP _____

How many copies? _____   Amount enclosed _____
       Price per book............................ $19.95
       Postage & handling..........................2.00
       Total $21.95
Please make checks payable to:
       STANGL PUBLISHING COMPANY
Mail orders to: Stangl Publishing Company
               808 W. Second St.
               Ottumwa, IA 52501

"HEART SMART - SUGAR WISE COOKBOOK"   ORDER BLANK

NAME _____

ADDRESS_____

CITY & STATE _____   ZIP _____

How many copies? _____   Amount enclosed _____
       Price per book............................ $19.95
       Postage & handling..........................2.00
       Total $21.95
Please make checks payable to:
       STANGL PUBLISHING COMPANY
Mail orders to: Stangl Publishing Company
               808 W. Second St.
               Ottumwa, IA 52501

"HEART SMART - SUGAR WISE COOKBOOK"   ORDER BLANK

NAME _____

ADDRESS_____

CITY & STATE _____   ZIP _____

How many copies? _____   Amount enclosed _____
       Price per book............................ $19.95
       Postage & handling..........................2.00
       Total $21.95
Please make checks payable to:
       STANGL PUBLISHING COMPANY
Mail orders to: Stangl Publishing Company
               808 W. Second St.
               Ottumwa, IA 52501